Respiratory
Pharmacology and
Pharmacotherapy

Series Editors:

Dr. David Raeburn
Discovery Biology
Rhône-Poulenc Rorer Ltd
Dagenham Research Centre
Dagenham
Essex RM10 7XS
England

Dr. Mark A. Giembycz
Department of Thoracic Medicine
National Heart and Lung Institute
Imperial College of Science, Technology and Medicine
London SW3 6LY
England

Clinical and Biological Basis of Lung Cancer Prevention

Edited by
Y. Martinet
F. R. Hirsch
N. Martinet
J.-M. Vignaud
J. L. Mulshine

Springer Basel AG

Editor:

Yves Martinet
Centre Hospitalier Universitaire de Nancy
Hôpital de Brabois
Service de Pneumologie A
54511 Vandoeuvre-lès-Nancy
France

Fred R. Hirsch
The Finsen Center
Department of Oncology 5074
Copenhagen University Hospital
Rigshospitalet
DK-2100 Copenhagen
Denmark

Nadine Martinet
INSERM U14
Unité de Recherche de Physipathologie Respiratoire
C.O. No 10
54511 Vandoeuvre-lès-Nancy
France

Jean-Michel Vignaud
Centre Hospitalier Universitaire de Nancy
Hôpital Central
Service d'Anatomie Pathologique
54035 Nancy
France

James L. Mulshine
National Cancer Institute / National Institutes of Health
Division of Clinical Sciences / Medicine Branch
Cell and Cancer Biology Department
Rockville, MD 20850-3300
USA

Library of Congress Cataloging-in-Publication Data

Clinical and biological basis of lung cancer prevention / edited by Y.
  Martinet ... [et al.].
    p.   cm. – (Respiratory pharmacology and pharmacotherapy)
  Includes bibliographical references and index.
  ISBN 978-3-0348-9829-4   ISBN 978-3-0348-8924-7 (eBook)
  DOI 10.1007/978-3-0348-8924-7
  1. Lungs – Cancer – Molecular aspects.   2. Lungs – Cancer -
  -Chemoprevention.   3. Lungs – Cancer – Prevention.   I. Martinet, Y.
  (Yves), 1948- .   II. Series.
  [DNLM: 1. Lung Neoplasms – prevention & control – congresses.
  2. Lung Neoplasms – diagnostis – congresses.   3. Lung Neoplasms-
  -genetics – congresses.   4. Smoking Cessation – congresses.
  5. Chemoprevention – congresses.   WF 658 C6405 1997]
  RC280.L8C535   1997
  616.99' 424 – dc21
  DNLM/DLC
  for Library of Congress

Deutsche Bibliothek Cataloging-in-Publication Data

Clinical and biological basis of lung cancer prevention / ed by Y.
Martinet ... – Basel ; Boston : Berlin : Birkhäuser, 1997
    (Respiratory pharmacology and pharmacotherapy)
    ISBN 978-3-0348-9829-4

© 1998 Springer Basel AG
Originally published by Birkhäuser Verlag Basel Switzerland in 1998
Softcover reprint of the hardcover 1st edition 1998

Printed on acid-free paper produced from chlorine-free pulp. TCF ∞

Cover design: Markus Etterich

ISBN 978-3-0348-9829-4

9 8 7 6 5 4 3 2 1

Contents

List of Contributors

Mark A. Akeson, Laboratory of Molecular Biology, National Institute on Deafness and other Communication Disorders, National Institutes of Health, 5 Research Court Room 2B28, Rockville, MD 20850, USA

Joseph Ayoub, Institut du cancer de Montréal and Centre de Recherche Louis-Charles Simard, Hôpital Notre-Dame, Montréal, Québec, Canada H2L 4M1; and Département de Médecine, Université de Montréal, Montréal, Québec, Canada H2L 4M3

James F. Battey, Laboratory of Molecular Biology, National Institute on Deafness and other Communication Disorders, National Institutes of Health, 5 Research Court Room 2B28, Rockville, MD 20850, USA

David G. Beer, Department of Surgery, University of Michigan, Ann Arbor, MI 48109-0510, USA

Dorina Belotti, Metastasis Research Laboratory, University of Liège, Tour de Pathologie 1, Bat. B23, Sart Tilman via, B-4000 Liège, Belgium

Simone Benhamou, Unit of Cancer Epidemiology, INSERM U351, Institut Gustave Roussy, 39 rue Camille Desmoulins, F-94805 Villejuif Cedex, France

Catherine Bonaïti-Pellié, Unit of Cancer Epidemiology, INSERM U351, Institut Gustave Roussy, 39 rue Camille Desmoulins, F-94805 Villejuif Cedex, France

Jacques Borrelly, Clinique Pneumologique Médico-Chirugicale, Université de Nancy, F-54511 Nancy, France

W. Edward C. Bradley, Centre de Recherche Louis-Charles Simard, Hôpital Notre-Dame, 1560 rue Sherbrooke Est, Montréal, Québec, Canada H2L 4M1; and Département de Médecine, Université de Montréal, Montréal, Québec, Canada H2L 4M3

Elisabeth Brambilla, Lung Cancer Research Group, Institut Albert Bonniot, Centre Hospitalier Universitaire, F-38043 Grenoble cedex 09, France

Vincent Castronovo, Metastasis Research Laboratory, University of Liège, Tour de Pathologie 1, Bat. B23, Sart Tilman via, B-4000 Liège, Belgium

Robert L. Dedrick, Biomedical Engineering and Instrumentation Program, National Center for Research Resources, National Institutes of Health, Bethesda, MD 20850, USA

Luigi M. De Luca, Laboratory of Cellular Carcinogenesis and Tumor Promotion, Division of Basic Science, National Cancer Institute, Bethesda, MD 20850, USA

Ray J. Donelly, Cardiothoracic Centre, Thomas Drive, Liverpool L14 3PE, UK

Yener S. Erozan, The Johns Hopkins University Medical Institutions, Baltimore, MD 21205, USA

Bénédicte Etienne, INSERM CJF 93-08, Hôpital Louis Pradel, F-69394 Lyon Cedex 03, France

John K. Field, Molecular Genetics and Oncology Group, Clinical Dental Sciences, The University of Liverpool, Liverpool L69 3BX, UK and Roy Castle International Center for Lung Cancer Research, 200 London, Road, Liverpool L3 9TA, UK

Franca Formelli, Istituto Nazionale Tumori, I-20133 Milan, Italy

Hirota Fujiki, Saitama Cancer Center Research Institute, Ina, Kitaadachi-gun, Saitama 362, Japan

Francoise Galateau-Salle, Laboratoire d'Anatomie Pathologique, Université de Caen, F-14033 Caen, France

Adi F. Gazdar, The Hamon Center for Therapeutic Oncology Research and Department of Pathology, University of Texas Southwestern Medical Center, 5323 Harry Hines Boulevard, Dallas, TX 75235-8593, USA

Robert Gemmill, University of Colorado Health Sciences Center, 4200 East 9th Avenue, Box B171, Denver, CO 80262, USA

John R. Gosney, Department of Pathology, The University of Liverpool, Liverpool L69 3BX, UK

Nigel Gray, Division of Epidemiology and Biostatistics, European Institute of Oncology, I-20133 Milan, Italy

Marc S. Greenblatt, Hematology/Oncology Unit, Fletcher Allen Health Care, MCHV Campus-Patrick 534, 111 Colchester Ave., Burlington, VT 05401, USA

Ellen R. Gritz, Department of Behavioral Science, M.D. Anderson Cancer Center, University of Texas, Houston, TX 77030, USA

Samir M. Hanash, Department of Pediatrics, University of Michigan, R4558 Kresge I, Ann Arbor, MI 48109-0510, USA

Curtis C. Harris, Laboratory of Human Carcinogenesis, National Cancer Institute, National Institutes of Health, Bethesda, MD 20892, USA

Mark R. Helmich, Laboratory of Molecular Biology, National Institute on Deafness and other Communication Disorders, National Institutes of Health, 5 Research Court Room 2B28, Rockville, MD 20850, USA

Fred R. Hirsch, Department of Oncology, Finsen Center, Rigshospitalet, 9 Blegdamsvej, DK-2100 Copenhagen, Denmark

Albert Hirsh, Service de Pneumologie, Hôpital Saint-Louis, F-75010 Paris, France

Michael Hogan, Genometrix, 3608 Research Forest Dr. Suite B7, The Woodlands, TX 77381, USA

Waun K. Hong, Department of Thoracic/Head and Neck Medical Oncology, The University of Texas M. D. Anderson Cancer Center, 1515 Holcombe Boulevard, Houston, TX 77030, USA

Daniel R. Jacobson, Medical and Research Services, New York Department of Veterans Affairs Medical Center, 423 E. 23 Street, New York, NY 10010, USA

Robert T. Jensen, Digestive Diseases Branch, National Institute of Diabetes and Digestive and Kidney Diseases, National Institutes of Health, Rockville, MD 20850, USA

Atsumasa Komori, Saitama Cancer Center Research Institute, Ina, Kitaadachi-gun, Saitama 362, Japan

Tomoko Kozu, Saitama Cancer Center Research Institute, Ina, Kitaadachi-gun, Saitama 362, Japan

Glenn S. Kroog, Laboratory of Molecular Biology, National Institute on Deafness and other Communication Disorders, National Institutes of Health, 5 Research Court Room 2B28, Rockville, MD 20850, USA

Rork Kuick, Department of Pediatrics, University of Michigan, R4558 Kresge I, Ann Arbor, MI 48109-0510, USA

Stephen Lam, Cancer Imaging Department, British Columbia Cancer Agency, and University of British Columbia, 111-2775 Heather Street, Vancouver, BC V5Z 3J5, Canada

Barbara Lamb, Department of Pediatrics, University of Michigan, R4558 Kresge I, Ann Arbor, MI 48109-0510, USA

Caroline Leroux, INSERM CJF 93-08, Hôpital Louis Pradel, F-69394 Lyon Cedex 03, France

Tirantafillos Liloglou, Molecular Genetics and Oncology Group, Clinical Dental Sciences, The University of Liverpool, Liverpool L69 3BX, UK; and Roy Castle International Center for Lung Cancer Research, 200 London, Road, Liverpool L3 9TA, UK

Robert Loire, INSERM CJF 93-08, Hôpital Louis Pradel, F-69394 Lyon Cedex 03, France

Richard Lubin, Unité 301 INSERM, Institut de Génétique Moléculaire, Paris, France and Pharmacell, Hôpital Saint-Louis, F-75010 Paris, France

Monique Lyon, INSERM CJF 93-08, Hôpital Louis Pradel, F-69394 Lyon Cedex 03, France

Calum E. MacAulay, Cancer Imaging Department, British Columbia Cancer Agency, and University of British Columbia, 601 West 10, Vancouver, BC V5Z 4E6, Canada

Béatrice Marie, Service d'Anatomie Pathologique, Centre Hospitalier Universitaire de Nancy, Hôpital Central, Avenue du Maréchal de Lattre de Tassigny, F-54035 Nancy Cedex, France

Jean-Pierre Martin, INSERM U295, Faculté de Médecine-Pharmacie de Rouen, Avenue de l'Université, BP 97, F-76803 Saint Etienne de Rouvray Cedex, France

Alfredo Martinez, Cell and Cancer Biology Department, National Cancer Institute, National Institutes of Health, 9610 Medical Center Drive, Rockville, MD 20580-3300, USA

Nadine Martinet, INSERM U14, CO No. 10, F-54511 Vandoeuvre-lès-Nancy, France

Yves Martinet, Clinique Pneumologique Médico-Chirugicale, Université de Nancy, F-54511 Vandoeuvre-lès-Nancy, France; and INSERM U14, CO No. 10, F-54511 Vandoeuvre-lès-Nancy, France

Johane Morin, Institut du cancer de Montréal and Centre de Recherche Louis-Charles Simard, Hôpital Notre-Dame, Montréal, Québec, Canada H2L 4M1

Jean-Francois Mornex, INSERM CJF 93-08, Hôpital Louis Pradel, F-69394 Lyon Cedex 03, France

James L. Mulshine, Intervention Section, Cell and Cancer Biology Department, Medicine Branch, Division of Clinical Sciences, National Cancer Institute, 9610 Medical Center Drive, Rockville, MD 20850-3300, USA

Karim Nabil, INSERM U14, CO No. 10, F-54511 Vandoeuvre-lès-Nancy, France

Yoshihiro Nambu, Department of Surgery, University of Michigan, Ann Arbor, MI 48109-0510, USA

Ingrid R. Nielsen, Department of Behavioral Science, M.D. Anderson Cancer Center, University of Texas, Houston, TX 77030, USA

John K. Northup, Laboratory of Cell Biology, National Institute of Mental Health, Rockville, MD 20850, USA

Sachiko Okabe, Saitama Cancer Center Research Institute, Ina, Kita-adachi-gun, Saitama 362, Japan

Vali A. Papadimitrakopoulou, Department of Thoracic/Head and Neck Medical Oncology, The University of Texas M.D. Anderson Cancer Center, 1515 Holcombe Boulevard, Houston, TX 77030, USA

Ugo Pastorino, Thoracic Surgery, Royal Brompton Hospital, Sydney Street, London SW3 6NP, UK

Andrea Pavirani, Transgène SA, 11 Rue de Molsheim, F-67082 Strasbourg Cedex, France

Evelyne Picard, Service d'Anatomie Pathologique, Centre Hospitalier Universitaire de Nancy, Hôpital Central, Avenue du Maréchal de Lattre de Tassigny, F-54035 Nancy Cedex, France

Wendy Prime, Molecular Genetics and Oncology Group, Clinical Dental Sciences, The University of Liverpool, Liverpool L69 3BX, UK and Roy Castle International Center for Lung Cancer Research, 200 London, Road, Liverpool L3 9TA, UK

Bruce Richardson, Department of Internal Medicine, University of Michigan, Ann Arbor, MI 48109-0510, USA

Helen Ross, Molecular Genetics and Oncology Group, Clinical Dental Sciences, The University of Liverpool, Liverpool L69 3BX, UK and Roy Castle International Center for Lung Cancer Research, 200 London, Road, Liverpool L3 9TA, UK

Enrique Rozengurt, Imperial Cancer Research Fund, 44 Lincoln's Inn Fields, London WC2A 3PX, UK

Annie J. Sasco, Programme of Epidemiology for Cancer Prevention, International Agency for Research on Cancer, World Health Organization, Institut National de la Santé et de la Recherche Médicale, 150 cours Albert Thomas, F-69372 Lyon Cedex 08, France

Christian Schatz, Transgène SA, 11 Rue de Molsheim, F-67082 Strasbourg Cedex, France

Irene E. Schauer, Department of Biochemistry, Biophysics and Genetics, University of Colorado Health Sciences Center, 4200 East Ninth Avenue, Denver, CO 80262, USA

Robert A. Sclafani, Department of Biochemistry, Biophysics and Genetics, University of Colorado Health Sciences Center, 4200 East Ninth Avenue, Denver, CO 80262, USA

Frank Scott, Molecular Genetics and Oncology Group, Clinical Dental Sciences, The University of Liverpool, Liverpool L69 3BX, UK and Roy Castle International Center for Lung Cancer Research, 200 London, Road, Liverpool L3 9TA, UK

Michael J. Seckl, Imperial Cancer Research Fund, 44 Lincoln's Inn Fields, London WC2A 3PX, UK; and Department of Medical Oncology, Charing Cross Hospital, London W6 8RF, UK

Janeric Seidegård, The Wallenberg Laboratory, University of Lund and Astra Draco AB, S-221 00 Lund, Sweden

Jöelle Siat, Clinique Pneumologique Médico-Chirugicale, Université de Nancy, F-54511 Nancy, France

Eisaburo Sueoka, Saitama Cancer Center Research Institute, Ina, Kitaadachi-gun, Saitama 362, Japan

Naoko Sueoka, Saitama Cancer Center Research Institute, Ina, Kitaadachi-gun, Saitama 362, Japan

Thierry Soussi, Unité 301 INSERM, Institut de Génétique Moléculaire, F-75010 Paris, France; and UMR218 CNRS, Institut Curie, 26 rue d'Ulm, F-75238 Paris Cedex 05, France

Masami Suganuma, Saitama Cancer Center Research Institute, Ina, Kitaadachi-gun, Saitama 362, Japan

Yukiko Tada, Saitama Cancer Center Research Institute, Ina, Kitaadachi-gun, Saitama 362, Japan

Didier H. Thoraval, Department of Pediatrics, University of Michigan, R4558 Kresge I, Ann Arbor, MI 48109-0510, USA

Melvyn S. Tockman, The H. Lee Moffitt Cancer Center & Research Institute, University of South Florida, 12902 Magnolia Drive, Tampa, FL 33612-9497, USA

Philip Tønnesen, Medical Department of Pulmonary Diseases, Gentofte University Hospital, Niels Andersensvej, DK-2900 Hellerup, Denmark

André Toulouse, Institut du cancer de Montréal and Centre de Recherche Louis-Charles Simard, Hôpital Notre-Dame, Montréal, Québec, Canada H2L 4M1

Jean Tredaniel, Service de Pneumologie, Hôpital Saint-Louis, F-75010 Paris, France

Jean-Michel Vignaud, Service d'Anatomie Pathologique, Centre Hospitalier Universitaire de Nancy, Hôpital Central, Avenue du Maréchal de Lattre de Tassigny, F-54035 Nancy Cedex, France; and INSERM U14, CO No. 10, F-54511 Vandoeuvre-lès-Nancy, France

Xin W. Wang, Laboratory of Human Carcinogenesis, National Cancer Institute, National Institutes of Health, Bethesda, MD 20892, USA

William H. Westra, The Johns Hopkins University Medical Institutions, Baltimore, MD 21205, USA

Katharina Wimmer, Department of Pediatrics, University of Michigan, R4558 Kresge I, Ann Arbor, MI 48109-0510, USA

Ignacio I. Wistuba, The Hamon Center for Therapeutic Oncology, University of Texas Southwestern Medical Center, 5323 Harry Hines Boulevard, Dallas, TX 75235-8593, USA; and Department of Pathology, Pontificia Universidad Catolica de Chile, Santiago, Chile

Ying Ying, Institut du cancer de Montréal and Centre de Recherche Louis-Charles Simard, Hôpital Notre-Dame, Montréal, Québec, Canada H2L 4M1

Judith Youngson, Molecular Genetics and Oncology Group, Clinical Dental Sciences, The University of Liverpool, Liverpool L69 3BX, UK and Roy Castle International Center for Lung Cancer Research, 200 London, Road, Liverpool L3 9TA, UK

Gérard Zalcman, Service de Pneumologie, Hôpital Saint-Louis, F-75010 Paris, France

Jun Zhou, Intervention Section, Cell and Cancer Biology Department, Medicine Branch, Division of Clinical Sciences, National Cancer Institute, 9610 Medical Center Drive, Rockville, MD 20850-3300, USA

Tatyana A. Zhukov, The Johns Hopkins University Medical Institutions, Baltimore, MD 21205, USA

Foreword

Foreword To The Workshops on Prevention and Early Detection of Lung Cancer – Clinical Aspects and Biological Basis of Lung Cancer Prevention Sponsored by the International Association for the Study of Lung Cancer (IASLC)

In 1996, the IASLC sponsored two workshops on lung cancer prevention. One focused on clinical studies and was held at Elsinore (Denmark) from June 22–25, 1996 and the other focused on basic studies and was held in Nancy (France) from October 20–22, 1996. Although it is not the most common cancer in developed countries, lung cancer is the leading cause of cancer deaths in these countries. Active tobacco smoking is responsible for 85–87% of cases and passive tobacco exposure accounts for another 2–3% of cases. Despite this knowledge, attempts to decrease tobacco usage have largely failed and lung cancer mortality continues to rise.

The cure rate for lung cancer is very low, ranging from 5% in many countries to 14% in the United States. The primary reason for the low cure rate is the fact that there are no known effective screening or early detection measures and in about 85% of cases the disease has already metastasized by the time of diagnosis. Systemic therapies cannot cure metastatic disease. Thus, the focus of these workshops was to present the latest basic and clinical studies on prevention and early detection.

The development of new screening and prevention strategies was difficult in the past when there were no known differences between normal, malignant and dysplastic bronchial epithelial cells. Recent studies have demonstrated a variety of genetic and biologic differences which will lead to new strategies in the near future. The large number of genetic changes which have been found to occur in premalignant lesion is surprising. There are mutations and deletions of many tumor suppressor genes. In other instances, such tumor suppressor genes are silenced by DNA methylation. Growth factors and the signal pathways by which they cause proliferation are being described and offer new potential prevention targets. The cell cycle is usually deregulated in lung cancer cells either by loss of the retinoblastoma (Rb) protein (SCLC) or by functional loss of Rb by overexpression of cyclin D1 and loss of P16. New avenues for developing prevention and screening strategies are being opened up by the delineation of these abnormalities.

Lung cancer invades and metastasizes readily and tumor angiogenesis develops universally. MMP inhibitors and anti-angiogenesis agents are a logical extension of this knowledge. Abnormalities in retinoic acid receptor expression may account for the effect of retinoids on lung cancer prevention.

Premalignant precursors of cells destined to become malignant are being detected at an earlier stage by using biologic markers such as monoclonal antibodies and by using sophisticated genetic studies of sputum and bronchial biopsies which rely on techniques such as FISH and PCR. In addition, a new fluorescence-based bronchoscopy technique opens the possibility of identifying premalignant lesions.

Gene and antisense strategies to prevent lung cancer are benefitting from new delivery systems to the airways involving direct injection or aerosolization.

At the clinical workshop, the use of the genetic and biologic abnormalities described above as intermediate biomarkers was described. In addition, the potential utility of a variety of new chemoprevention agents was described. It remains to be determined whether these new agents will actually change the expression of various intermediate markers.

Clinical trials using various vitamin A analogs and green tea have given some promising early results. Confirmatory trials of vitamin A analogs are underway in Europe and the USA and results are eagerly awaited. These studies used resected stage I patients as the high risk patients for study.

Based on the results of studies presented at these meetings, there is reason for optimism regarding the potential to develop useful screening and early detection, as well as prevention measures based on the new knowledge of the differences between normal bronchial epithelium, dysplastic epithelium and expressed lung cancer.

Paul A. Bunn
Heine H. Hansen

Preface

Y. Martinet, F.R. Hirsch, N. Martinet, J.M. Vignaud, J.L. Mulshine

Lung cancer is a disease with enormous public health implications as it is now the leading cause of cancer mortality throughout the world. The International Association for the Study of Lung Cancer (IASLC) is a body of clinical and basic science investigators who are united in their efforts to improve the outcome for this lethal disease. The composition of the IASLC has always been diverse and all professionals with an interest in improving lung cancer outcome have always been welcomed by the Association. The wisdom of that inclusive membership policy is brought into sharp focus in addressing the needs of lung cancer prevention. Two recent IASLC Workshops on Lung Cancer Prevention have involved a remarkably wide range of professional skills. From government ministers to electronic engineers who design biochips, the participants in the meetings reflect the reality that the answer to the principal cancer epidemic of the twentieth century is going to require the committed involvement of many. Through the two Workshops, a balance has been struck between considering public health approaches to tobacco control and population-based screening, along with consideration of the evolving clinical evaluation of chemoprevention approaches and the biology of lung carcinogenesis. The Workshop in Elsinore (Denmark) was weighted towards clinical issues, with intensive consideration of smoking and tobacco control. One reason for the Danish location was the concern of senior Danish cancer investigators that the potential of lung cancer prevention was not receiving sufficient attention in Scandinavia. This sentiment was echoed by the French leadership of the Nancy (France) Workshop, and a vibrant element of both meetings was the international sharing of perspectives and successful directions. The deliberations surrounding the unification of Europe have profound impact on tobacco control issues, and these were discussed in depth. The science of smoking cessation is evolving as new pharmacological tools are moving into clinical evaluation. The current series of court cases in the United States also appear to have the potential for a major impact on smoking. The rising problem of youth smoking has worldwide implications and represents a consensus priority.

The current impact of molecular diagnostics is profound and this was reviewed in great depth at the more basic science-oriented Workshop in Nancy. Rapidly evolving diagnostic technologies are revolutionizing basic scientific investigation of cancer, and the expectation is that this trend will soon spill over into clinical medicine. The evolution of economical diagnostic platforms to allow for direct bronchial epithelial evaluation in high risk populations promises to improve the diagnostic lead-time for this disease. The hope is that enough progress will occur to permit lung cancer detection in advance of clinical cancer so that the early disease can be addressed while it is still confined to the site of origin.

The approach of chemoprevention, that is, trying to intervene in the early phase of carcinogenesis prior to any subjective clinical manifestation of a cancer, is also capturing greater research interest. Investigators responsible for conduct and reporting the initial lung cancer chemoprevention trials outlined their experiments. New candidate drugs and the clinical validation of new agents were reviewed in detail. The interactive aspect of the Workshops was particularly evident in these sessions, as the molecular tools that are being developed for early cancer detection might also have application as tools for monitoring the success of chemoprevention. Promising new intervention approaches include an array of vaccines and molecular tools. Redirecting the administration of conventional chemoprevention agents from oral to aerosolized administration has great appeal and may result in the reduction of cancer when integrated with the use of the new diagnostic technologies. A persistent concern of conference members was whether progress in successful early lung cancer intervention would happen quickly enough. The ethical dilemma of diagnosing a serious condition for which effective treatment was not available was a significant problem that dominated many discussions. Redoubled chemoprevention research efforts are required to avoid this situation.

The intensity and enthusiasm displayed at these two stimulating fora are a surprising development in considering a disease where progress has been so elusive. The manuscripts produced for this book all capture aspects of new possibilities. If the tenor of these Workshops is grounded in reality, then the next decade of lung cancer research will be an era of unprecedented opportunity. To realize this, the dialogue and directions begun at these meetings must be carefully nourished and IASLC's pioneering role in fostering this process must continue.

Clinical and Biological Basis of Lung Cancer Prevention
ed. by Y. Martinet, F. R. Hirsch, N. Martinet, J.-M. Vignaud
and J. L. Mulshine
© 1998 Birkhäuser Verlag Basel/Switzerland

CHAPTER 1
Prevention and Early Detection of Lung Cancer – Clinical Aspects

Fred R. Hirsch[1],* and James L. Mulshine[2]

[1] *Department of Oncology, Finsen Center, Rigshospitalet, Copenhagen, Denmark*
[2] *Cell and Cancer Biology Department, Medicine Branch, Division of Clinical Sciences, National Cancer Institute, NIH, Rockville, Maryland, USA*

1. Introduction

In the absence of significant reductions in the mortality rate of lung cancer, the International Association for the Study of Lung Cancer (IASLC) has attempted to nurture development in the area of lung cancer prevention. This has principally been accomplished through a series of workshops, where investigators working on aspects of prevention research share their experience with lung cancer investigators interested in developing expertise in prevention research. In the first IASLC workshop, conducted in November 1993 in Potomac, MD, three major areas of interest were defined including issues with tobacco consumption, early detection and early clinical intervention and the deliberations from that meeting were published [1]. This meeting set the stage for a proactive smoking-oriented agenda at the Seventh World Conference on Lung Cancer held in Colorado Springs, Colorado in 1994. This IASLC membership endorsed a ten point tobacco policy that aligned the organizations with other major public health groups in regard to tax and public education issues [2]. A distinctive aspect of the IASLC document was a statement of support for the farmers and other industries dependent on tobacco commerce for their economic live-

---

* Author for correspondence.

lihood. Support of these workers' efforts to transfer nontobacco-related jobs, may ultimately permit faster reduction in tobacco consumption. Also, since the IASLC is an organization of health care professionals, the obligation of health care workers to remain informed about smoking issues and to educate patients and to support tobacco control public health measures was emphasized. Finally, since the effects of tobacco in causing cancer will be manifested for decades after the cessation of smoking continued research to improve the diagnosis and treatment of lung cancer will be essential to reduce lung cancer mortality.

The present chapter presents a consensus from the recent IASLC workshop that was conducted in Elsinore, Denmark during the summer of 1996. The aims of the workshop were:

1. To collect and discuss the available information in the topics of prevention, clinical intervention and early detection of lung cancer.
2. To clarify the state of the art and set guidelines for future studies.
3. To stimulate research and encourage new scientists into that research area.

This forum further developed the vision of the anti-smoking strategy as outlined in this report. The location of this workshop in Europe brought the regional smoking issues into sharp focus. Under the informed leadership of Doctors Nigel Gray and Ellen Gritz, the smoking-related discussion benefited from the excellent outline of current smoking issues before the European ministers. This critical message was supported by the independent comments of Dr Gordon McVie, who is the director of the Cancer Research Campaign in the United Kingdom. These issues were communicated to the workshop attendees in an impassioned appeal from the membership to do what they could to address this public health crisis. Due to the importance of these issues the deliberations of the workshop in this regard were captured in a previous report in the journal; *Lung Cancer*, that is reproduced with editorial comment for this chapter [3]. While the basic science and translational issues were the principal focus of the subsequent IASLC workshop scheduled for Nancy, France in October of 1996, some of the relevant diagnostic and translational issues were discussed in the Elsinore workshop. The intention in having two workshops in close temporal proximity was to concentrate on complementary areas. Given the recent interest not only in smoking control but also on translating laboratory leads into clinical trials, the intense level of clinical and research interest suggested that the two meetings could be coordinated to have additive benefit. The present book is an effort to capture the importance of the interaction between clinical and basic research in this fast-moving area. The consensus from the three main sessions are presented below:

2. Smoking Prevention
(Chairs: Nigel Gray and Ellen Gritz)

The workshop focused on defining recommendations for future public health policy beyond the issues outlined in the IASLC Policy Statement in 1994 [2]. Since the workshop was conducted in Europe, tobacco control issues that were the subject of European community discussions emerged as major areas of concern as outlined in Table 1. The progressive unification of the European community poses both a challenge and an opportunity for improved tobacco control measures. Efforts to coordinate actions were considered to be important so that the message to the public about smoking was consistent. The regional differences in measures to address smoking control were also significant. By enunciating IASLC positions, medical professionals in countries with less proactive tobacco control approaches have a guideline to use in formulating new strategies.

In addition to the global (political) issues described above specific measures for the individual health care provider to consider implementing within their own practice were proposed as listed:

1. Health care providers, particularly physicians, dentists, and nurses have a professional and ethical obligation to discourage tobacco use in their patients. This obligation includes discouraging initiation in young people who have not yet begun to smoke, motivating smokers who are not ready to stop and providing assisstance to those who are ready to make an attempt to quit. Providers can demonstrate their responsibility in their own behaviour as well, as summarized in Table 2.

Table 1. Proposed tobacco control issues for the european union

1. Harmonise taxes (standardize national tax rates) on tobacco on the highest EU taxation rate. Dedicate the revenues raised to smoking prevention and control, health care delivery, research into disease, interventions, policy and economic transition (for tobacco industry-affected workers).
2. Eliminate passive smoking by banning smoking in schools and other settings which children frequent, health care settings (part of accreditation) and public transportation (passenger and exposed employees). Smoking should be prohibited in all workplaces.
3. Reduce youth access by enforcing a minimum age of 18 years for purchase of cigarettes, requiring identification for purchase, imposing strong penalties for violation by vendors, introducing licensing of cigarette sales vendors, and banning vending machine sales of cigarettes. It is noted that the right to drink alcohol, to drive and to vote occurs at this age.
4. Regulate nicotine in cigarettes by setting a low maximum permissible level (e.g. 0.5 mg nicotine) and by banning reapplication of nicotine during the manufacturing process.
5. Regulate tobacco advertising and promotion by eliminating sports sponsorship, coupon and merchandise giveaways and banning the appearance of tobacco billboards or other visible emblems during electronic media programming.
6. Mandate effective health warning labels by making these clear and visible (e.g. Canadian and Australian examples), by utilizing a multiple warning rotational system, and by printing a hazardous ingredient list on the package and on advertisements.
7. Reimburse behavioral and pharmacological treatment for smoking cessation, using criteria developed by the Agency for Health Care Policy and Research (AHCPR).

Table 2. Basic measures for health practitioners to reduce smoking activity

1. Strive for a smoke-free profession.
2. Never use tobacco in presence of patients.
3. Make professional meetings smoke-free.
4. Enforce smoke-free regulations in hospitals and practice site.
5. Use professional organizations to develop a strong anti-smoking policy and advocacy position.

2. Health care providers should provide state-of-the-art assistance to patients and family members. Such assistance includes the four A model developed by the U.S. National Cancer Institute, and the evidence-based "Smoking Cessation Clinical Practive Guideline" recently published by the Agency for Health Care Policy and Research (AHCPR). These guidelines contain patient-oriented material, advice guidelines for primary care providers, and more detailed information for the smoking cessation specialist. Based on a meta-analysis of the last 16 years of clinical research on smoking cessation interventions, the main recommendations are summarized in Table 3. For successful smoking cessation efforts, it is useful to incorporate social support from the family and friends to reinforce new healthy behaviour. New and improved delivery systems for nicotine compel the medical community to reconsider the value of these tools in helping individuals to stop smoking. The efficacy of nicotine replacement therapy (NRT) has been established with transdermal patch and polacrilex (gum). Newer formulations are proving successful in clinical evaluation so that the pharmacological intervention component is far stronger than in the past. Patients should also be encouraged to view smoking relapse as a valuable learning experience rather than a failure, as research shows that multiple relapses occur before successful, longterm smoking cessation.

3. Physicians and other health care professionals should seek opportunities to speak out against tobacco use and its associated disease and dependence consequences. In speaking out physicians should take note of

Table 3. The Agency for Health Care Policy and Research (AHCPR) recommendations for health care professionals.*

1. Every person who smokes should be offered smoking cessation treatment at every office visit.
2. Clinicians should ask and record the tobacco-use status of every patient.
3. Cessation treatments even as brief as 3 minutes a visit are effective.
4. More intense treatment is more effective in producing longterm abstinence from tobacco.
5. Nicotine replacement therapy (nicotine patches or gum), physician-delivered social support, and providing coping skills training are the three most effective components of a smoking cessation treatment.
6. Health care systems should make institutional changes that result in systematic identification of, and intervention with, all tobacco users at every visit.

* The AHCPR Clinical Practice Guideline, number 18, Smoking Cessation is available from the AHCPR Publication Clearinghouse (USA) by phone at +1-800-358-9295.

current international policy issues which include the need for abolition of all forms of tobacco promotion, for increased tobacco taxes, for controls on tobacco accessibility to children, for limits on tar content to 12 mg per cigarette (as is current in Europe), for stronger health warnings, and finally for better product information. Such opportunities may occur in media interviews and in public lectures delivered in schools and other community settings. The mortality and morbidity burden of tobacco should be compared to exposures that the lay public is commonly concerned about (e.g. air pollution, food additives, illegal drug use).

4. Primary prevention of smoking initiation in youth is particularly important because of the rising incidence of smoking among teenagers in many countries in Europe, the U.S. and developing nations. Since 90% of smoking begins before age 19, family practitioners and pediatricians should intervene preventively with children, especially during the most vulnerable teen years, and with their parents. Parents serve an important function as role models; they also protect their children against exposure to environmental tobacco smoke (passive exposure), which is especially important for children with respiratory disorders such as asthma.

5. Individuals at highest risk for smoking-related tumors should be targeted for the most intensive interventions. Vulnerable populations include: patients with smoking related prior cancers; other smoking related diseases (e.g. coronary artery disease, chronic obstructive pulmonary disease and other respiratory diseases, vascular diseases, etc.); chronic heavy smokers; survivors of any cancer site who continue to smoke; and genetically susceptible individuals (once reliable and valid biomarkers are etablished). Furthermore, intensive smoking cessation treatment (combining behavioral and pharmacotherapy), delivered by clinical specialists, could be integrated into chemoprevention trials which recruit former, but not current smokers. One design suggestion would be to provide such treatment during the run-in period and to incorporate smoking cessation as an eligibility criterion. Booster treatments to maintain abstinence could be made readily available. Research might also examine the relationship of nicotine dependence, smoking cessation and chemoprevention efficacy, involving genetic, behavioral and biological variables and predictors and endpoints.

3. Clinical Intervention for Pre-invasive Lung Cancer
(Chairs: Ugo Pastorino and Gary J. Kelloff)

Chemoprevention is the use of specific compounds to prevent, inhibit, or reverse the lengthy (frequently 20–40 years) process of carcinogenesis, before invasive disease develops. Lung carcinogenesis potentially provides significant opportunities for chemoprevention based on the well-known exposure risks (e.g. smoking and industrial chemicals) and the long pre-neoplastic period. The challenge is to design clinical trials for successfully evaluating intervention strategies in high-risk cohorts given the long time period required for carcinogenesis and the relatively low incidence of resulting cancers. A range of agents are in active clinical evaluation that show preliminary promise [4, 5]. The objective of this working group was to present a consensus on clinical trial designs that are most useful for evaluating chemopreventive interventions in lung.

3.1. Cohorts

The general opinion among the group was that the next generation of chemo-preventive intervention trials should be represented by small studies con-ducted in former smokers with the aim of defining optimal drug regimen, dose, duration and toxicity, using intermediate biomarkers of cancer as surrogate endpoints for efficacy. Two reasons were cited as a rationale to restrict chemoprevention trials to individuals who had stopped smoking. First was a concern that the benefit of new intervention agents may be obscured in a population that continues to smoke. Second individuals taking chemo-prevention drugs may feel that they may safely continue to smoke. Even the most optimistic investigators doubted the ability of chemoprevention agents to neutralize the harmful effects of smoking completely. Large-scale preven-tion trials, particularly those using retinoids and carotenoids, should there-fore be preferentially offered to former smokers. Intervention in current smokers should be restricted to small, well-controlled pilot studies, with preference for drugs such as detoxifiers, e.g. oltipraz, N-acetyl-l-cysteine (NAC), in combination with intensive smoking cessation programs.

3.2. Agents

Retinoids have undergone extensive preclinical and clinical testing in pre-vention and therapy. Various retinoids have shown significant activity in randomized trials by reversing premalignant lesions of the oral cavity, cervix, and skin, and preventing tumors of the upper aerodigestive tract and skin [4]. Among these compounds, 13-cis-retinoic acid is the most extensively studied in the clinic [6]. More general application of these approaches is limited by clinical toxicity. Several directions have been taken to address this problem, including dose reduction and combination therapy without agents such as vitamin E. New delivery systems including liposomes and topical application through aerosol inhalation, are currently being tested. Fenretinide is the second promising retinoid [7]. Longterm clinical testing has demonstrated a favorable profile in terms of tolerability and toxicity. The most significant side effects are hyporetinolemia and night blindness, but both can be well managed by drug holidays. Confirmation on the efficacy of the selected 200 mg/day dose has been provided by inhibition of oral leucoplakia. In addition, fenretinide appears to be a more potent inducer of apoptosis than previously studied retinoids [8]. The role of retinyl palmitate will be clarified by the large, ongoing EUROSCAN trial [9]. Current retinoid research is focused on nuclear receptor-specific compounds to improve pharmacological profiles in terms of both activity and toxicity. Recent large randomized trials have shown no benefit of beta-carotene on lung cancer prevention, and a potential harmful effect in current smokers. A longer follow-up is needed to assess the ultimate results of such intervention, especially in nonsmokers. Based on preclinical and some clinical data, there is now greater interest in other carotenoids such as alpha-carotene and lycopene. Other potentially interesting compounds for chemoprevention include N-acetyl-l-cystein, olipraz and phenethyl isothiocyanate, which work by enhancement or induction of detoxifying enzymes. The EUROSCAN trial will provide definitive data on efficacy and safety on NAC [9]. Phase II studies will evaluate clinical efficacy of oltipraz and phenethyl isothiocynate. Other promising agents with pre-clinical and early data include folate (with vitamin B12), tea polyphenols, selenium, nonsteroidal anti-inflammatory drugs and several antioxidants.

3.3. Biomarkers

The application of specific biomarkers is critical for chemoprevention research. Two major roles of biomarkers of cancer prevention are identifi-cation of optimal cohorts for intervention and the intermediate assessment of chemoprevention efficacy [10]. The higher the a priori risk of the pro-posed clinical trial, the smaller the requisite study size or duration and study cost. Biomarker evaluation of study candidates may define such high risk subjects. The use of intermediate endpoint markers as surrogates of clinical endpoints is essential since the most relevant clinical endpoint, of death due to cancer, requires long study durations. The use of intermediate endpoints which have been validated to parallel cancer mortality would permit a preliminary prevention trial to be conducted on a much shorter time frame. Candidate biomarkers include genetic, histological and other phenotypic tissue changes associated with multistep lung carcinogenesis. Future studies should incorporate molecular biomarkers for correlation against endpoints to identify validated intermediate endpoint marker.

4. Diagnostic Aspects

The diagnostic issues were the focus of intense discussion throughout the course of the workshop. This interest may in part reflect an evolving under-standing of molecular carcinogenesis as well as a growing array of powerful diagnostic tools that are accelerating the process of discovery in the area of tumor biology. In the context of the workshop, the orientation of the participants was the charge to discuss a rational process of establishing clinically useful applications of the burgeoning number of biochemical and molecular targets to identify and monitor early lung cancer in a clinical setting.

The challenge of more effective detection of lung cancer is related to the vast at-risk population (including the millions of current and former smokers), the long duration of risk (lifelong) as well as the relative frequency of diagnosing a lung cancer at a single point in time (usually a rate of less than 100 cases per 100 000 persons). Considering effective lung cancer detection in the United States, where the risk population includes at least ninety four million current and former smokers, the logistics of implementing population-based detection strategies are formidable. Thoughtful consideration of the requirements of an effective early detection approach are critical to address the growing concern about the economic impact of such health care interventions [11].

Fortunately diagnostic technology is rapidly expanding with assay platforms that may be more efficient and economical, making the screening of populations more feasible. This technology has not been refined to deal with the small clinical specimens with low numbers of informative cells that one would routinely expect in an early detection setting, but the enormous financial commitment of the diagnostic industry may allow the development of this type of tool to proceed rapidly. In addition numerous less glamorous issues will have to be addressed, to optimize clinical specimen acquistion handling and storage as well as data handing and reporting procedures. Clinical trials will be required to validate the actual cost-utility of newly proposed diagnostic technology. The implementation of diagnostic markers for early detection leads to the consideration of other useful applications of markers. From a statistical perspective, it is axiomatic that a diagnostic test works best when the probability of finding a positive outcome is high. From a "Baysean" perspective measures to increase the *a priori* risk of a defined population serve to improve the prospects for successful validation of a diagnostic tool. The higher risk profile of a particular population also allows for more economical study sizes. As a result a science of risk assessment has emerged in the epidemiological world and the integration of that field into clinical practice was a major topic of discussion. Many of the same markers to be considered for early detection usage could also be used for risk assessment to define more compact study sizes for early detection trials. By extension some of the same detection or risk markers, which presumably reflect aspects of the biology of lung cancer, could be used to monitor the success of interventions intended to arrest the progression of early lung cancer. An observation that emerged through the course of the workshop was that morphology was not correlated to the expression of many markers that suggest the presence of early stage lung cancer, so that the need for molecular tools to monitor the early stages of lung cancer is evident. A greater overall focus on the nature of the premalignant phase of cancer emerged from the workshop. The pathology participants focused on refining the classical morphological criteria for preneoplasia, especially for small cell and adenocarcinoma lesions. While in the course of the workshop deliberations long lists of candidate markers were enumerated, the process of appropriate marker validation was also considered. In particular, the consensus was that panels of markers would require highly efficient assay platforms to allow for economical multiplexed assay analysis. The diagnostic infrastructure development will occur largely in an industry setting. Fortunately there was strong representation of the diagnostic manufacturing community at the workshop so that a realistic discussion about the likely evolution of these approaches was possible. While the focus of this workshop was clearly lung cancer, there was a general understanding that the development challenges for preventive approaches to this disease shared features with the challenges that would have to be addressed with other major cancers. The fundamental importance of the issues charged the conduct of the meeting and led to informal discussion sessions that continued into the night.

In addition to direct assay costs are other, potentially more important costs. These include both the monetary and physical costs of the downstream management identified in the screening process. These issues have figured prominently in the discussions of both breast and prostate cancer screening. Systematic consideration of the components of those decision analyses was thoroughly discussed. For both prostate cancer and breast cancer a positive screening test evokes a major invasive and costly therapeutic intervention. Today for lung cancer screening the same type of invasive surgical intervention would be the first option. However, with the evolution of chemoprevention approaches, what if an effective and less toxic alternative emerged?

Cost-benefit analysis of lung cancer screening is conditional upon the context of the proposed clinical management algorithm. The workshop was an opportunity to hear about the future of diagnostic technology as well as the evolving chemoprevention options. The impetus to develop economical and effective chemoprevention strategies would enable a shift in management strategies from dealing with advanced disseminated lung cancer to detecting and interrupting lung cancer progression prior to lethal metastatic progression. The interaction of the diagnostic management and the intervention research issues was constantly evident and supported the integrated focus of the workshop.

5. Early Detection
(Chairs: Elisabeth Brambilla and Ilona R. Linnoila)

Better methods of lung cancer early detection are fundamental to a paradigm shift allowing routine management of truly early (premetastatic) lung cancer. Longstanding evidence suggests that invasive lung cancer is the end result of a multistep process [12] in which progressive molecular changes accompany and even precede morphological changes [13]. Due to the exquisite specificity or selectivity biomarkers may be suitable as tools to phenotype the premalignant stage of cancer. However, greater knowledge of the genetic etiology would facilitate the selection of genetic markers most appropriate for evaluation in clinical management of early cancer. Current directions for biomarker research includes the evaluation of tools to select populations for prevention clinical trials and for the identification of additional informative biomarkers for early cancer detection. The assumption that a normal appearing cell is completely genetically normal is eroding. With smoking, the entire bronchial epithelium is the target of carcinogens as conveyed in the concept of the field effect [14, 15]. Information is emerging to suggest that numerous molecular events frequently precede cytomorphological changes. Aims for early cancer management therefore should be to identify the core molecular determinants of field effects and devise suitable methods of intervention [16]. Clearly our knowledge is rudimentary, the steps in clonal progression of the cancer between pre- and postinvasion are not fully defined. Issues such as whether a random biopsy in a high risk individual could yield information about the status of the rest of the organ epithelium need to be systematically evaluated in clinical studies. Another prevention research approach is to do multiple biopsies in order to evaluate how broad is the cancerization field in regard to genetic damage.

The types of specimens on which to test markers include bronchial biopsies, bronchial brushings (with or without fluorescence bronchoscopy), sputum, bronchial washings, and bronchioloalveolar lavage. Further technological developments are required for new assays to get meaningful clinical information easily from few cells, such as exfoliated bronchial cells in a sputum specimen. Whether these few cells will be representative of the abnormal clonal population in the cancerization field is being evaluated in at least two ongoing clinical trials. Normal DNA from blood or plasma as well as fresh tissues could be evaluated to compare normal DNA with DNA from preneoplastic or neoplastic lesions. This type of information could lead to better understanding of the genetic composition of individuals who eventually succumb to cancer. An emerging area of diagnostic pathology is the development of risk assessment markers, since these tools may be used to identify patients at higher risk of developing cancer.

Risk assessment research frequently complements early detection research in helping to identify the populations most at-risk for developing a cancer, that would be suitable cohorts for early cancer screening trials. Biological considerations can be used in selecting markers for clinical application [17]. Potential markers for progression of initiated clones can be stratified in many ways. Markers can be classified as: 1) morphological changes; 2) immunocytochemical markers for differentially expressed proteins; 3) markers for genomic instability; 4) markers of epigenetic change (abnormal methylation); 5) gene mutations.

Morphological markers include histopathological changes (which is currently the gold standard) and morphometric analysis of nuclear morphology and nucleolar organizers. Among immunocytochemical markers which detect abnormally expressed proteins are hnRNP A2/B1, p53, epidermal growth factor receptor, proliferation markers (PCNA, Ki 67), markers of apoptosis (bcl-2, bax), differentiation markers, and markers of abnormal maturation including secretory proteins, enzymes, proteases, retinoic acid receptors, and loss of blood group antigens. Markers of genetic changes include genomic instability, aneuploidy, loss of heterozygosity (LOH) of frequently altered loci, gene amplification (new candidates could originate from comparative genomic hybridization studies), and microsatellite instability. Another class of genetic change frequently seen in cancer is oncogene mutation. An example of an epigenetic phenomenon is abnormal methylation (hypermethylation of 5′ end of genes inhibiting transcription). The biomarkers can be divided into two types according to their specificity for tumor progression.

Generalized markers which reflect genetic damage may not be exclusively on the pathway of cancer. Early histopathological changes like hyperplasia, metaplasia, low grade dysplasia, morphometric change and expression of proliferation markers, as well as differentially expressed proteins such as enzymes, proteases, retinoic acid receptors, apoptotic factors, and telomerase activity, can be considered as generalized biomarkers. As to whether growth factor and growth factor receptor autocrine loops (EGF-R, c-erb2-R, GRP-R, IGF-R, PAM-R) belong to the first generalized or more specific markers needs further comparison between different cohorts of patients with and without history of cancer. The second type of markers are specific markers that identify genetic abnormalities definitively on an irreversible pathway to cancer. Oncogene activation (*ras* mutation, *myc* amplification, cyclin D1 amplification) and inactivation of identified tumor suppressor genes, are examples of specific markers for tumor progression. Other specific markers include inactivation of tumor suppressor genes detected using LOH for their specific chromosomal loci and identification of abnormal alleles or protein products: 3p LOH at 3p14, 3p25 and 3p21 (FHIT for Fragile Histidine Triad); 9p/p16 (LOH for 9p21, immunohistochemistry for p16 expression and methylation study for p16 methylation); 17p/p53 (LOH for 17p13 deletion detected by sequencing, SSCP; immunostaining for p53 mutation; 13q/Rb (LOH 13q14, immunohistochemistry to detect Rb loss of expression); 5q21 (LOH). Establishing a defined sequence of expression for particular markers may improve clinical application of particular biomarkers and can be applied to identify the field cancerization. Other, late markers can be utilized as markers for cancer progression.

Our knowledge of the chronology of these different genetic events is only partial. 3p and 9p LOH as well as general aneuploidy can be considered as early markers for initiation and promotion. Mutations of *ras* or *p53* as well as *Rb* are currently regarded by some as late genetic molecular abnormalities more predictive of progression and invasion. These hypotheses should be evaluated in larger clinical trials. Correlating histopathological changes with marker phenotypes is of interest since this is the mainstay of current diagnosis for invasive carcinoma. The correlation of genetic damage with preinvasive morphological changes could be challenging as evidence mounts that extensive genetic damage precedes morphological change. So far most lung biology studies have concentrated on proximal airways. Understanding of the morphological changes involved in preneoplastic peripheral lesions for adenocarcinoma is poor and requires more morphological and molecular study.

Workshop participants enumerated the criteria for clinically applying new markers and these validation steps are listed in Table 4. An important theme that was echoed throughout the workshop was that the development of effective early lung cancer detection markers does not diminish the fundamentally important role played by smoking cessation in the management of this disease. However, the number of lung cancer cases arising in aging former smokers is now approaching the number of lung cancer cases arising in current smokers. Early detection and effective chemoprevention may be the most promising clinical approach to benefit former smokers. If one is optimistic about the rapid improvement of early detection tools validated with high positive predictive value emerging from already ongoing clinical trials, then another concern is how these early detected cohorts are going to be managed clinically. This possibility warrants enhanced research efforts to develop chemoprevention alternatives to control lung cancer confined to the bronchial tree. Only with coordinated clinical management strategies appropriate to the early stage of lung cancer will the optimal benefit of effective early lung cancer detection be realized.

In addition, further research on elucidating useful intermediate end-point biomarkers to monitor the success of chemoprevention measures should be encouraged. Currently there are no reliable means to evaluate disease progression and response to establish the benefit of clinical interventions. This

Table 4. Considerations in validating a marker for clinical application

1. Clearly define the particular clinical application (early diagnosis, progression marker, metastatic marker).
2. The following criteria should be fulfilled: the marker must be expressed by a large proportion of clinical specimens from individuals who eventually develop lung cancer (retrospective study on archived material); the marker must allow stratification of individuals by clinical risk, the marker must be expressed at high enough levels to allow detection, detectable in small samples by technologically feasible methods (feasible in this context means the assay should have low cost and high throughput capacity).
3. Prospective clinical trials to rigorously define the performance characteristics of the new marker imply that comprehensive databases (clinical, epidemiological, genetic susceptibility) should be included in the trial design.

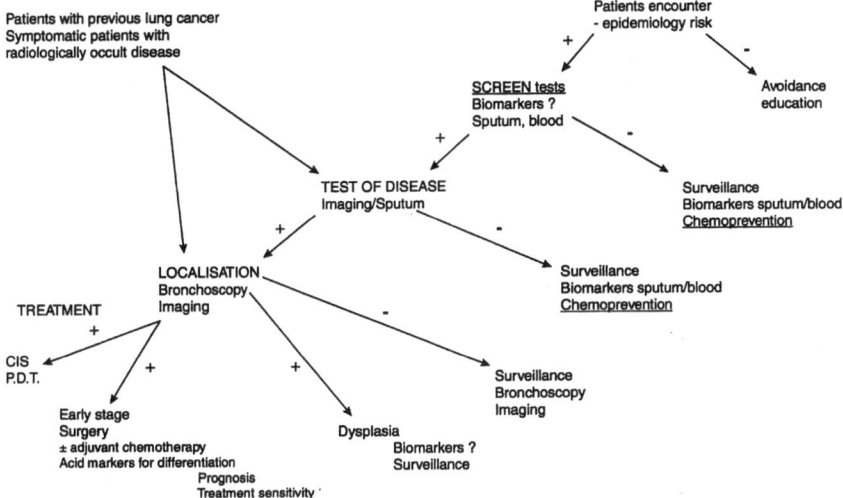

Figure 1. P.D.T.: Photodynamic therapy.

is an important new application in which biologically-defined markers can play a fundamental role.

It is highly unlikely that any single marker will have sufficient sensitivity, specificity and positive predictive value to stratify all patients. Thus, algorithms based on panels of markers will have to be developed and validated for use in patient management. New technologies may allow for multiple marker determinations to be performed with acceptable costs on routine clinical specimens. A proposal for how the early detection issues can be phased in with clinical management of patients while applying the paradigm shift into early detection in oncology is summarized in Figure 1.

The meeting was adjourned and the dialogue about the opportunities to move to a more prevention-oriented approach to lung cancer care moved to Nancy, France in October 1996, due to the intense interest in this promising new area. The group shared a sense of optimism about developing research opportunities that may finally translate into significant improvements in lung cancer outcomes.

References

1. Battey JF, Brown PH, Gritz ER, Hong WK, Johnson BE, Karp DD, Mulshine JL, Shaw GL, Shopland BR, Sunday ME, Szabo E (1995) Primary and secondary prevention of lung cancer: An international association for the study of lung cancer workshop. *Lung Cancer* 12: 91–103.
2. Tobacco policy recommendations of the international association for the study of lung cancer (IASLC): a ten point program. (1994) *Lung Cancer* 405–407.
3. Hirsch FR, Brambilla E, Gray N, Gritz E, Kelloff G, Linnoila RI, Pastorino U, Mulshine JL (1997) Prevention and early detection of lung cancer – clinical aspects. *Lung Cancer* 17: 163–174.

4. Lippman S, Benner S, Hong WK. (1994) Cancer chemoprevention. *J Clin Oncol* 12: 851.
5. Kelloff GJ, Boone CW (1995) Cancer chemopreventive agents: drug development status and future prospects. *J Cell Biochem Suppl* 22: 1–259.
6. Hong WK, Lippman SM, Itri LM, Karp DD, Lee JS, Byer RM, Schantz SP, Kramer AM, Lotan R, Peters LJ (1990) Prevention of second primary tumors in squamous cell carcinoma of the head and neck with 13-cis-retinoic acid. *N Engl J Med* 323: 795.
7. Costa A, Formelli F, Chiesa F, Decensi A, DePalo G, Veranesi U (1994) Prospects of chemoprevention of human cancers with the synthetic retinoid, fenretinide. *Cancer Res* 54: 2032S–2037S.
8. Oridate N, Lotan D, Xu X-C, Hong WK, Lotan R (1996) Differential induction of apoptosis by all-trans-retinoic acid and N-(4-hydroxyphenul) retinamide in head and neck squamous cell carcinoma cell lines. *Clin Cancer Res* 2: 855–863.
9. DeVries N, Van Zandwijk N, Pastorino U (1991) The EUROACAN Study. *Br J Cancer* 64: 985–989.
10. Szabo E, Mulshine JL (1996) Lung cancer prevention: historical and future perspectives. *In*: Aisner J, Arrigada R, Green MR, Martini N, Perry MC (eds) *Comprehensive textbook of thoracic oncology*. Baltimore: Williams and Wilkins, p. 90–104.
11. Jones R (1996) The impact of molecular medicine on health services. *Nature Med* 2: 959.
12. Saccomanno G, Archer VE, Auerbach O, Kuschner M, Beckler PA (1965) Cancer of the lung: the cytology of sputum prior to the development of carcinoma. *Acta Cytol* 9: 413–423.
13. Yakubovskaya MS, Spiegelman V, Luo FC, Malaev S, Salnev A, Zborovskaya I, Gasparyan A, Polotsky B, Machaladze Z, Trachtenberg AC, Belitsky GA, Ronai Z (1995) High frequency of K-ras mutations in normal appearing lung tissues and sputum of patients with lung cancer. *Int J Cancer* 63: 810–814.
14. Slaughter DP, Southwick HW, Smejkal W (1953) "Field cancerization" in oral stratified squamous epithelium. *Cancer* 6: 963–968.
15. Auerbach O, Hammond EC, Garfinkel L (1979) Changes in the bronchial epithelium in relation to cigarette smoking 1955–1960 vs. 1970–1977. *N Engl J Med* 300: 381–386.
16. Mulshine JL, Zhou J, Treston AM, Szabo E, Tockman MS, Cuttitta F (1997) New approaches to the integrated management of early lung cancer. *Hem Oncol Clin N Am.* 11: 253–252.
17. Harris CC, Hollstein M (1993) Clinical implications of the p53 tumor-suppressor gene. *N Engl J Med* 329: 1318.

Clinical and Biological Basis of Lung Cancer Prevention
ed. by Y. Martinet, F.R. Hirsch, N. Martinet, J.-M. Vignaud
and J.L. Mulshine
© 1998 Birkhäuser Verlag Basel/Switzerland

CHAPTER 2
Smoking Prevention and Cessation

Philip Tønnesen[1,*], Ellen R. Gritz[2], Nigel Gray[3] and Ingrid R. Nielsen[2]

[1] *Medical Department of Pulmonary Diseases, Gentofte University Hospital,
Hellerup, Denmark*
[2] *Department of Behavioral Science, M.D. Anderson Cancer Center, University of Texas,
Houston, Texas, USA*
[3] *Division of Epidemiology and Biostatistics, European Institute of Oncology, Milan, Italy*

1. Introduction

The most important etiological factor in the development of lung cancer is
smoking, which accounts for approximately 80 to 85% of all lung cancer
cases. Tobacco use is also a major contributor to the incidence of chronic
respiratory disease (80 to 90%) and myocardial infarction (23 to 40%) [1]
and has been strongly correlated with other cancers (e.g. oral, laryngeal
and bladder cancers). Approximately one-third of all cancer deaths is attributed to tobacco [2].

Thus, tobacco smoking has a great impact on morbidity and mortality.
Peto et al. forecast that in this century 60 million people will die in devel-
oped countries as a result of smoking [2]. Tobacco smoking is a pandemic.
While there has been a decrease in the prevalence of smoking in developed

---

* Author for correspondence.

countries, there has been an increase in prevalence in developing countries. If the present trend continues, globally, a dramatic increase in smoking-related deaths will occur in the next 25 years.

The World Health Organization (WHO) has established goals to reduce tobacco related morbidity and mortality [3]. The three major target areas include prevention, smoking cessation and passive smoking. Prevention efforts include activities to discourage initiation of tobacco use, particularly among youth. This will reduce morbidity and mortality rates; however, changes will not be seen until the year 2015 because lung cancer usually takes 20 to 30 years to develop. Encouraging smokers to make attempts to quit and ensuring that adequate cessation resources exist is critical. Avoiding involuntary exposure to environmental tobacco smoke (ETS) protects the health and rights of children and adults.

2. Smoking Prevention and Cessation

2.1. Public Health Policy and Regulations

Preventing young people and others from starting to smoke is a very important element in the struggle against tobacco use. Ninety-two percent of adult smokers in the US tried their first cigarette and 77% became daily smokers before the age of 21 [4]. Smoking cessation is only part of the picture. Changing public policy and regulations are required, although tobacco issues are highly politicized. For example, the tobacco industry has a very powerful lobby which opposes restrictive regulation. Additionally, many national governments raise substantial revenues from tobacco monopolies or sales taxes on cigarettes.

Important elements in a national strategy to prevent and reduce smoking are presented in Table 1, which is based on elements discussed at a recent IASLC workshop (June 1996) combined with relevant elements from other reports [3, 5]. Taxation is very important because increases in cigarette prices decrease the number of young people who start smoking and also encourages some individuals to quit. Legislation aimed at eliminating tobacco advertising is another important tool, in conjunction with regulations to reduce access to cigarettes for minors and policies to prohibit smoking in public places and in workplaces. Lobbying by antismoking activists in the political arm of professional organizations (e.g. the American Public Health Association) at national and international levels is important. Globally, it is important to regulate international sales of tobacco products to countries which have no protections (e.g. advertising restrictions) related to the use of tobacco.

Table 1. National Tobacco Public Health Policy Programmes on Tobacco Control

1. Stimulate, support and coordinate national tobacco control activities by maintenance of a national focal point.
2. Establishment of a national coordinating organization on tobacco and health aspects.
3. Tobacco taxes that increase faster than the growth in prices and incomes. (In EU: Harmonize taxes on tobacco at the highest EU taxation rate).
4. Governments should reduce support for tobacco farming and develop strategies to provide economic alternatives to tobacco agricultural workers. (The EC subsidization plan should be rapidly phased out).
5. A portion of tobacco taxes should be used to finance tobacco control measures and research into smoking-related diseases and smoking prevention.
6. Banning all forms of tobacco advertizing, promotion and sponsorship, (eliminating sports sponsorships, free gifts of coupons and merchandise and banning tobacco billboards and other visible emblems during electronic media programming).
7. A legal requirement for strong, varied warnings on packets of cigarettes. Making health warning labels visible, using a multiple warning rotation system.
8. Restriction of access to tobacco products including a prohibition on sale of tobacco products to young people (<18 years), banning vending machine sales of cigarettes, banning tax-free sale of tobacco in airports etc.
9. Limitations on the level of tar and nicotine permitted in manufactured tobacco products (e.g. a nicotine delivery of <0.5 mg).
10. Mandatory reporting of the levels of toxic constituents in the smoke of manufactured tobacco products.
11. Eliminate passive smoking in workplaces, public transport, public buildings, schools and kindergartens.
12. Monitoring of trends in smoking and other forms of tobacco use, tobacco-related diseases, and effectiveness of national control actions.
13. Health care providers and institutions should set a good example by not smoking themselves, by making institutions smoke-free and by providing smoking cessation treatment.
14. Effective programmes of education and promotion aimed at smoking prevention and cessation.
15. Voluntary organizations should be involved in smoking prevention and cessation. Ex-smokers might be very useful in these programmes.
16. Effective and widely available support for cessation of smoking, focusing on self-help programmes. Initiate cessation programmes in the electronic media. Reimburse behavioural and pharmacological treatment for smoking cessation.

2.2. Health Care Providers

Health care providers, particularly physicians, dentists and nurses, have a professional as well as an ethical obligation to discourage tobacco use by their patients (Table 2) [3]. Many professional organizations have stressed the importance of reducing smoking to reduce premature death worldwide. The American College of Chest Physicians, American Thoracic Society, Asia Pacific Society of Respirology, Canadian Thoracic Society, European Respiratory Society and International Union Against Tuberculosis and Lung Diseases have stated in an official report that the physician has a responsibility to play a strong and active role in seeking to reduce smoking [6]. Providers can demonstrate their responsibility in their own behavior as well, by 1) striving for a smoke-free profession; 2) never using tobacco in the presence of their patients; 3) making professional meetings smoke-free;

Table 2. Health Care Providers' (HCP) responsibility regarding smoking

1. HCP should discourage tobacco use in their patients.
2. HCP should deliver state-of-the-art assistance to patients and family members.
   (NCI model: Ask, Advise, Assist and Arrange for followup).
3. Physicians and other health care professionals should make antismoking statements in
   media and community (schools).
4. Promote smoking prevention in young people, especially by the family practitioner and
   dentists. Parents serve as important role models.
5. Promote the involvement of professional organizations on the local, state and national
   level. Encourage meetings about smoking-related topics.
6. Individuals at high risk for smoking-related tumors should be targeted for more intensive
   interventions.
7. Doctors and all other health care providers should serve as role models by not smoking
   at all.
8. Introduce and support local policy initiatives; public health advice will have the largest impact.
9. All patients should have a smoking history recorded regularly and this should lead to
   regular counseling. Brochures and other self-help material about smoking cessation
   should be delivered to patients.
10. HCP should be updated about smoking-related topics (diseases, prevention, cessation)
    by participating in regular educational courses.

4) enforcing smoke-free regulations in their hospitals and practices; and
5) using their professional organizations to develop a strong antismoking
policy and advocacy position.

The involvement of physicians in smoking prevention and cessation has
grown slowly over time and varies substantially between specialities, as
well as between nations. While physicians receive training in the adverse

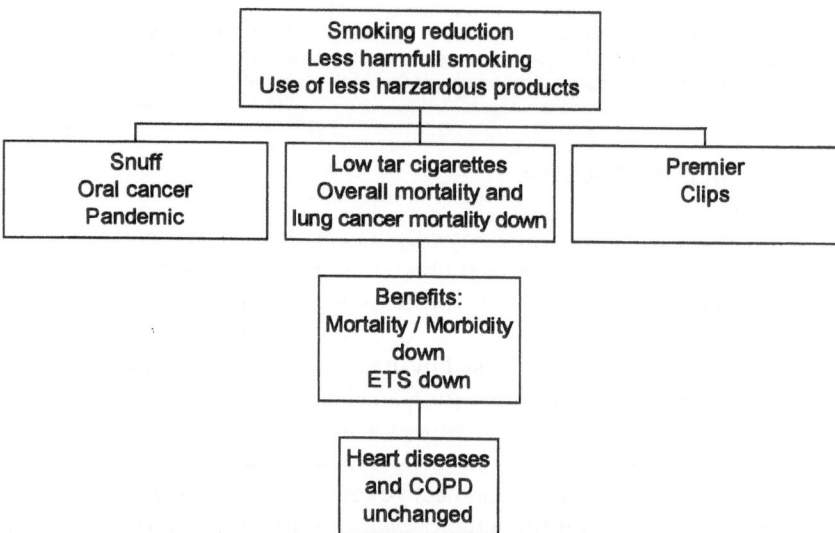

Figure 1. Schematic presentation of smoking reduction. Premier and Clips = ultra low tar
cigarettes.

pathophysiological consequences of tobacco use, most are not adequately trained in providing smoking cessation counseling [7]. In addition, physicians often believe that cessation counseling takes too much time, and they become discouraged if their patients fail to quit smoking [7]. Physicians, particularly in many European countries, have been limited by few available, effective treatment resources. Engaging other health care providers (e.g. nurses or psychologists) to promote smoking cessation is important. Incorporating information about smoking cessation in medical school curricula and in continuing medical education is essential.

2.3. Clinical Guidelines

Health care providers should deliver state-of-the-art assistance to help their smoking patients to quit. The Agency for Health Care Policy and Research [8] in the US has recently published guidelines for successful smoking cessation treatment based on meta-analyses and a comprehensive and systematic literature review of smoking cessation interventions spanning 1978 to 1994 [8].

These guidelines contain patient-oriented material, advice guidelines for primary care providers, and detailed information for smoking cessation specialists.

Smoking cessation methods range from no professional contact (i.e. self-help) to minimal professional contact (i.e. brief advice from primary health provider) to intensive contact (i.e. group or individual counseling). Intervention strategies may include general skill-building (e.g. coping skills, relapse prevention techniques); addressing components known to affect quitting (e.g. weight/diet); and behavioral strategies (e.g. contingency contracting).

The major findings and recommendations from the AHCPR Smoking Cessation Guideline Panel (1996) include [8]:

1. Effective smoking cessation treatments be available and every patient who smokes should be offered one or more of these treatments.
2. It is essential that clinicians determine and document the tobacco-use status of every patient treated in a health care setting.
3. Brief cessation treatments are effective, and at least a minimal intervention should be provided to every patient who uses tobacco.
4. A dose-response relation exists between the intensity and duration of treatment and its effectiveness. In general, the more intense the treatment, the more effective it is in producing long-term abstinence from tobacco.
5. Three treatment elements, in particular, are effective, and one or more of these elements should be included in smoking cessation treatment:
   Nicotine Replacement Therapy (nicotine patches or gum)
   Social support (clinician-provided encouragement and assistance)
   Skills training/problem solving (techniques of achieving and maintaining abstinence).

6. Effective reduction of tobacco use requires that health care systems make institutional changes that result in systematic identification of, and intervention with, all tobacco users at every visit.

2.3.1. Assessing nicotine dependence: Cigarette smoking is governed by social, psychological, habitual and behavioral factors as well as by nicotine addiction. Quitting smoking requires far more than willpower. The importance of nicotine dependence is underscored by the findings that nicotine replacement doubles outcome in smoking cessation trials [8, 9]. Withdrawal symptoms begin hours after quitting, peak at approximately 7 days, and then gradually decrease over 4 to 12 weeks. The nicotine withdrawal syndrome may include the following: dysphoric or depressed mood; insomnia; irritability; frustration or anger; anxiety; difficulty in concentrating; restlessness; decreased heart rate; and increased appetite or weight gain [10]. Nicotine dependence should be assessed and recorded for every smoker using the Fagerstrom Tolerance Questionnaire (FTQ) or the modified Fagerstrom Test for Nicotine Dependence (FTND) (Table 3) [11].

2.3.2. Addressing barriers to smoking cessation: There are some basic principles related to successful smoking cessation that are important for the physician to consider [12]: patients must stop smoking completely at quit day (even 1 or 2 cigarettes per day during the first 2 weeks of cessation are usually followed by relapse); use of nicotine replacement therapy lessens withdrawal symptoms and improves cessation outcomes; followup should be arranged to prevent relapse (which is highest during the first 3 to 6 weeks and then gradually declines, similar to other addictions); if the patient relapses, encourage him/her to make another quit attempt (the average 12-month success rate reported in most studies is 15 to 25%).

2.3.3. Addressing high risk populations: Individuals at highest risk for smoking-related tumors should be targeted for the most intensive interventions. Vulnerable populations include patients with smoking-related prior

Table 3. Clinical guidelines for Health Care Providers for smoking cessation treatment

1. Every person who smokes should be offered cessation treatment at every visit to the practice.
2. Clinicians should ask and record the tobacco-use status of every patient (also use carbon monoxide measurements).
3. Cessation treatments even as brief as 3 minutes per visit are effective.
4. More intensive treatment is more effective in producing longterm abstinence from tobacco.
5. Nicotine replacement therapy (nicotine patches and gum), clinician-delivered social support, and skills training are the three most effective components of smoking cessation treatment.
6. Health care systems should make institutional changes that result in the systematic identification (and intervention) of all tobacco users at every visit.

cancers; other smoking-related diseases (e.g. coronary heart disease, chronic obstructive pulmonary disease (COPD), vascular diseases); chronic heavy smokers; survivors of any cancer site who continue to smoke; and genetically susceptible individuals (once reliable and valid biomarkers are established). Furthermore, intensive smoking cessation treatment (combining behavioral and pharmacotherapy), delivered by clinical specialists, could be integrated into chemoprevention trials which recruit former, but not current smokers. One design suggestion would be to provide such treatment during the run-in period and to incorporate smoking cessation as an eligibility criterion for randomization in such clinical trials. Booster treatments to maintain abstinence could be made readily available. Research might also examine the relationship of nicotine dependence, smoking cessation and chemoprevention efficacy, involving genetic, behavioral and biological variables as predictors and endpoints.

2.4. Pharmacotherapy: Nicotine Replacement Therapy

The effect of nicotine in the brain is complex and not fully explored. Nicotine binds to cholinergic nicotinic receptors in the brain, in the limbic system and the cortex [13]. The physiological effects of nicotine include both stimulant (behavioral arousal and stimulation of the sympathetic nervous system) and sedative effects. Nicotine stimulates the release of neurotransmitters such as β-endorphins which may result in feelings of relaxation including reduced anxiety and tension [14].

The rationale for nicotine substitution is as follows: When quitting smoking, the administration of nicotine decreases withdrawal symptoms in the first months, thus allowing the subject to cope with the behavioral and psychological aspects of smoking. With the nicotine replacement products used today, lower nicotine levels are attained compared to smoking (i.e. the high peak plasma levels of nicotine reached during smoking are not achieved). Nicotine replacement products are reduced gradually (usually over 2 to 6 months) when withdrawal symptoms are lessened due to decreased dependence.

Results reported in a recent meta-analysis of 53 trials with 17,703 subjects, who received various forms of NRT (gum, patch, nasal spray and inhaler), indicated that the nicotine replacement therapy doubled long-term (6 to 12 months) quit rates [15]. The odds ratio for success of nicotine replacement therapy compared with controls was 1.71 (95% CI, 1.56−1.87). The odds ratio for the different nicotine replacement products were: 1.61 for gum; 2.07 for patch; 2.92 for nasal spray; and 3.05 for inhaler. No studies have directly compared the efficacy of different forms of nicotine administration. However, historical data from three trials by Hjalmarson in Sweden [16−19] using similar designs and adjunctive group therapy found remarkable consistency in 12-month success rates for nico-

Table 4. Fagerström Test for Nicotine Dependence (FTND)

Questions	Answers	Points
1. How soon after you wake up do you smoke your first cigarette?	Within 5 min 6−30 min 31−60 min 61 min +	3 2 1 0
2. Do you find it difficult to refrain from smoking in places where it is forbidden, e.g. in church, at the library, in the cinema etc.?	Yes No	1 0
3. Which cigarette would you hate most to give up?	The first one in the morning All others	1 0
4. How many cigarettes per day do you smoke?	10 or less 11−20 21−30 31 or more	0 1 2 3
5. Do you smoke more frequently during the first hours after waking than during the rest of the day?	Yes No	1 0
6. Do you smoke if you are so ill that you are in bed most of the day?	Yes No Total score: Heavily nicotine addicted >6	1 0 0−10

tine gum (29%), nicotine nasal spray (27%), and nicotine inhaler (28%) with placebo rates of 16%, 15% and 18%, respectively (Table 4). The nicotine replacement products described above are self dosing systems to be used *ad libitum*, in contrast to the patch, which "infuses" about 1 mg of nicotine per hour at a constant rate.

2.4.1. Nicotine chewing gum: Nicotine is bound to an ion-exchange resin in the gum base, and bicarbonate is added to attain an alkaline pH in the mouth in order to facilitate absorption of nicotine. To reduce side effects due to swallowed nicotine, proper patient instruction is important. Gum users should chew a piece only 5 to 10 times until they can taste the nicotine, then let the gum rest in the cheek for a few minutes, and then chew again to expose a new surface of the gum. The gum can be chewed for 20 to 30 minutes. About 0.8 to 1.0 mg of nicotine is absorbed from a piece of 2-mg nicotine gum and 1.2 to 1.4 mg of nicotine from a 4-mg piece [20]. With use of nicotine gum throughout the day, blood levels of one-third (for 2-mg gum) and two-thirds (for 4-mg gum) of the nicotine obtained through smoking are achieved [21, 22, 23].

A basic advantage of the gum is the ability to self-titrate the dose, as opposed to the patch, which delivers a fixed dose. Thus, it is possible to use a piece of gum whenever wanted or needed during the day. The principal disadvantage of gum use is potential underdosing, which might explain the

Table 5. Success rate in % from three placebo-controlled trials with nicotine chewing gum, nasal spray and inhaler by Hjalmarson [16]

Modality:	Gum		Nasal Spray		Inhaler	
Treatment:	Nicotine	Placebo	Nicotine	Placebo	Nicotine	Placebo
Subjects:	n = 106	n = 100	n = 125	n = 123	n = 123	n = 124
6 weeks	77	52	53	27	46	33
3 months	53	30	41	20	37	23
6 months	37	20	35	15	35	19
12 months	29	16	27	15	28	18

Differences between nicotine and placebo significant at at least $p < 0.05$.

lack of effect in several trials. The approximate dose equivalent for most nicotine patches is 20 pieces of the 2-mg gum, whereas the mean number of pieces of gum consumed daily is only around 5 to 6 in most studies [12]. Thus, underdosing is a plausible explanation for the lack of efficacy in several studies [23–26].

From these observations, it would be logical to attempt to raise the consumed dose either by increasing the number of pieces of gum chewed or by using the higher dose gum (4-mg). In four studies comparing the two, the 4-mg gum was superior to the 2-mg gum for short-term outcome [27–30]. Another way to increase the amount of consumed gum might be to administer the gum in fixed dosage schedules, as shown by Killen et al. [31].

Side effects of the gum consist mainly of mild, transient local symptoms in the mouth, throat and stomach due to swallowed nicotine (nausea, vomiting, indigestion and hiccups). After adequate instruction most smokers can learn to use the gum properly. However, without instructions many will discontinue use or underdose themselves. The constant chewing might produce side effects such as oral or throat soreness, ache in muscles of mastication, hypertrophy of the masseter muscles and loss of dental fillings.

Among subjects who used ≥ 6 pieces of gum daily for one year, success rates ranged from 0 to 25% [32]. Gradual reduction of nicotine gum use seems to be possible in many quitters without relapse to smoking. In the Lung Health Study, among 3,094 smokers who were followed for 5 years, the use of the 2-mg gum appeared safe and did not produce cardiovascular problems or other adverse effects even in subjects who continued to smoke and still used nicotine gum [33].

We suggest that the smoker be instructed to stop smoking completely, use the nicotine gum on a fixed schedule (every hour, from early morning, for at least 8 to 10 hours) and use extra pieces of gum whenever needed. The 2-mg gum can be used for low to medium dependent smokers (i.e. smokers scoring less than 6 on the Fagerstrom Scale), while highly dependent smokers (scoring 6 or more) should start with the 4-mg gum. If the subject uses more than 15 pieces of the 2-mg gum per day, it may be appropriate to switch to the 4-mg gum.

The optimal duration of treatment is not known; however, in most studies the gum has been used for at least 6 to 12 weeks and up to one year. Individualization of treatment duration is recommended.

2.4.2. Nicotine transdermal patch: This is a fixed nicotine delivery system which releases about 1 mg of nicotine per hour for 16 hours (daytime patch) or for 24 hours (24-hours patch). Nicotine substitution is about 50% of the smoking level (21 mg patch/24 hours and 15 mg patch/16 hours). It is much easier to administer the patch and to use it compared to the gum, but it is not possible to self-titrate [34]. The recommended treatment duration is 8 to 12 weeks. In a multicenter smoking cessation trial from the US examining the effect of 0,7-mg, 14-mg and 21-mg nicotine patches, a dose response effect to increasing nicotine dosages was reported [35]. Two large placebo-controlled trials comprising 600 and 1,686 smokers have recently been published [36, 37]. A one year success rate of 9.3% in the active patch group versus 5.0% in the placebo patch group was reported in first study [36] and a 3-month success rate of 14.4% versus 8.6% in the other [37]. Among eight studies examining long-term smoking cessation success, five showed a significant outcome in favor of the nicotine patch [34].

Side effects are mainly mild local skin irritation, occurring in 10 to 20% of subjects. In only 1.5 to 2% of subjects, treatment had to be terminated due to more persistent and severe skin irritation at the location of the nicotine patch [34].

Due to its ease of use, the patch may be the first choice of nicotine delivery systems today. The patch has also been effective when combined with minimal supportive behavioral therapy. The findings from the two large trials in general practice [36, 37] are also very encouraging. Transdermal nicotine replacement does increase success in smoking cessation with minimal adjunctive support. Thus, the patch could also be administered by the busy clinician in most hospitals.

2.4.3. Nicotine inhaler: Each inhaler contains about 10 mg of nicotine and can release approximately 5 mg nicotine. In clinical use, each inhaler releases approximately 1.5 to 2.0 mg of nicotine and the number of inhalers used daily averages 5 or 6. Thus, nicotine levels comparable to those found during use of the 2-mg nicotine gum are attainable (i.e. relatively low concentrations). Few controlled trials have been conducted with a nicotine inhaler. The efficacy and safety of the nicotine inhaler in a double-blind, clinical smoking cessation trial has been examined [38]. The first published study was a 1-year randomized, double-blind, placebo-controlled trial which enrolled 286 smokers. The success rate for smoking cessation was 28% and 12% after 6 weeks, and was 15% and 5% at 12 months ($P < 0.001$), for active versus placebo respectively. The mean nicotine substitution based on determinations after 1 to 2 weeks of therapy was 38 to 43% of smoking levels. The treatment was well accepted and no serious adverse events were reported. In this low intervention setting, the nicohaler appeared safe to use and increased success in smoking cessation. Three other studies have confirmed the above finding with odds ratios in favor of active treatment of 1.6, 2.2 and 1.6 [18, 19, 39]. Another randomized trial (n=223) showed the nicotine inhaler to be significantly ($P<0.01$) superior to placebo particularly among short-term quitters (<3 months). Reported side-effects included mouth/throat irritation and coughing [39]. The inhaler may replace some of the habit patterns associated with smoking (by oral and handling reinforcement) along with providing nicotine replacement.

2.4.4. Nicotine nasal spray (NNS): The NNS consists of a multidose, hand-driven pump spray with nicotine solution. Each puff contains 0.5 mg nicotine, thus a 1 mg dose is delivered if both nostrils are sprayed as recommended. The NNS is a strong and rapid means of delivering nicotine into the human body with a pharmacokinetic profile closely approximating cigarettes. After a single dose of 1 mg nicotine, the peak level is reached within 5 to 10 minutes with average plasma trough levels of 16 ng/ml. Three published studies with the nicotine nasal spray indicate that the 1-year success rates for active NNS versus placebo, were 26% and 10% [17], 27% and 15% [40], and 27% and 17% [41] respectively. Nicotine substitution with the NNS was 40% after 1 month, but 79% in the long-term users after 1 year [40].

During use of the NNS, weight gain was reduced as compared to placebo. This strong spray induces localized side effects such as sneezing, nasal secretion and irritation, and congestion, watery eyes and coughing. For up to 5% of the subjects these side effects were rated as unacceptable, but most symptoms decrease within a few days after the spray is initiated. NNS seems to be effective but difficult to use as a primary tool. Highly nicotine-dependent smokers might be the target group for this delivery mode of nicotine.

2.4.5. Nicotine combinations: Laboratory studies have shown that the combination of nicotine gum and patch might relieve withdrawal symptoms to the same degree as when smoking [42]. Combinations of different delivery forms of nicotine should be tested to evaluate potential side effects, and determine which combination approach is more efficacious. Of course, different combinations may be more appropriate for different clinical populations (heavy versus light smokers, oral cancer patients versus COPD patients, etc.). At the present, use of the nicotine patch to provide a systemic level of nicotine in combination with the use of 1 to 6 pieces of nicotine chewing gum as needed during the day appears to be safe.

2.5. Other Pharmacotherapy

In addition to nicotine replacement therapy, other drugs have been used for smoking cessation, including clonidine, antidepressants, anxiolytics/benzodiazepines, and silver acetate. Clonidine and buspirone have been shown to improve cessation rates [43, 44] but no recommendations were made in the AHCPR smoking cessation guidelines because most of the trials failed to meet the clinical selection criteria for meta-analysis or revealed inconsistent beneficial effects for smoking cessation [8]. Bupropion (Welbutrin), an antidepressant drug, will probably soon be approved in the US for smoking cessation [45].

2.6. Behavioral/Psychological Interventions

Varying degrees of psychological or behavioral therapy have been used as adjunctive therapy. The use of counseling/psychosocial interventions, where individual sessions last 10 minutes or more, markedly increase cessation rates relative to no-contact intervention; however, brief counseling interventions (sessions lasting 3 to 10 minutes) also increase cessation rates over no-contact interventions [8]. These interventions may be delivered by a variety of clinicians and health care personnel. A dose-response relationship exists between person-to-person contact and successful cessation rates [8].

Recommendations for the content of smoking cessation interventions are also included in the AHCPR guideline [8]. While the strength of evidence was somewhat inconsistent, the following recommendations were made: smoking cessation interventions should help smokers recognize and cope with problems encountered in quitting (problem solving/skills training) and should provide social support as part of the treatment. Smoking cessation interventions that use some type of aversive smoking procedure (e.g. rapid smoking, rapid puffing) increase cessation rates and may be used with smokers who desire such treatment or who have been unsuccessful using other methods [8].

Other interventions include acupuncture, hypnosis, negative affect and cue exposure (i.e. exposing smokers to smoking cues without the opportunity to smoke). The evidence was inadequate to support hypnosis, and a meta-analysis comparing active vs control acupuncture concluded that acupuncture was no more effective than placebo [8, 46]. Similarly, insufficient evidence existed to indicate that addressing negative affect and cue exposure treatment improved cessation rates.

3. Conclusion

Cigarette smoking is one of the leading causes of preventable death and disability in the world. Health professionals play a vital role in promoting smoking cessation and in discouraging initiation of tobacco use. Assessing smoking status should become as routine as assessing vital signs. Intervention with all smoking patients is critical if reductions in morbidity and mortality are to be achieved. While nicotine replacement therapy greatly enhances cessation outcomes, cessation counseling and behavioral strategies are important adjuncts for maintaining long-term smoking cessation. Health care providers should take advantage of the excellent resources now available which provide effective smoking cessation models that can be easily incorporated into clinical practice [7, 8, 47].

References

1. USDHHS (1990) *The Health Benefits of Smoking Cessation: A Report of the Surgeon General,* DHHS CDC 90-8416. US Department of Health and Human Services, Public Health Service, Centers for Disease Control, Center for Chronic Disease Prevention and Health Promotion, Office on Smoking and Health, Rockville, Maryland, USA.
2. Peto R, Lopez AD, Boreham J, Thun M, Herth C (1994) *Mortality from tobacco in developed countries 1950–2000.* Oxford University Press.
3. WHO (1995) *Guidelines for controlling and monitoring the tobacco epidemic.* Pre-publication draft. WHO, Geneva.
4. CDC (1994) Reasons for tobacco use and symptoms of nicotine withdrawal among adolescent and young adult tobacco users. *Morbidity and Mortality Weekly Report* 43(41): 745–750.
5. IASLC Workshop (1996) *Prevention and early detection of lung cancer. Clinical aspects.* Proceedings, Elsinore, Denmark.
6. American College of Chest Physcians, American Thoracic Society, Asia Pacific Society of Respiralogy, Canadian Thoracic Society, European Respiratory Society International Union Against Tuberculosis and Lung Diseases (1995) Smoking and health: A physician's responsibility. A statement of the joint committee on smoking and health. *Eur Respir J* 8: 1808–1811.
7. USDHHS (1994) *Tobacco and the Clinician Interventions for Medical and Dental Practice,* NCI 94-3693. US Department of Health and Human Services, Public Health Service, National Institutes of Health, Rockville, Maryland, USA.
8. Fiore MC, Bailey WC, Cohen SJ, Goldstein MG, Gritz ER, Heyman RB, et al. (1996) *Smoking Cessation. Clinical Practice Guideline No 18,* AHCPR 96-0692. US Department of Health and Human Services, Public Health Service, Agency for Health Care Policy and Research.
9. Fiore MC, Smith SS, Jorenby DE, Baker TB (1994) The effectiveness of the nicotine patch for smoking cessation. *JAMA* 271(24): 1940–1947.
10. APA (1994) *Diagnostic and Statistical Manual of Mental Disorders – IV.* American Psychiatric Association, Washington D.C.
11. Fagerström KO, Heatherton TF, Kozlowski LT (1991) Nicotine addiction and its assessment. *Ear, Nose and Throat* 69: 763–768.
12. Tønnesen P (1994) Smoking cessation programs. *In*: Hansen HH (ed.): *Lung Cancer,* Kluwer Ac. Pb., pp 75–89.
13. Corrigall WA (1991) Understanding brain mechanisms in nicotine reinforcement. *Br J Addiction* 86: 507–510.
14. Lynch BS, Bonnie RJ (eds) (1994) *Growing Up Tobacco Free-Preventing Nicotine Addiction in Children and Youths,* National Academy Press, Institute of Medicine, Washington, D.C.
15. Silagy C, Mant D, Fowler G, Lodge M (1994) Meta-analysis on efficacy of nicotine replacement therapies in smoking cessation. *Lancet* 343: 139–142.
16. Hjalmarson A (1984) Effect of nicotine chewing gum in smoking cessation: A randomized, placebo-controlled, double-blind study. *JAMA* 252: 2835–283.
17. Hjalmarson A, Franzon M, Westin A, Wiklund O (1994) Effect of nicotine nasal spray on smoking cessation. *Archs Intern Med* 154: 2567–2572.
18. Hjalmarson A, Nilsson F, Sjostrom L, Wiklund O. The nicotine inhaler in smoking cessation: A double-blind randomized clinical evaluation. In manuscript.

19. Hjalmarson A. Smoking Cessation. Evaluation of supportive strategies with special reference to nicotine replacement therapy (Thesis), Goteborg University, 1996.
20. Benowitz NL (1988) Toxicity of nicotine: Implications with regard to nicotine replacement tharapy. *In:* Pomerleau OF, Pomerleau CS (eds): *Nicotine replacement. A critical evaluation.* Alan R. Liss, Inc, New York, pp 187–218.
21. McNabb ME, Ebert RV, McCusker K (1982) Plasma nicotine levels produced by chewing nicotine gum. *JAMA* 248: 865–868.
22. McNabb ME (1984) Chewing nicotine gum for 3 months: What happens to plasma nicotine levels? *Can Med Assoc J* 131: 589–592
23. Tønnesen P, Fryd V, Hansen M, Helsted J, Gunnersen AB, Forchammer H, Stockner M (1988) Two and four mg nicotine chewing gum and group counseling in smoking cessation: An open, randomized, controlled trial with a 22 month follow-up. *Addict Behav* 13: 17–27.
24. Malcolm RE, Sillett RW, Turner JAMcM, Ball KP (1980) The use of nicotine chewing gum as an aid to stopping smoking. *Psychopharmacologia* 70: 295–296.
25. Fee WM, Stewart MJ (1982) A controlled trial of nicotine chewing gum in a smoking withdrawal clinic. *Practitioner* 5; 226: 148–151.
26. Fagerström KO (1982) A comparison of psychological and pharmacological treatment in smoking cessation. *J Behav Med* 5: 343–351.
27. Tønnesen P, Fryd V, Hansen M, Helsted J, Gunnersen AB, Forchammer H, Stockner M (1988) Effect of nicotine chewing gum in combination with group counseling on the cessation of smoking. *N Engl J Med* 318: 15–18.
28. Puska P, Bjorkqvist S, Koskela K (1979) Nicotine containing chewing gum in smoking cessation: A double-blind trial with half year follow-up. *Addict Behav* 4: 141–146.
29. Blöndal T (1989) Controlled trial of nicotine polacrilex gum with supportive measures. *Arch Intern Med* 149: 1818–1821.
30. Kornitzer M, Kittel F, Draimaix M. Bourdoux P (1987) A double-blind study of 2 mg versus 4 mg nicotine gum in an industrial setting. *J Psychosom Res* 31: 171–176.
31. Killen JD, Fortmann SP, Newman B, Varady A (1990) Evaluation of a treatment approach combining nicotine gum with self-guided behavioral treatments for smoking relapse prevention. *J Consult Clin Psychol* 58: 85–92.
32. Hughes JR, Gust SW, Keenan R, Fenwick JW, Skoog K, Higgins ST (1991) Long-term use of nicotine vs placebo gum. *Arch Intern Med* 151: 1993–1998.
33. Murray RP, Bailey WC, Daniels K, Bjornson WM, Kurnow K, Connett JE, Nides MA, Kiley JP (1996) Safety of nicotine polacrilex gum used by 3,094 participants in the lung health study. *Chest* 109: 438–445.
34. Fagerström KO, Säwe U, Tønnesen P (1992) Therapeutic use of nicotine patches: Efficacy and safety. *J Smoking-Related Dis* 3: 247–261.
35. Transdermal Nicotine Study Group. Transdermal nicotine for smoking cessation. (1991) *JAMA* 22: 3133–3138.
36. Russell MAH, Stableton JA, Feyerabend C, Wiserman SM, Gustavsson G, Säwe U, Connor P. (1993) Targeting heavy smokers in general practice: randomised controlled trial of transdermal nicotine patches. *Br Med J* 306: 1308–1312.
37. Imperial Cancer Research Fund General Practice Research Group: Effectiveness of a nicotine patch in helping people to stop smoking: results of a randomised trial in general practice. (1993) *Br Med J* 306: 1304–1308.
38. Tønnesen P, Nørregaard J, Mikkelsen K, Jørgensen S, Nilsson F (1993) A double-blind trial of a nicotine inhaler for smoking cessation. *JAMA* 269: 1268–1271.
39. Schneider NG, Olmstead R, Nilsson F, Vaghaiwalla Mody F, Franzon M, Doan K (1996) Efficacy of a nicotine inhaler in smoking cessation: a double-blind, placebo-controlled trial. *Addiction* 91(9): 1293–1306.
40. Sutherland G, Stapleton JA, Russell MAH, Jarvis MJ, Hajek P, Belcher M, Feyerabend C (1992) Randomised controlled trial of a nasal nicotine spray in smoking cessation. *Lancet* 340: 324–329.
41. Blondal T, Franzon M, Westin A, Olafsdottir I, Gudmundsdottir S, Gunnarsdottir R (1993) Controlled trial of nicotine nasal spray with long term follow-up. (Abstract) *ARRD* 147: A806.
42. Fagerström KO, Schneider NG, Lunnel E (1993) Effectiveness of nicotine patch and nicotine gum as individual versus combined treatment for tobacco withdrawal symptoms. *Psychopharmacology* 110: 251–257.

43. UDHHS (1988) US Department of Health and Human Services. *The Health Consequences of Smoking: Nicotine Addiction: A Report of the Surgeon General,* DHHS CDC 88-8406. Public Health Service, Centers for Disease Control, Center for Chronic Disease Prevention and Health Promotion, Office on Smoking and Health, Rockville, Maryland, USA.
44. Glourlay SG, Stead LF, Benowitz NL (1997) A meta-analysis of clonidine for smoking cessation. *The Cochrane Library* 1.
45. Gawin F, Comptom M, Byck R (1989) Buspirone reduces smoking. *Arch Gen Psychiat* 46: 288.
46. White AR, Rampes H (1997) Acupuncture in smoking cessation. *The Cochrane Library* 1.
47. Glynn TJ, Manley MW (1991) *How to Help Your Patients Stop Smoking. A National Cancer Institute Manual for Physicians.* NIH 92-3064. Smoking, Tobacco and Cancer Program, Division of Cancer Prevention and Control, National Cancer Institute.

Clinical and Biological Basis of Lung Cancer Prevention
ed. by Y. Martinet, F. R. Hirsch, N. Martinet, J.-M. Vignaud
and J. L. Mulshine
© 1998 Birkhäuser Verlag Basel/Switzerland

CHAPTER 3
Clinical Pharmacology of Vitamin A and Retinoids

Ugo Pastorino[1] and Franca Formelli[2]

[1] *Department of Thoracic Surgery Royal Brompton Hospital, London, UK*
[2] *Istituto Nazionale Tumori, Milan, Italy*

1 Vitamin A (Retinol)
2 All-*Trans* Retinoic Acid
3 13-*cis* Retinoic Acid
4 Fenretinide (4HPR)
References

1. Vitamin A (Retinol)

Natural vitamin A (all-*trans* retinol, retinal, and retinyl esters; Figure 1) is essential for vision, reproduction and maintenance of differentiated epithelia and mucus secretion in humans and higher animals [1]. *Trans*-retinoic acid shares only a part of these functions, being unable to support vision and

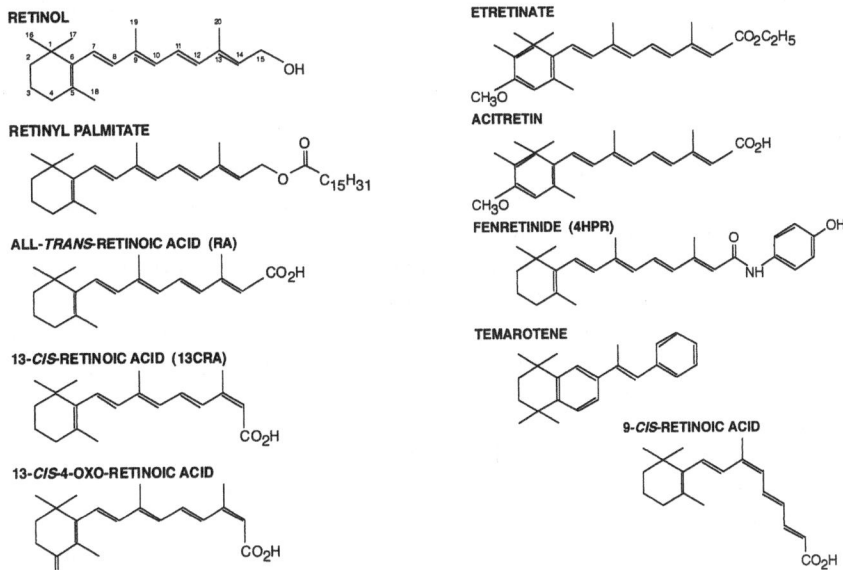

Figure 1. Chemical structure of different retinoids.

reproduction; so animals maintained on retinoic acid as their only source of vitamin A are both blind and sterile [2, 3]. Retinol is stored in the liver in large amounts (over 90% of the total capacity), which normally exceed the one-year physiological requirement, and is then released into the plasma and transported bound to a specific retinol-binding protein (RBP). The process of mobilization is mainly controlled by the liver, although according to new studies recycling from peripheral tissues and extravascular spaces may also be relevant [4]. Consequently, retinol plasma levels are maintained stable except in extreme conditions (chronic dietary deficiency, high dose supplementation).

Pharmacokinetics of orally administered retinol are controlled by a tight homeostatic mechanism, and the administration of moderate doses of vitamin A failed to show any significant change of retinol plasma levels in a number of studies. A randomized double-blind trial on 376 volunteers revealed that oral administration of retinyl palmitate at moderate dosage (10,000 to 36,000 IU daily) could induce a slight but significant increase of basal retinol level, about 2% for every 10,000 IU [5]. In a pilot study on cancer patients, higher doses of oral retinol (up to 200,000 IU/m^2 daily) produced a rapid increase of retinyl palmitate, with a mean time to peak plasma concentration of nearly 4 hours and an initial phase halflife of 2 hours [6]. However, plasma retinol concentration was increased only in patients with low initial levels. Plasma halflife of retinyl palmitate, when retinol was given at the daily dose of 25,000 IU, ranged between 15 and 22 hours [7]. In our experiments, based on 307 patients randomized to receive retinyl palmitate or control, a daily dose of 300,000 IU was associated with a significant increase of the average values of plasma retinol and RBP (greater than 30% and 60% respectively) after 12 months of treatment [8].

Although it has never been properly evaluated, intestinal absorption rate in humans is commonly estimated as 50% to 60% of total dietary retinol. However, several factors may influence the pharmacology of oral vitamin A supplementation, such as the chemical structure (alcohol, esters) or the type of preparation (oily solution, emulsion). For instance, a retrospective study on human toxicity data has estimated that the absorption and storage rate of emulsified retinol may be as high as 80%, compared to only 20% for oily solutions [9]. Chemical and physical properties, may also be implicated in the pattern of liver toxicity as well as the bioavailability of the substance in extrahepatic tissues. The difference may be prominent between natural substances such as retinol, which are almost entirely vehiculated as chylomicrons in the general circulation through the lymphatic system, and retinoic acid which is directly transported to the liver through the portal system [10]. *In vitro* experiments on HL-60 cells, showing growth inhibition and differentiation after exposure of leukemic cells to chylomicron retinyl esters, represent an indirect confirmation of the biological and clinical relevance of extrahepatic uptake of chylomicron retinyl esters [11].

In our randomized trial using emulsified retinyl palmitate at high dose for a period ranging from 12 to 24 months, we could demonstrate neither a significant impairment of liver function nor an objective liver toxicity, as assessed by standard hematochemical tests. Average values of liver enzymes (serum SGOT and GPT), measured every month up to 24 months of treatment, were nearly identical in randomized controls compared to treated individuals, with only a limited proportion of patients (10 to 20%) showing serum levels above the normal range in both groups [12]. On the other hand, retinyl palmitate administration caused a remarkable increase of serum triglycerides, becoming statistically significant at 12 months of treatment, with average values in excess of 60% compared with baseline levels. Such a significant increase of serum triglycerides was not associated with clinical symptoms or objective signs of cardiovascular damage, and spontaneously reverted to normal values soon after completion of the treatment. Cholesterol levels were less strikingly modified, and the differences in mean values were not significant between the two groups. Renal function tests, glucose fasting levels, hemoglobin values, RBC, WBC and lymphocyte counts were not affected by retinyl palmitate administration. These observations underline the need of properly controlled studies, with prospective randomized setting, for an accurate assessment of the side-effects associated with longterm retinol administration.

2. All-*Trans* Retinoic Acid

Research into the pharmacology of all-*trans* retinoic acid (RA) has been boosted by the clinical challenge of treatment for acute promyelocytic leukemia (APL) [13]. In fact, induction treatment with all-*trans* RA alone could achieve complete remissions in a high proportion of patients with APL, but in the majority of cases the disease recurred after a few months and these patients appeared to be resistant to further treatment at higher doses [14, 15].

After administration of a single oral dose, peak plasma concentrations of all-*trans* RA are reached within 1 to 3 hours, with a halflife of approximately 40 minutes [16, 17] (Table 1). Continuous daily dosing of patients with APL has been associated with a progressive decrease in plasma drug

Table 1. Plasma elimination halflives of various retinoids administered orally to humans

	Halflife in hours	Reference
All-*trans*-retinoic acid (ATRA)	0.8 ± 0.1	[17]
13-*cis*-retinoic acid (13CRA)	10 (6.7 – 36.5)	[18]
Fenretinide (4HPR)	27 ± 4	[19]
Acitrecin	50 (36 – 96)	[20]
Etretinate	2500	[21]

concentrations, and even a two-fold increase in the oral dose did not significantly increase the plasma AUC values [22]. The decrease in Cp_{max} and AUC values was associated with an approximately 10-fold increase in urinary excretion of 4-oxo retinoic acid metabolites. The extent of isomerization to 13-*cis* retinoic acid was minimal in plasma.

In a study of patients with non-small cell lung cancer, the median AUC value appeared to be substantially lower than in patients with APL. This observation led to the classification of cancer patients into "normal" or "rapid" catabolizers, based on whether the AUC on the initial day of dosing was greater or less than the median value of 250 ng·hr/ml [23]. Patients who were rapid catabolizers had significantly lower endogenous plasma retinoid levels than the normal catabolizers. Further studies have shown that a major pathway of metabolic degradation of all-*trans* RA was oxidation by cytochrome P450 enzymes, and that accelerated retinoid catabolism could be blocked by inhibitors of cytochrome P450 oxidases such as ketoconazole or liarozole [24].

It appears that clinical resistance to all-*trans* RA in APL occurs rapidly and universally, but also that it may be reversible after drug treatment has been discontinued for several months [25]. These observations have led to the hypothesis that continuous exposure to this natural retinoid rapidly induces a variety of metabolic processes, ultimately resulting in the reduction of the effective intranuclear concentrations of the ligand to levels that are inadequate to initiate or maintain cellular differentiation.

3. 13-*Cis* Retinoic Acid

The interest in the use of synthetic retinoids in oncology is largely due to the results obtained with 13-*cis* retinoic acid (13CRA) in oral premalignant and malignant diseases. In oral leukoplakia, 13CRA has induced complete clinical and pathological remission in a high proportion of patients [26]. In patients treated for a prior head and neck cancer, 13CRA was effective in preventing the occurrence of second primary tumours [27]. However, two major problems became evident with this drug: the limited tolerability of side-effects with high doses, and the recurrence of leukoplakia when the treatment was stopped. In chemoprevention trials very few patients were able to tolerate the dose of 1 mg/kg for periods greater than 6 months. More recent experiments with low-dose maintenance (0.5 mg/kg) following full-dose induction appeared to be better tolerated [28], and new prospective trials have selected a daily dose of 30 mg.

After a single oral dose of 0.5 mg/kg of 13CRA, mean peak plasma concentration was 250 ng/ml (range 0–740), time to peak plasma concentration 4 hours (range 2–6 hr). After 4 mg/kg p.o. mean peak plasma concentration was 1160 ng/ml (range 828–1950) and time to peak plasma concentration 3 hours (range 1.5–6 hr) [29]. A marked difference in gastrointestinal absorption was probably responsible for the great variation of peak plasma levels (up to 10-fold) in patients receiving the same dose [30]. A lag time of up to 2 hours was reported prior to the onset of intestinal absorption, as well as marked secondary and tertiary concentration peaks consistent with enterohepatic circulation of 13CRA [31]. The pharmacokinetics of multiple doses of 13CRA were tested in 10 patients treated with 40 mg daily for 25 days [18]. Peak plasma concentration after 25 days of treatment was similar to the one observed after the first dose (310 ± 184 ng/ml versus 262 ± 139 ng/ml), time to peak plasma levels was 3.1 versus 2.9 hours, and halflife 9.2 versus 10.4 hours. On the contrary, the concentration of metabolite 13-*cis*-4-oxo-retinoic acid showed a tendency to increase with time. Mean ratio between the area under the curve (AUC 0-infinity) of 13-*cis*-4-oxo-retinoic acid and 13CRA rose from 3.4 ± 1 to 5.1 ± 1, and the halflife of the metabolite was 24.5 hours (range 16.5–49.5).

Data on the pharmacokinetics of chronic administration of 13CRA were obtained from patients who underwent longterm treatment (10 to 360 mg, for at least 2 months) for various dermatological diseases. Maximum drug concentration occurred 1 to 4 hours after drug administration; elimination halflife ranged from 10 to 23 hours for 13CRA and from 20 to 49 hours for 13-*cis*-4-oxo-13CRA; mean AUC ratio between the two substances resulted 3.1 ± 1 (1.7–5.4).

Overall, the available data suggest that plasma levels of 13CRA were relatively stable after multiple doses, and that a longterm pharmacokinetic profile can be predicted from single dose data.

Although animal data have demonstrated that oral administration of many retinoids, including 13CRA, causes significant and dose-proportional reduction of plasma retinol levels [32], clinical data on 13CRA are not conclusive. Some authors have reported no effect on plasma retinol levels after relatively high oral doses, ranging from 3mg/kg daily to 5 mg/kg daily [30]. Others have reported plasma retinol concentrations below the expected normal range in healthy individuals, after 1 to 28 days of treatment [29]. However, baseline levels were not evaluated in these patients and lower plasma retinol concentrations may well be attributable to the advanced neoplastic status rather than 13CRA administration.

4. Fenretinide (4HPR)

The pharmacokinetics of N-(4-hydroxyphenyl)retinamide (4HPR) have been studied in healthy volunteers [33] and in cancer patients [19, 34]. After oral administration, maximum blood concentrations of 4HPR occurred between 3 and 4 hours, whereas the concentrations of its main metabolite N-(4-methoxyphenyl)retinamide (4MPR) occurred between 8 and

12 hours. The bioavailability of 4HPR, as of other retinoids, has been shown to be enhanced by administering it with food, and to be influenced by the composition of meals [35].

Following single oral doses of 25 to 600 mg in healthy subjects, a linear relationship between dose and C_{max} and between dose and AUC was found for both 4HPR and 4MPR [33]. In these subjects the mean elimination halflife of 4HPR was 16 to 20 hours and the halflife of 4MPR was 22 hours. Similar values were found in cancer patients treated with a single oral dose of 300 mg: the halflives of 4HPR and of 4MPR were 13.7 and 23.0 hours, respectively [34].

After multiple daily doses of 150 and 300 mg for 28 days, no significant differences in the pharmacokinetics of 4HPR between the first and the last dose were found and the halflife was found to be 27.2 hours. The metabolite 4MPR showed evidence of accumulation, since the AUC after multiple dosing was higher than for the single dose. No unchanged compound, 4MPR or conjugates were detected in urine, indicating biliary excretion [33].

Monitoring of 4HPR pharmacokinetics during longterm administration have been performed in breast cancer patients who participated in the initial phase I study [34] or received the drug for 5 years within the phase III chemoprevention trial [19]. After 5 months of daily treatment with 100, 200 and 300 mg/day doses, a linear relationship was found between the doses administered and the plasma concentrations of both 4HPR and 4MPR. The daily administration of a dose of 200 mg for 5 years resulted in 4HPR plasma concentrations of approximately 1 µmol/l which remained steady for the whole period [19]. After 5 years of treatment, the halflives of 4HPR and of 4MPR were 27 and 54 hours respectively, similar to those found after 28 days.

In contrast to all-*trans* RA, constant concentrations and constant halflives of 4HPR suggest that the pharmacokinetics of this retinoid do not change during longterm treatment. At 6 and 12 months after drug discontinuation, the concentrations of 4HPR were at the limit of detectability (0.01 µmol/l) whereas those of 4MPR were five times higher.

A relevant pharmacological effect of 4HPR, reported in rats as well as in humans, is the rapid decrease in the plasma concentrations of both retinol and its plasma transport protein RBP [34, 36, 37]. The reduction, which is reversible, occurs after a single dose and is proportional to the dose administered. This effect was associated with impaired dark adaptation in 4HPR-treated patients [38–40]. With daily doses of 200 mg 4HPR, baseline retinol levels were reduced by 71%. As a consequence of these observations, a 3-day treatment interruption at the end of each month was introduced to increase plasma retinol concentrations and allow sufficient storage of retinol in the retina. With this modification of the treatment schedule, mean retinol reduction was limited to 38% [19]. Lower retinol levels persisted throughout the 5-year treatment period but reversal to baseline retinol concentrations was observed in all the patients, shortly after discontinuation. Studies performed on the mechanisms responsible for reduction of retinol levels by 4HPR have shown that this effect is associated with the high binding affinity of this retinoid to RBP and to its interference with the RBPtransthyretin(TTR) complex formation [32].

References

1. Goodman DS (1984) Vitamin A and retinoids in health and disease. *N Engl J Med* 310: 1023−1031.
2. Dowling JE, Wald J (1960) The biological function of vitamin A acid. *Proc Natl Acad Sci USA* 46: 587−608.
3. Thompson JN, Howell JM, Pitt GAJ (1964) Vitamin A and reproduction in rats. *Proc R Soc Lond* 159: 510−535.
4. Blomhoff R, Green MH, Green JB, Berg T, Norum KR (1991) Vitamin A metabolism: new perspectives on absorption, transport and storage. *Physiol Rev* 71: 951−990.
5. Wald NJ, Cuckle HS, Barlow RD, Thompson P, Nanchahal K, Blow RJ, Brown I, Harling CC, McCulloch WJ, Morgan J, Reid AR (1985) The effect of vitamin A supplementation on serum retinol and retinol-binding protein levels. *Cancer Letters* 29: 203−213.
6. Goodman GE, Alberts DS, Peng YM, Beaudry J, Leigh SA, Moon T (1984) Plasma kinetics of oral retinol in cancer patients. *Cancer Treat Rep* 68: 1125−1133.
7. Plezia PM, Alberts DS, Peng YM, Xu MJ, Sayers S, Davis BT, Surwit EA, Meyskens F (1989) The role of serum and tissue pharmacology studies in the design and interpretation of chemoprevention trials. *Preventive Medicine* 18: 680−687.
8. Infante M, Pastorino U, Chiesa G, Bera E, Pisani P, Valente M, Ravasi G (1991) Laboratory evaluation during high-dose vitamin A administration: a randomised study on lung cancer patients after surgical resection. *J Cancer Res Clin Oncol* 117: 156−162.
9. Korner WF, Vollm J (1975) New aspects of the tolerance of retinol in humans. *Int J Vit Nutr Res* 45: 363−372.
10. Fidge NH, Shiratori T, Ganguly J, Goodman DS (1968) Pathways of absorption of retinal and retinoic acid in the rat. *J Lipid Res* 9: 103−109.
11. Wathne KO, Norum KR, Smeland E, Blomhoff R (1988) Retinol bound to physiological carrier molecules regulates growth and differentiation of myeloid leukemic cells. *J Biol Chem* 263: 8691−8695.
12. Pastorino U, Chiesa G, Infante M, et al. (1991) Safety of high-dose vitamin A. Randomized trial on lung cancer chemoprevention. *Oncology* 48: 131−137.
13. Warrell RP Jr (1993) Acquired retinoid resistance in acute promyelocytic leukemia: new mechanisms, strategies, and implications. *Blood* 82: 1949−1953.
14. Huang ME, Ye YC, Chen JR, et al. (1988) Use of all-*trans* retinoic acid in the treatment of acute promyelocytic leukemia. *Blood* 72: 567−572.
15. Fenaux P, Le Dely MC, Castaigne S, Archimbaud E, Chomienne C, Link H, et al. (1993) Effect of all-*trans* retinoic acid in newly diagnosed acute promyelocytic leukemia: results of a multicenter randomized trial. *Blood* 82: 3241−3249.
16. Lefebvre P, Thomas G, Gourmel B, Agadir A, Castaigne S, Dreux C, et al. (1991) Pharmacokinetics of oral all-*trans* retinoic acid in patients with acute promyelocytic leukemia. *Leukemia* 5: 1054−1058.
17. Muindi J, Frankel S, Huselton C, DeGrazia F, Garland W, Young CW, et al. (1992) Clinical pharmacology of oral all-*trans* retinoic acid in patients with acute promyelocytic leukemia. *Cancer Res* 52: 2138−2142.
18. Brazzell RK, Vane FM, Ehmann CW, Colburn WA (1983) Pharmacokinetics of isotretinoin during repetitive dosing to patients. *Eur J Clin Pharmacol* 24: 695−702.
19. Formelli F, Clerici M, Campa T, Di Mauro MG, Magni A, Mascotti G, Moglia D, De Palo G, Costa A, Veronesi U (1993) Five-year administration of fenretinide: pharmacokinetics and effects on plasma retinol concentrations. *J Clin Oncol* 11: 2036−2042.

20. Wiegand UW, Busslinger AA, Chou RC, Jensen BK (1993) The pharmacokinetics of acitretin in humans: an update. *In:* Livrea MA, Packer L (eds): *Retinoids. Progress in research and clinical application,* M. Dekker, Inc., New York, pp 617–628.
21. Massarella JW, Vane FM (1985) Etretinate kinetics during chronic dosing in severe psoriasis. *Clin Pharmacol Ther* 37: 439–446.
22. Muindi J, Frankel SR, Miller WH Jr, Jakubowski A, Scheinberg DA, Young CW, et al. (1992) Continuous treatment with all-*trans* retinoic acid results in a progressive decrease in plasma concentrations: implications for relapse and retinoid "resistance" in acute promyelocytic leukemia. *Blood* 79: 299–303.
23. Rigas JR, Francis PA, Muindi JRF, Huselton C, DeGrazia F, Kris MG, Young CW, Warrell RP Jr (1993) Constitutive variability in catabolism of the natural retinoid, all-*trans* retinoic acid, and its modulation by ketoconazole. *J Natl Cancer Inst* 85: 1921–1926.
24. Miller VA, Rigas JR, Muindi JRF, Tong WP, Venkatraman E, Kris MG, Warrell RP (1994) Modulation of all-*trans* retinoic acid pharmacokinetics by liarazole. *Cancer Chemother Pharmacol* 34: 522–526.
25. Warrell RP Jr, de The H, Wang Z-Y, Degos L (1993) Acute promyelocytic leukemia. *N Engl J Med* 329: 177–189.
26. Hong WK, Endicott J, Itri L, et al. (1986) 13-cis-retinoic acid in the treatment of oral leukoplakia. *New Engl J Med* 315: 1501–1505.
27. Hong WK, Lippman JM, Itri L, et al. (1990) Prevention of second primary tumors with isotretinoin in squamous cell carcinoma of the head and neck. *N Engl J Med* 323: 795–801
28. Lippman SM, Batsakis JG, Toth BB, Weber RS, Lee JJ, Martin JW, Hays GL, Goepfert H, Hong WK (1993) Comparison of low-dose isotretinoin with beta carotene to prevent oral carcinogenesis. *N Engl J Med* 328: 15–20.
29. Kerr IG, Lippman ME, Jenkins J, Myers C (1982) Pharmacology of 13-cis-retinoic acid in humans. *Cancer Res* 42: 2069–2073.
30. Goodman GE, Alberts DS, Peng YM, Beaudry J, Einspahr J, Leigh S, Miles NJ, Davis TP, Meyskens FL (1983) Pharmacokinetics and phase I trial of retinol and 13-cis-retinoic acid. *In:* Modulation and mediation of cancer by vitamins, pp 311–316, Karger, Basel.
31. Khoo KC, Reik FD, Colburn WA (1982) Pharmacokinetic profile of isotretinoin following a single oral dose to normal man. *J Clin Pharmacol* 22: 395–402.
32. Berni R, Clerici M, Malpeli G, Cleris L, Formelli F (1993) Retinoids: *in vitro* interaction with retinol-binding protein and influence on plasma retinol. *FASEB J* 7: 1179–1184.
33. Desiraju RK, Scott V, Nayak RK, Minn FL (1985) Pharmacokinetics of fenretinide in healthy volunteers. *Clin Pharmacol Ther* 37(2): 190.
34. Peng YM, Dalton WS, Alberts DS, Xu MJ, Lim H, Meyskens FL (1989) Pharmacokinetics of N-4-hydroxyphenyl-retinamide and the effect of its oral administration on plasma retinol concentrations in cancer patients. *Int J Cancer* 43: 22–26, 1989. Erratum: *Int J Cancer* 44: 567.
35. Doose DR, Minn FL, Stellar S, Nayak RK (1992) Effects of meals and meal composition on the bioavailability of fenretinide. *J Clin Pharmacol* 32: 1089–1095.
36. Formelli F, Carsana R, Costa A, Buranelli F, Campa T, Dossena G, Magni A Pizzichetta M. (1989) Plasma retinol level reduction by the synthetic retinoid fenretinide: a one year follow-up study of breast cancer patients. *Cancer Res* 49: 6149–6152.
37. Dimitrov NV, Meyer CJ, Perloff M, Ruppenthal MM, Phillipich MJ, Gilliland D, Malone W, Minn FL (1990) Alteration of retinol-binding-protein concentrations by the synthetic retinoid fenretinide in healthy human subjects. *Am J Clin Nutr* 51: 1082–1087.
38. Kaiser-Kupfer MI, Peck GL, Caruso RC (1986) Abnormal retinal function associated with fenretinide, a synthetic retinoid. *Arch Ophtalmol* 104: 69–70.
39. Costa A, Malone W, Perloff M, Buranelli F, Campa T, Dossena G, Magni A, Pizzichetta M, Andreoli C, Del Vecchio M, Formelli F, Barbieri A (1989) Tolerability of the synthetic retinoid fenretinide (HPR). *Eur J Cancer Clin Oncol* 25: 805–808.
40. Decensi A, Torrisi R, Polizzi A, Gesi R, Brezzo V, Rolando M, Rondanina G, Orengo MA, Formelli F, Costa A (1994) Effect of the synthetic retinoid fenretinide on dark adaptation and the ocular surface. *J Natl Cancer Inst* 86: 105–110.

Clinical and Biological Basis of Lung Cancer Prevention
ed. by Y. Martinet, F.R. Hirsch, N. Martinet, J.-M. Vignaud
and J.L. Mulshine

CHAPTER 4
Early Lung Cancer Detection

Elisabeth Brambilla

Lung Cancer Research Group, CSF INSERM 97-01 Institut Albert Bonniot, Grenoble, France and Laboratoire de Pathologie Cellulaire, Hôpital A. Michallon, Grenoble, France

1. Introduction

Lung cancer is a highly lethal global problem. The disease is too often detected only at a terminal stage, when treatment by even the best current methods is insufficient. Better methods of early lung cancer detection are fundamental for a shift to the routine management of truly early (preinvasive) lung cancer. This should be based on two main concepts: 1) A large body of evidence is accumulating which suggests that invasive lung cancer is the end result of a multistep process, in which progressive molecular changes accompany or even precede morphological changes. Genetic changes, because of their exquisite specificity or selectivity, are ideally suited as markers of premalignancy. However, a knowledge of the genetic etiology is required before the markers can be used. It is usually assumed that a phenotypically normal cell is completely genetically normal. 2) The entire epithelium is the target of carcinogens and this is the basis of the field effect concept. Early detection should therefore aim to identify the field effect and devise suitable methods of intervention. Our knowledge is still rudimentary: the clonal/multifocal relationship between pre- and postinvasion is still being investigated. Could a random biopsy yield information for the rest of the field? This is still a matter of discussion. Multiple biopsies should be performed in order to evaluate how broad the cancerization field is as regards genetic damage.

We have known for thirty years, that improvement in outcome requires the ability to identify the disease while it is still localized in the airways. Enhanced understanding of tumor biology and preneoplasia should help to optimize early lung cancer detection, and to select the best from among all of the possible biological markers.

2. Natural History of Carcinogenesis

Lung tumors, both central (squamous and small cell carcinomas) and peripheral (adenocarcinoma), are thought to develop through sequentially appearing morphological and molecular changes, driven by underlying somatic genetic changes. The real frequency of these morphological preneoplastic changes (dysplasia of increasing degrees of severity, and carcinoma *in situ* (CIS)) is difficult for a surgical pathologist to appreciate (Auerbach, 1961) [1]. They are observed by chance in the vicinity of a surgically treated lung cancer, or in a bronchial biopsy taken surgery, or in bronchial biopsies taken from the vicinity of an obvious obstructive tumor by fiberoptic bronchoscopy. Without searching from them, we detected these lesions in 80 patients over five years out of ≈ 1000 patients from whom a diagnostic lung sample was taken. The real frequency is undoubtedly higher, as shown by fluorescent fiberoptic directed bronchial biopsies, which detected dysplasias in 40% of smokers (including 12% with severe dysplasia), and in 25% of ex-smokers (6% severe dysplasias) who had no longer been smoking for 10 years [2].

The stepwise horizontal progression of these morphological lesions is likely to follow highly variable progression rates according to the initial genetic lesions. Vogelstein and others have demonstrated that most tumors undergo a multistep set of genetic events (10 to 20) during their evolution [3]. It is possible that hyperplasia, metaplasia (early changes preceeding dysplasia) and dysplasia itself could bypass further steps and follow a vertical progression to invasion. This would hamper the predictive value of any morphological step except the late ones such as CIS. Clearly, our knowledge of the sequence of molecular events in lung cancer and their relationship to morphological changes is rudimentary. In heavy smokers exhibiting metaplasia, half revert to normal after stopping smoking, which make it difficult to distinguish between reactive reversible and tumorigenic irreversible morphological changes.

The genetic changes, because of their remarkable specificity and selectivity, are ideally suited as markers of premalignancy. However, the definition of a genetically normal cell has not been established. Is a mutation possible in any normal cell? Is a set of mutations specific for malignancy?

The "field cancerization" theory states that much of the epithelium of the upper aerodigestive tract has been mutagenized as the result of exposure to carcinogens (such as cigarette smoke) and is at risk of developing one or more cancers. The high incidence of preneoplastic lesions found in lung cancer, and the high risk of developing second primaries, favors this theory. Two parallel concepts have been proposed by different groups from their studies. The first hypothesis is that inside this "carcinogen-exposed" field, distinct multifocal clones develop with different genotypes. This has been claimed in head and neck as well as in lung carcinoma with regard to p53 and 3p mutations [4–7]. This theory of multiclonal premalignancies in the cancerization field supports the use of genetic markers in the differential diagnosis of recurrence of metastasis versus second primaries in the lung. 3p loss of heterozygosity (LOH) was found in 93 % of alveolar preneoplastic lesions observed in the vicinity of invasive cancers (type II cell hyperplasia, atypical alveolar hyperplasia, alveolar bronchiolization) (I. Linnoila – Workshop communication): discordant 3p LOH between preneoplasia and tumor was found in several cases. In contrast, Pamela Rabbits [8, 9] and other workers [10, 11] found the same genetic lesions with regard to 3p, 9p or p53 in physically distant lesions in almost all the cases they studied. P. Rabbits presented evidence that allele loss on chromosome 3 appears as early as squamous metaplasia and precedes p53 mutation [12]. Damage to chromosome 3 was sequential in the pattern of allele loss and much more discrete in dysplasia than in corresponding invasive tumors. 3p loss progressed continuously from the small interstitial deletions in metaplasia or early dysplasia to a wide allelic loss in invasive carcinoma of the same patients. Pamela Rabbits et al. [9] could also demonstrate the clonal relationship between low grade metaplasia, bronchial dysplasia of increasing severity and high grade CIS and invasive carcinoma in one patient with p53 mutation. Using a plaque assay to detect in preneoplasia the specific p53 mutation cloned from the invasive cancer of the patient, the same p53 mutation as in the tumor was found in a small proportion of cells in an adjacent squamous metaplasia. This was also reported on the margin of invasive carcinoma of the head and neck [13]. Moreover, two dysplasia samples from the same site examined in the same patient after 9 months showed one p53 mutation on one allele in the first biopsy and the addition of a second mutation to the second allele in the second biopsy, thus demonstrating increasing genetic damage during clonal expansion in longitudinal samples from the same patient [9]. This does not contradict the multifocal/ multiclonal theory. Rabbits et al. could also demonstrate the clonal relationship of samples of squamous metaplasia and squamous carcinoma, collected in the same patient from different sites at the same time. These samples showed the same pattern of clonal development as those collected over time, suggesting that the analysis of simultaneously collected samples of different grades is a legitimate approach to the study of lung tumor progression, since adjacent or distant lesions are on the same pathway of lung tumor development. This model of progression was confirmed in head and neck carcinoma, where chromosomal losses progressively increase at each histopathological step from hyperplasia to dysplasia to CIS to invasive cancer [14]. Adjacent areas of tissue with different histopathological changes shared common genetic changes, but with additional genetic alterations in the more severe histopathological lesions. Moreover, normal-appearing epithelial cells surrounding preinvasive or microinvasive lesions shared common genetic lesions with those primary lesions.

From studies of the field cancerization process in the upper aerodigestive tract, it can be concluded that lesions adjacent to invasive carcinoma arise from a single progenitor clone, and additionally, distant lesions in the field often share the same genetic lesions as regards 3p deletion and p53 mutation. That they are located on the same parent allele was confirmed by the demonstration that these different lesions displayed the same pattern of X-chromosome inactivation, as assessed by the clonality of the methylation site located at a repeat polymorphic site near the androgen receptor gene. This demonstrated that all the cells had inactivated the same X-chromosome by hypermethylation, and so belong to the same clone, in contrast with a population of normal cells which have randomly inactivated one or other of the paternal or maternal alleles [15]. Based on these findings, the local and multifocal phenomenon of field cancerization could involve subsequent migration of clonally related preneoplastic cells.

3. Evaluation of the Field Cancerization Process

Information is emerging to suggest that numerous molecular events such as 3p allelic loss, aneuploidy and genomic instability precede cytomorphological changes. New unpublished data indicate that 50 % of the normal epithelia of smokers contain mutations (A. Gazdar, unpublished data). 3p LOH also appears to be an early event in hyperplasia and metaplasia of the alveolar compartment. Aims for early detection should therefore be to identify the core molecular determinants of field effect and devise suitable methods of intervention. Future chemoprevention trials, which would benefit from the development of markers, could identify individuals at very high risk of developing lung cancer. Such biomarkers should ideally identify the cancerization field, allow determination of the intensity of genetic damage and the cancerization process, and enable the impact of chemoprevention on the genetic damage and on lung cancer incidence to be measured.

Potential markers for evaluation of the field of cancerization (risk assessment research) can be classified as follows:

1. Morphological changes;
2. Immunohistochemical markers for abnormal or differentially expressed proteins;
3. Markers for genomic instability;
4. Identification of mutations/deletions of specific genes which are responsible for the lung tumor phenotype;
5. Epigenetic phenomena such as abnormal phosphorylation or methylation.

3.1. Morphological Markers

The only diagnostic tool currently available to localize premalignant cellular alterations and early bronchial cancer is conventional white light fiberoptic bronchoscopy. However, even for centrally located CIS, only 30% of the lesions are visible to an experienced endoscopist. Dysplasia and CIS are difficult to detect because they are composed of only a few cell layers (0.2 to 1 mm thick) and often less than 1 mm in surface diameter. Detection of precancerous and cancerous tissues with fluorescent light can be based on the fact that they are less autofluorescent in the green wavelength than normal tissues, and abnormal areas can be identified on the basis of altered tissue autofluorescence. Moderate and severe dysplasia and CIS which are considered as true preinvasive lesions, are 80% detected with this type of fluorescent endoscopy with a 28% false positive rate (S. Lam, unpublished data). To reinforce the suggestion that morphological markers of premalignancy could include early lesions, half of these "false positives" may in fact be true positives. This is suggested by molecular genetic analysis of the bronchial biopsies for LOH at different sites. Thus, fluorescence bronchoscopy may be an important tool to pick out significant lesions with molecular genetic abnormalities that are commonly associated with lung cancer, even when the lesion may appear to be benign low grade atypia according to conventional morphological criteria. Abnormal fluorescence was also found to correlate with the degree of change by quantitative morphometry of the bronchial tree. Most importantly, the same area can be revisited and biopsied precisely in subsequent examination, as was demonstrated in a pilot study using a chemopreventive intervention with Sialor, which showed that fluorescence examination can be used to manage the effect of chemoprevention treatment [2].

Histological diagnosis of neoplasia and preneoplasia is currently the most reliable standard of diagnosis [16]. Preneoplastic lesions are well recognized for squamous cell carcinoma with general acceptance of the concept that the normal pseudostratified ciliated bronchial/bronchiolar epithelium progresses through a spectrum of changes including basal cell hyperplasia, squamous metaplasia, varying degrees of mild, moderate and severe dysplasia to CIS and microinvasive carcinoma. Squamous dysplasia and CIS do not necessarily progress to invasive carcinoma, and could even regress to normal mucosa [17]. Evidence has accumulated to suggest that precursor lesions exist for adenocarcinoma [18–20]. However, the concept of preneoplasia for adenocarcinoma is not as clearly defined as it is for squamous cell carcinoma. The terminology and criteria used for these lesions in the published studies are not consistent, which makes it difficult to compare data. Reproducibility in diagnosis of alveolar dysplasia called atypical alveolar hyperplasia (AAH) has been identified as a very difficult problem. These lesions have been called bronchioloalveolar adenoma, atypical bronchioloalveolar cell hyperplasia, atypical alveolar cuboidal cell hyperplasia, alveolar epithelial hyperplasia, and atypical adenomatous hyperplasia (AAH). In general AAH is defined as a lesion which resembles bronchioloalveolar carcinoma (BAC), but falls short of criteria for malignancy. The distinction between AAH and BAC is subtle and can be very difficult to make. Some have defined a spectrum of low and high grade AAH. As more elaborate and expensive techniques are applied to these lesions, it is very important that the data be interpreted and reported using consistent terminology and criteria. Although the preneoplastic lesions of a squamous dysplasia and CIS are well defined for squamous cell carcinoma, AAH is becoming accepted as a preneoplastic lesion for adenocarcinoma. More precise and standardized criteria need to be applied, and these will be part of the new WHO classification of lung cancer to be completed in 1998. While AAH and squamous CIS have been described in some cases of small cell carcinoma and large cell carcinoma, preneoplastic lesions are not well recognized for these tumors.

Morphological markers also include ploidy and nuclear morphometry on Feulgen-stained cells, analysing the content of DNA and structural and textural nuclear features, in order to identify those that distinguish preneoplastic from neoplastic and normal cells. The nucleolar organizer region, shown by silver staining, may also be a morphological marker.

3.2. Immunohistochemical (IH) Markers to Detect Abnormal Proteins

Abnormally expressed proteins detectable by IH are of several types. Typical is the immunostaining of p53 protein stabilized by missense mutation. A loss of protein expression, resulting from tumor suppressor gene inactivation, typifies loss of Rb, and P16 (CDK^{INK4}) protein expression. The proliferation markers (PCNA, Ki67 or MIB1, Cyclins), are typically overexpressed in preneoplasia; the markers of apoptosis (*Bax*, *Bcl2* and the *Bcl2* family of genes such as Bclx-S, or -L,...) which dictate the cells susceptibility to death, can show a desequilibrium between apoptotic and antiapoptotic factors; growth factor ligands and receptors (EGF-receptor, Her2-Neu (*c-erb2*), GRP and GRP-receptor, IGF-like and receptor, adrenomedullin and receptor ...) can be overexpressed. The differentiation proteins provide markers for abnormal differentiation. Secretory protein (CC10), enzymes (peptidyl glycine alpha-amidating mono-oxygenase (PAM), proteases, telomerases), loss of HLA I or II histocompatibility complex protein and of blood group antigens, expression of tumor specific antigen P31 (hRNP), and expression of CEA, are some of these abnormally expressed differentiation proteins.

Type II cell hyperplasia in a cancerization field with or without atypia was shown to express peptidyl amidating enzyme (PAM) an enzyme necessary for amidation of peptidic growth factors, pointing to its possible role as an autocrine growth factor in metaplastic and dysplastic alveoli [21].

CC10 was shown to be a sign of metaplasia of alveolar epithelium [22]. It remains to be demonstrated that PAM and CC10 expression are related to the cancerization process.

One of the most accurate of these markers (88%) is overexpression of a 31 kD protein, recently characterized as homologous to the pre-mRNA binding heterogenous nuclear ribonuclear protein, hn-RNP, A2, B1 [23, 24]. Immunodetection of this protein by an antibody (703D4) is highly sensitive even in the absence of morphological change, by distinguishing cells which concentrate hn-RNP above the background of its normally low cellular expression. Because it is usually present at low levels in normal cells, hn-RNP cannot yet be considered definitively as a specific maker for the cancer pathway.

Telomerase, a ribonuclear protein polymerase enzyme associated with "immortality", has been focused on in lung and head and neck preneoplasia [25, 26], and obviously has a place in early detection strategies. Telomerase activity is present in the vast majority of invasive cancers of the lung (small cell and non small cell lung cancer SCLC and NSCLC) and of the head and neck. It can be detected by in situ hybridization for RNA components and, at the level of protein activity on telomeres using a PCR-based enzyme assay. Activation of telomerase of low level occurs early and can even be detected in normal bronchial cells of patients with NSCLC. However, a tendency towards high levels of expression was seen in severe dysplasia and CIS adjacent to invasive carcinoma. It can be regarded as a new tool for early detection or detection of preneoplasia on exfoliated cells as shown with oral rinses [26]. In this study, 23% of patients with head and neck squamous cell carcinoma had detectable telomerase activity compared with less than 5% in normal control patients. Whether these changes of telomerase activity can be modulated by chemoprevention agents is currently determined.

Matrix degrading proteases are involved in the majority of lung cancers. Urokinase plasminogen activator (UPA) and metalloprotease MMP3 have been studied. UPA and MMP3 mRNA and proteins are detected in more than 80% of lung cancers (more often in NSCLC than in SCLC and neuroendocrine tumors) and correlate with tumor progression [27]. They have been demonstrated in preneoplastic lesions, using both *in situ* hybridization and immunohistochemistry, adjacent to carcinoma. They were assumed to be secreted by epithelial cells in preinvasive lesions, and by contrast mostly by stromal cells in corresponding microinvasive and invasive lesions [28]. Detection of those proteases in bronchial biopsies and shed cells in sputum could find a place in early detection strategies.

Susceptibility markers for lung cancer are provided by differentially expressed proteins. Differential susceptibility to lung cancer is the key to the application of molecular epidemiology of lung cancer. Some constituents of tobacco smoke (polycyclic aromatic hydrocarbon (PAHs) and N-nitrosamine) are metabolically activated *in vivo* to form highly reactive intermediates. These can complex with DNA to form DNA adducts. Quantitative measurements of DNA and protein adducts to estimate exposure to environmental toxins are the basis of the molecular epidemiology of lung cancer. Moreover, inherited variations in the capacity to metabolize environmental carcinogens may predispose certain individuals to develop cancer. These are aryl-hydrocarbone-hydrolase, glutathione-s-transferase μ and debrisoquin-hydoxylase. Recent studies have not confirmed an excess risk of lung cancer among extensive debrisoquin metabolizers [29].

3.3. Genomic Instability

Aneuploidy is a general marker for lung cancer and could well occur before invasion. DNA measurement (Feulgen staining quantitation and flow cytometry) can broadly estimate abnormal DNA content. Premature chromosome condensation is a technique used to examine the constitution of "normal" lung cells in the field of lung tumors and was found to be abnormal in normal cells distant from the tumor. FISH analysis is a very powerful approach to detect specific chromosomal imbalance. Using the technique on chromosomes (CISH) with DNA probes for the centromeric regions of chromosome 7, 9 and 17, it is possible to appreciate the degree of genetic instability in exfoliated cells in bronchoscopy brushings [30], or even in section of bronchial biopsies [31, 32]. This technique allows counting of the chromosome copies per cell *in situ*. With the assumption that normal cells are diploid (<2% trisomy 7 in normal patients, <1% trisomy 2) one can assess the genetic instability in high risk patients. The fraction of polysomic cells in the tissue samples and their spatial arrangement indicates a clonal outgrowth and suggests a more active ongoing tumorigenesis process. This allows quantification of the degree of clonal change in the tissue, independently of the particular probe used, which proves that the assay detects the presence of generalized genetic changes throughout the lung. Spatial analysis of the tissue suggest the presence of multiple clonal or subclonal outgrowths which can be quantified on a random biopsy, because it reflects a generalized accumulation of genetic changes rather than those specific to tumor development. The evaluation of changes in the degree of ongoing instability or the degree of accumulated clonal outgrowth in the tissue following chemopreventive intervention might provide intermediate markers for response [33].

A similar CISH analysis of trisomy 7 was used in smokers and ex-uranium miners, on bronchial epithelial cells obtained by bronchoscopy brushing of normal-appearing airways in cancer-free patients [30]. Trisomy 7, which is present in more than 50% of NSCLC, was found in some specimens of cancer-free patients, with or without cytologic abnormalities. This suggests that some cancer-free smokers and miners harbour premalignant lesions in their bronchial tree, indicated by an increase in the number of cells having an extra chromosome 7.

Microsatellite alteration is another clue to assess genomic instability and clonal outgrowth. Tandem repeat DNA sequences (known as microsatellites) represent a very common and highly polymorphic class of genetic elements, which are susceptible to widespread instability, as demonstrated by expansion or deletion of repeat elements in neoplastic tissues. These microsatellite alterations are propagated with cell division and clonal expansion. Thus, some microsatellite alterations typical of tumors will enable us to detect clonal proliferations and serve as markers for cancer screening. Sidransky has shown that a search for the most susceptible microsatellite markers (tri- and tetranucleotides) can allow identification of "clonal cells" in body fluids such as urine, sputum and saliva [34].

3.4. Evidence of Clonality

Evidence of clonality relies on studies of specific genes leading to cancer progression. Specific genetic changes include LOH at sites where tumor suppressor genes map: 3p (*FHIT* and others), 9p (9p21 for *p16*, *CDK^{INK4}*), 17p (17p13 for *p53* gene and others), 13q (13q14 for retinoblastoma gene and others). LOH in tumors represents one "hit" which inactivates one allele of the tumor suppressor genes. The second hit can be loss of the second allele (homozygous deletion), mutation of the remaining allele, or hypermethylation. Concordant lesions indicate a complete inactivation of a tumor suppressor gene. Eighty percent of tumor cells with LOH at these specific sites have a mutation detectable in the remaining allele (at least for 13q14, 9p21, and 17p13). However, some discordance is observed in preneoplastic lesions where LOH (17p, 9p) is more frequent than inactivation of corresponding tumor suppressor gene alleles, suggesting that LOH could precede the inactivation of the second allele in these lesions, or that LOH targets another tumor suppressor gene at the same chromosomal location.

LOH at 3p loci occur at four distinct regions located ab 3p25, 3p21.3–21.2, and more proximal deletions at 3p12 and 3p14.2 regions. The 3p14.2 light band contains the most active aphidicolin-induced fragile site of the human genome, the FRA3B. The human *FHIT* gene spans this fragile site [35]. *FHIT* (fragile histidine triad) is a member of the histidine triad gene family and encodes a protein with 69% similarity with the diadenosine tetraphosphate asymmetrical hydrolase, which cleaves the diadenosine tetraphosphate into ATP and AMP. Gabrielle Sozzi [36] reported an analysis of 59 tumors and 11 cell lines of small cell and non-small cell types for alterations of the *FHIT* gene, using nested RT-PCR and sequencing. Eighty percent of small cell lung tumors and cell lines and about 40% of non-small cell tumors and cell lines show abnormal RNA transcripts of *FHIT* after nested PCR. Moreover, loss of one *FHIT* allele, evaluated by microsatellite polymorphism analysis, was observed in 76% of primary tumors of both small cell and non-small cell types. This finding suggests that inactivation of the *FHIT* gene could have occurred by loss of one allele and altered expression of the remaining one, and plaids for a critical role of *FHIT* in lung carcinogenesis. Thus, FRA3B deletion and *FHIT* gene abnormalities could be used as molecular markers for early lung cancer detection and identification of high risk patients. Whether *FHIT* is the crucial gene or a "bystander" at FRA3B deletion has been proved conclusively, by the absence of protein expression in neoplasia and preneoplasia (CIS).

Amplification of proto-oncogenes is a genetic lesion specific for cancer. Known oncogenes susceptible to amplification in lung cancer are the *myc* family of oncogene (c-, L-, N-*myc*), c-*erb*-b2-*Neu* (P185), Cyclin D1 (amplification at 11q13, not yet demonstrated in lung cancer). Other candidate genes for amplification and deletion will be enlighted by comparative genomic hybridization studies, which could identify new oncogenes and tumor suppressor genes.

Another clue for clonality is *ras* gene mutations, which are present in about 30 to 50% of lung adenocarcinoma (mainly in smokers) and some of their relevant bronchioloalveolar preneoplasia. *Ras* gene is not mutant in other types of tumor or squamous preneoplasia. *Ras* mutations have been detected in sputum one year in advance of a diagnosis of lung cancer [34].

Specific genomic damage accumulation can finally be determined by looking for DNA adducts (32p post-labelling-antibodies), or at sites for the mutational activity of specific carcinogens like BP (benzo-a-pyrene)-induced adduct at codon 157 of *p53* gene [37]. Mitochondrial DNA changes, surrogate gene mutations (5S rRNA), and occasional chromosomal non disjunction are part of the specific genomic alterations due to exogenous carcinogens.

3.5. Epigenetic Phenomena

Epigenetic phenomena include several means of tumor suppressor gene "silencing". Many tumor suppressor genes achieve inactivation without obvious mutation or homozygous deletion. Hypermethylation occurs commonly to inactivate the potent p16 (CDK-Inhibitor of CDK4-CDK6-cyclin D1 kinases, which allow Rb phosphorylation at the G1S boundary. Loss of p16 protein expression releases a constraint on Rb phosphorylation and provides loss of control at the G1 checkpoint. Thus, *p16* inactivation in tumors, especially lung and head and neck tumors, occurs through *p16* loss of one allele (LOH at 9p21) accompanied by loss or mutation of the remaining allele, or methylation of its 5' end. This methylation phenomenon occurs in 25% of lung cancer *in vivo*. *p16* hypermethylation is typical of cancer since it has never been shown in normal or non-neoplastic tissue. Thus, its detection in preneoplasia or early cancer is a potential means of early detection. Screening for *p16* inactivation would however necessarily include *p16* detection, by IH, to assess loss of *p16* expression, which reflects any type of genetic alteration involved in *p16* inactivation. Phosphorylation could inactivate tumor suppressor genes without silencing them, but as a post translational regulation (p53-Rb). Rb gene protein product is commonly inactivated in tumors through inappropriate phosphorylation, as the result of *p16* inactivation or of overexpression of cyclin D1. These epigenetic phenomena on Rb protein have not yet been demonstrated in preneoplastic lesions.

Several questions remain to be solved, once all these potential markers are listed and identified. The first involves the type of specimen on which to test markers. Bronchial biopsies are ideal material, obtained with or without fluorescence bronchoscopy. Directed bronchial bushing and washing, sputum and bronchioloalveolar lavage samples can be used for early detection. Further technological developments are required for new assays to obtain meaningful clinical information easily from only a few exfoliated bronchial cells in a sputum specimen. Whether these few cells will be representative of the abnormal clonal population in the cancerization field is currently under evaluation in at least two clinical trials. Highly sensitive methods allow detection of $1-10^{5-6}$ mutant cells (e.g. *ras* mutation), raising the possibility that any single mutant cell could be eventually eliminated by sociobiological environmental controls. How to combine information obtained with these highly sensitive methods with risk assessment has to be evaluated when developing alternative methods such as microarray technology on a few exfoliated cells. Normal DNA from blood and plasma as well as fresh tissues could be used to compare normal DNA with DNA from preneoplastic or neoplastic lesions. Serum and plasma also transport clonal DNA which could be of use in the identification of a preclinical tumor. However, clonal DNA in the circulation mostly occurs late in tumor progression [15]. Finally, the presence of autoantibodies in the sera of 50% of patients bearing mutant stabilized p53, questions the capacity of the use of this determination as a biomarker for a preinvasive state [38]. It is obviously included among tests for early detection of occult neoplasia.

4. Stratification and Chronology of Markers

Potential molecular markers for clonal expansion can be devided in two types according to their specificity for cancer progression.

1) Generalized markers reflect genetic damage, instability, and molecular alterations which may not exclusively be a pathway to cancer, and are reversible. These are part of the genetic and molecular alterations observed within the cancerization field.
2) Specific markers identify genetic abnormalities definitively on a irreversible pathway to cancer progression.

This distinction is obviously provisional and depends on further prospective studies including patients with cancer progression and control patients without history of cancer. The list of potential generalized biomarkers to evaluate field cancerization includes early histopathological changes like hyperplasia, metaplasia and low grade dysplasia, morphometric changes and proliferation markers as well as differentially expressed proteins (enzymes, proteases, retinoic acid receptors, apoptotic factors and telomerase activity). The question of whether growth factors and growth factor autocrine loops (EGF receptors (EGFR), c-erb-2R GRPR, IGFR, AMR) belong to the first generalized or more specific markers needs further comparison between cohorts of patients with and without history of cancer. As an example, EGFR is produced in metaplasia and dysplasia adjacent to CIS at equal or higher levels than in invasive carcinoma, in parallel with the increasing proliferation index. Moreover, EGFR upregulation is common to all squamous metaplasia and dysplasia encountered in patients with or without developing cancer, as experienced by the present author.

In contrast, oncogene activation (*myc* or cyclin D1 amplification, *ras* mutation) and inactivation of both alleles of identified or putative tumor suppressor genes, are examples of specific markers for tumor progression. LOH at specific sites for tumor suppressor genes, identification of genetic abnormalities of the remaining allele, or absence of protein product are also ways to detect specific markers. The following guidelines to tumor suppressor gene inactivation can be given: LOH could be searched for at multiple 3p regions: 3p25, 3p21, 3p12 and 3p14 associated with identification of *FHIT* mutation; *p16* inactivation could be detected by LOH at 9p21, immunohistochemistry for p16 expression, study of p16 mutation and methylation; *p53* inactivation can be studied by LOH at 17p13, immunohistochemistry to detect *p53* stabilizing mutation, SSCP single strand conformation polymorphism and sequencing; *Rb* inactivation could rely on LOH at 13q14, immunohistochemistry to detect Rb loss of expression, or even Western blot demonstrating abnormal phosphorylation.

Establishing a defined sequence of expression for particular markers may make possible the clinical application of particular biomarkers. Early markers can be applied to identify the field cancerization. Late markers could then be used for cancer progression and early detection of clinically occult cancers. However, our knowledge of the chronology of these different genetic events is sparse; 3p and 9p LOH as well as general aneuploidy and aneusomy can be considered as early markers for clonal expansion; 3p and 9p deletions precedes *p53* mutation. Mutation of *p53* (and *ras* in preneoplastic lesions for adenocarcinoma), LOH at 5q and p16 loss of protein expression are currently regarded by some as rather late genetic molecular abnormalities, more predictive of progression to invasion. As a matter of fact, there is a high discrepancy between 9p21 and 13q14 rate of LOH in preneoplastic lesions as compared to corresponding P16 and Rb loss of protein expression, which may indicate other tumor genes at these sites. An alternative strategy is to develop genetic assays that reflect, on a random biopsy, the extent of an ongoing process of genetic instability. If the genetic change is proceeding at a high rate on this random biopsy (aneusomy ...), there would be an increased possibility that specific genetic changes (for tumor development) occur somewhere in the tissue field [39].

A tempting hypothesis from the overall results, which has the attraction of embracing apparently discordant theories of field cancerization, is that loss of several chromosomes (3p, 9p), aneuploidy and aneusomy (trisomy 7) allow cell transformation, replacement and spreading of clonally related cells, insuring horizontal stepwise progression. In contrast, *p53* mutation, high telomerase activity and matrix degrading enzymes could arise independently at each tumor focus, increasing the slope of progression towards invasion and "verticalization" of the multistep process. Alternatively, one or several transforming events including p53 mutation could occur early in a progenitor cell before migration or later, explaining both concordant or discordant *p53* mutations at different sites in the same patients. These hypotheses of the chronology of cancer development should be evaluated in larger clinical trials.

Correlating histopathological changes with marker phenotypes is of interest since this is the mainstay of current diagnosis for invasive carcinoma. Evidence is mounting that extensive genetic damage precedes morphological change and correlation of these could be a further challenge. So far, most of the lung biology studies have concentrated on proximal airways. The morphological changes involved in preneoplastic peripheral lesions for adenocarcinoma are poorly understood and require more morphological and molecular study. The definition of a preneoplastic lesion will soon include both histology and genetic/molecular pathology, and we hope that this combination will provide a better predictor for risk of progression.

5. Selection and Validation of New Lung Cancer Markers

The main objective is to identify a strategy for the selection and validation of biomarkers of preclinical lung cancer that will allow stratification of patients and the selection and implementation of rational management approaches.

5.1. New Validation of Markers

For clinical application of a new marker, the validation steps include:

1) A clear definition of the particular clinical application (early diagnosis, progression marker, metastatic marker, intermediate endpoint and treatment response);

2) The marker must be expressed by a large proportion of clinical specimens which eventually develop lung cancer (retrospective study on
   archived material);
3) The marker must allow stratification of individuals by clinical risk,
   must be expressed at high enough levels to allow detection, must be
   detectable in small samples by technologically feasible methods
   (feasible in this context means the assay should have low cost and high
   throughput capacity).

Prospective clinical trials are necessary to define the performance characteristics of any new marker rigorously, which implies that a comprehensive
data base (demography, smoking history, environmental or occupational
exposure, clinical, epidemiological and genetic susceptibility) and other
potentially confounding variables (medical history, social status, family
history) should be included in the trial design.

Specimens to include when possible in this approaches for marker
validation are normal DNA, blood plasma, serum, fresh frozen and patho-
logically characterized affected tissues associated with adjacent or distant
normal tissue, formalin-fixed paraffin-embedded tissues (also including
pathological and adjacent or distant normal tissue) and sputum.

5.2. Strategy

Clinical application of early lung cancer detection markers does not dilute
the fundamentally important role played by smoking cessation in the management of this disease. However, the number of lung cancer cases arising
from former smokers is now approaching the number of lung cancer cases
arising from current smokers. Early detection and effective chemoprevention may be the most promising clinical approach to benefit former
smokers. If we can be optimistic about rapid improvement and early detection tools validated with high positive predictive value emerging from
already ongoing clinical trials, a separate concern is how those early detected cohorts are going to be managed clinically. This warrants enhanced
research efforts to develop chemoprevention alternatives to control lung
cancer confined to the bronchial tree. Only with a coordinated clinical
management strategy appropriate to the early stage of lung cancer will the
optimal benefit of effective early lung cancer detection be realized [40].

Further research to elucidate useful intermediate biomarkers to monitor
the success of chemoprevention measures should be encouraged. There is
currently no reliable evaluation of disease progression and response to use
which could establish the benefit or duration of clinical intervention.
Among other things, this calls for a more active and thorough programme
of sputum analysis and more early and systematical recognition of preneoplastic lung lesion using fluorescent endoscopy. This is an important new
application in which biologically defined markers can play a fundamental

role. Currently existing markers should be used as tools to select populations of cells or tissue specimens that represent the disease and for the identification of new and more specific biomarkers as well as targets for intervention. The expression of an intermediate endpoint biomarker should reflect disease progression and predict the response to various options for clinical intervention.

It is highly unlikely that any single marker will have sufficient sensitivity, specificity and predictive value to stratify all patients according to risk for lung cancer progression. Algorhythms, based on panels of markers will have to be developed and validated for use in patient management. New technologies may allow for multiple marker determinations to be performed (at acceptable cost) on routine clinical specimens.

Enhanced understanding of tumor biology and of the preneoplastic stage should not replace or divert attention away from detection of clinical malignancy. Some markers, expressed both by the archived sputum cells (with the earliest morphological changes) and also by a subsequent tumor, could enable recognition of all the invasive but occult malignancies. For example, 703D4 immunodetection of hn-RNP could predict lung cancer in 68% (positive predictive value) within 1 to 2 years, a sensitivity greater than cytological detection [24]. Continued followup of clinical populations is necessary to define the ultimate performance characteristics of these antibodies.

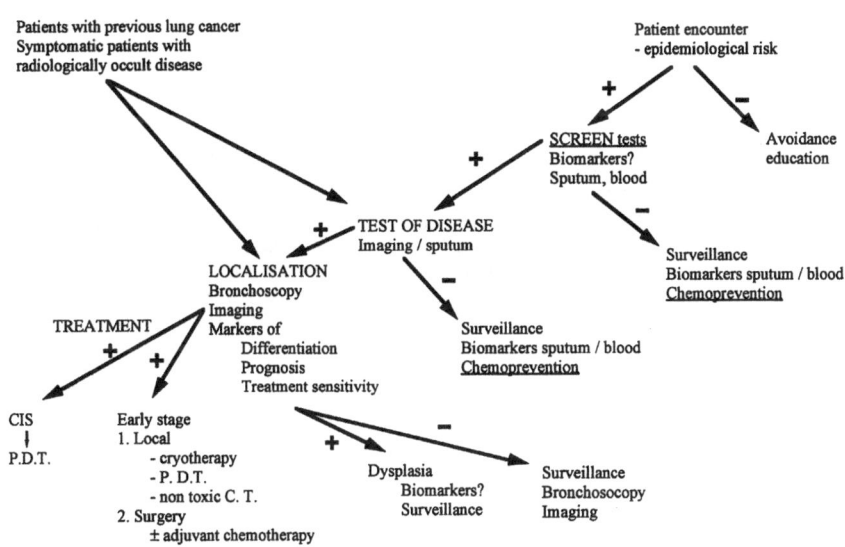

(P.D.T. : Photodynamic Therapy
C. T. : Chemotherapy)

Figure 1

In order to move important new molecular markers into a clinical setting that will help the health service, it is imperative that this research is carried out in a clinical environment where the relevant specimens are generated. The specimens also need to be subjected to a quality control procedure to provide the most accurate information which in time will be useful for health care. Early detection of lung cancer is a major challenge and involves a wide spectrum of research technologies and this effort is a model for early detection of epithelial cancers. This challenge requires a cross-disciplinary approach, between fundamental research and the clinical environment.

Planning should begin now, for trials to determine whether localization (e.g. by fluorescent endoscopy, segmental washing and brushings, or PET scanning) followed by local surgical, radiation or photodynamic therapy has an advantage over chemoprevention with several promising new agents. A proposal for how the early detection issues can be phased in with the clinical management of patients, while moving towards early detection in oncology, is summarized in Figure 1 (E. Edell, unpublished data).

It is now believed that molecular and genetic characteristics of cells during the preclinical phase could provide us with an opportunity to intervene in the transformation process, by gene therapy, immunotherapy, pharmacological intervention in the methylation process and so on [41]. There is therefore a growing interest in integrating this knowledge with practical applications, commonly referred to as translational research, in order to benefit the ultimate users: the physicians and (most importantly) the patients.

Acknowledgments

We are grateful to Adi Gazdar for supervision of the manuscript, and Ilona Linnoila for advice.

This chapter is the summary of the workshop on the early detection of lung cancer held in Copenhagen (I.A.S.L.C. Workshop, Elisnor, June 1996). We are grateful for the contributions of the following people: Eric Edell, MD (USA); John Field, MD (England); Wilbur Franklin, MD (USA); Adi Gazdar, MD (USA); Kenneth Hirsch, MD (USA); Walter Hittelman, PhD (USA); John Lechner, MD; Ilona Linnoila, MD (USA); Yves Martinet, MD, PhD (France); Pamela Rabbits, PhD (England); David Sidransky, MD (USA); Gabriella Sozzi, MD (Italy); Sudhir Srivastava, PhD (USA); Melvyn Tockman, MD, PhD (USA); William Travis, MD (USA).

References

1. Auerbach O, Stout AP, Hammond EC, Garfinkel J (1961) Changes in bronchial epithelium in relation to lung cancer. *N Engl J Med* 265: 253–67.
2. Lam S, McAulay C, Hung J, et al. (1993) Detection of dysplasia and carcinoma in situ with lung imaging fluorescence endoscope device. *J Thorac Cardiovasc Surg* 105: 1035–1040.
3. Vogelstein B, Kinzler KW (1993) The multistep nature of cancer. *Trends Genet* 9: 138–141.
4. Chung KY, Mukhopadhyay T, Kim J, et al. (1993) Discordant p53 gene mutations in primary head and neck cancer and corresponding second primary cancer of the upper aerodigestive tract. *Cancer Res* 53: 1676–1683.

5. Noguchi M, Maezawa N, Nakanishi Y, Matsuno Y, Shimosato Y, Hirohashi S (1993) Application of the p53 gene mutation pattern for differential diagnosis of primary versus metastatic lung carcinomas. *Diagn Mol Pathol* 2: 29–35.
6. Nees M, Homann N, Dishcer H, et al. (1993) Expression of mutated p53 occurs in human distant epithelia of head and neck cancer patients: a possible molecular basis for the development of multiple tumors. *Cancer Res* 53: 4189–4196.
7. Sozzi G, Miozzo M, Pastorino U, et al. (1995) Genetic evidence for an independent origin of multiple preneoplastic and neoplastic lung lesions. *Cancer Res* 35: 135–140.
8. Chung GTY, Sundaresan V, Hasleton P, Rudd R, Taylor R, Rabbits P (1995) Sequential molecular genetic changes in lung cancer development. *Oncogone* 11: 2591–2598.
9. Chung G, Sundaresan V, Hasleton P, Rudd R, Taylor R, Rabbits P (1996) Clonal evolution of lung tumors. *Cancer Res* 56: 1609–1614.
10. Hung J, Kishimoto Y, Sugio K, et al. (1995) Allele specific chromosome 3p deletions occur at an early stage in the pathogenesis of lung carcinoma. *JAMA* 273: 558–563.
11. Kishimoto Y, Murakami Y, Shiraishi M, Hayashi K, Sekiya T (1992) Aberrations of the P53 tumor suppressor gene in human non-small cell carcinomas of the lung. *Cancer Res* 52: 4799–4804.
12. Chung G, Sundaresan V, Hasleton P, Rudd R, Taylor R and Rabbits P (1995) Sequential molecular genetic changes in lung cancer development. *Oncogene* 11: 2591–2598.
13. Brennan JA, Mao L, Hruban R, et al. (1995) Molecular assessment of histopathological staging in squamous-cell carcinoma of the head and neck. *N Engl J Med* 332: 429–435.
14. Califano J, Van-Der-Riet P, Westra W, Nawroz H, Clayman G, Piantadosi S (1996) Genetic progression model for head and neck cancer: implications for field canceration. *Cancer Res* 56: 2488–2492.
15. Bedi GC, Westra W, Gabrielson E, Koch W, Sidransky D (1996) Multiple head and neck tumors. Evidence for a common clonal origin. *Cancer Res* 56: 2484–2487.
16. Bennett WP, Colby TV, Travis WD, et al. (1993) P53 protein accumulates frequently in early bronchial neoplasia. *Cancer Res* 53: 4817–4822.
17. Auer G, Ono J, Nasiell M, et al. (1982) Reversibility of bronchial cell atypia. *Cancer Res* 42: 4241–4247.
18. Kodama T, Biyajima S, Watanabe S, Shimosato Y (1986) Morphometric study of adenocarcinomas and hyperplastic epithelial lesions in the peripheral lung. *Am J Clin Pathol* 85: 146–151.
19. Mori M, Tesuka F, Chiba R, et al. (1996) Atypical adenomatous hyperplasia and adenocarcinoma of the human lung. Their heterology in form and analogy in immunohistochemical characteristics. *Cancer* 77: 665–674.
20. Kitamura H, Kameda Y, Nakamura N et al. (1995) Proliferative potential and p53 overexpression in precursor and early stage lesions of bronchioloalveolar lung carcinoma. *Am J Pathol* 146: 876–887.
21. Martinez A, Treston AM, Saldise L, Montuenga LM, Linnoila RI (1996) Expression of peptidyl-glycine a-amidating mono-oxygenase (PAM) enzymes in morphological abnormalities adjacent to pulmonary tumors. *Am J of Pathol* 149: 707–716.
22. Jensen SM, Pass H, Jones JE, Steinberg S, Linnoila RI (1994) Clara cell 10kD protein mRNA in normal and atypical regions of human respiratory epithelium. *Intl J Cancer* 58: 629–637.
23. Zhou J, Mulshine JL, Unsworth EJ, et al. (1996) Purification and characterization of a protein that premits early detection of lung cancer. *J Biol Chem* 271: 10760–10766.
24. Tockman MS, Erozan YS, Gupta P, et al. (1994) The early detection of second primary lung cancers by sputum immunostaining. *Chest* 106: 385S–390S.
25. Hiyama K, Ishioka S, Shirotani Y, et al. (1995) Alterations in telomeric repeat length in lung cancer are associated with loss of heterozygosity in P53 and Rb. *Oncogene* 10: 937–944.
26. Califano J, Ahrendt SA, Meininger G, Westra WH, Koch WM, Sidransky D (1996) Detection of telomerase activity in orale rinses from head and neck squamous cell carcinom patients. *Cancer Res* 56: 5720–5722.
27. Bolon I, Devouassoux M, Robert C, Moro D, Brambilla C, Brambilla E (1997) Expression of urokinase type plasminogen activator, Stromelysin 1, Stromelysin 3 and Matrilysin genes in lung carcinomas. *Am J Pathol* 150: 1–11.

28. Bolon I, Brambilla E, Vandenbunder B, Robert C, Lantuejoul S, Brambilla C (1996) Changes in the expression of matrix proteases and of the transcription factor c-Ets-1 during progression of precancerous bronchial lesions. *Lab Invest* 75: 1–13.
29. Shaw GL, Falk RT, Deslauriers J, et al. (1995) Debrisoquine metabolism and lung cancer risk. *Cancer Epidemiol Biomarkers Prev* 4: 41–48.
30. Crowell RE, Gilliland FD, Temes RT, et al. (1996) Detection of trisomy 7 in non malignant bronchial epithelium from lung cancer patients and individuals at risk for lung cancer. *Cancer Epidemiol Biomarkers Prev* 5: 631A–637.
31. Shin DM, Hittelman WN, Hong WK (1994) Biomarkers in upper aerodigestive tract tumorigensis: A review. *Cancer Epidemiol Biomarkers Prev* 3: 697–709.
32. Dhingra K, Sneige N, Pandita TK, et al. (1994) Quantitative analysis of chromosome in situ hybridization signal in paraffin-embedded tissue sections. *Cytometry* 16: 100–112.
33. Hittelman WN, Lee JS, Cheong N, Shin DM, Hong WK (1991) The chromosome view of "field cancerization" and multi-step carcinogenesis. Implications for chemopreventive approaches. *In:* Pastorino V, Hong WK (eds): *"Chemoimmuno prevention of cancer".* Georg Thieme Verlag, Stuttgart, pp 41–47.
34. Mao L, Hruban RH, Boyle JO, Tockman M, Sidransky D (1994) Detection of oncogene mutations in sputum preceds diagnosis of lung cancer. *Cancer Res* 54: 1634–1637.
35. Otah M, Inoue H, Cotticelli MG, et al. (1996) The human FHIT gene, spanning the chromosome 3p14.2 fragile site and renal carcinoma associated translocation breakpoint, is abnormal in digestive tract cancers. *Cell* 84: 587–597.
36. Sozzi G, Veronese ML, Negrini M, et al. (1996) The FHIT gene at 3p14.2 is abnormal in lung cancer. *Cell* 85: 17–26.
37. Denissenko MF, Pao A, Tang MS, Pfeifer GP (1996) Preferential formation of benzo(a)pyrene adducts at lung cancer mutational hotspots in P53. *Science* 274: 430–432.
38. Lubin R, Zalcman G, Bouchet L, et al. (1995) Serum P53 antibodies as early markers of lung cancer. *Nature Med* 1: 701–702.
39. Hittelman WN, Kim HJ, Lee JS, et al. (1996) Detection of chromosome instability of tissue fields at risk: in situ hypbridization. *J Cell Biochemist* 25S: 57–62.
40. Mulshine JL, Scott F, Zhou J, et al. (1996) Development of molecular approaches to early lung cancer detection. *Semin in Radiation Oncol* 6: 72–75.
41. Srivastava S, Rossi SC (1996) Early detection research program at the NCI. *Int J Cancer* 69: 35–37.

Clinical and Biological Basis of Lung Cancer Prevention
ed. by Y. Martinet, F. R. Hirsch, N. Martinet, J.-M. Vignaud
and J. L. Mulshine

CHAPTER 5
Molecular Abnormalities in the Sequential Development of Lung Carcinoma

Ignacio I. Wistuba [1,3] and Adi F. Gazdar [1,2,*]

[1] *The Hamon Center for Therapeutic Oncology Research, University of Texas Southwestern Medical Center, Dallas, Texas, USA*
[2] *Department of Pathology, University of Texas Southwestern Medical Center, Dallas, Texas, USA*
[3] *Department of Pathology, Pontificia Universidad Catolica de Chile, Santiago, Chile*

1. Introduction

Lung cancer is the most frequent cause of cancer death in both men and women in the USA [1] and tobacco smoking is accepted to be the number one cause of this devastating disease [2, 3]. As with other epithelial tumors, lung carcinoma is believed to arise after a series of progressive pathological changes (preneoplastic lesions) in the bronchial epithelium, that develop and progress over a period of several years [4]. While the sequential preneoplastic changes have been defined for centrally arising squamous carcinoma [4], they have been poorly documented for large cell carcinomas, adenocarcinomas and small cell carcinomas. For squamous cell carcinomas, the morphological preneoplastic steps include hyperplasia, metaplasia, dysplasia and carcinoma *in situ* (CIS) [4]. Peripherally arising cancers (most adenocarcinomas and large cell carcinomas) also appear to be accompanied by hyperplastic and dysplastic changes in peripheral airway cells [5, 6]. Presumably, adenocarcinomas must go through a non-invasive (CIS) stage prior to becoming invasive. Although currently available

---

* Author for correspondence.

information obtained by extensive airway sampling is sketchy in regard to premalignant changes, the information that is available suggests that lung preneoplastic lesions are frequently extensive and multifocal throughout the lung, indicating a field effect ("field cancerization") by which much of the respiratory epithelium has been mutagenized, presumably form exposure to carcinogens [8, 9]. Thus, lung carcinoma may occur anywhere in the vast and anatomically complicated respiratory tree including the peripheral lung.

Advanced lung preneoplastic changes occur far more frequently in smokers than lifetime nonsmokers and increase in frequency with amount of smoking, adjusted for age [10, 11]. Although morphological recovery occurs after smoking cessation [10, 12], elevated lung cancer risk persists [13]. From the current smoking trends, it appears that former smokers will account for a growing percentage of all lung cancer patients. While the risk population has been defined to target the early detection and chemoprevention efforts (current and former heavy smokers, and patients who have been cured of cancer of the upper aerodigestive tract), the limitations of conventional morphological methods in identifying premalignant cell populations in the airways have led to a search for other biological properties of respiratory mucosa that may predict the future development of carcinoma. These markers (also referred to as "intermediate markers") include immunophenotypic changes in airway epithelium as well as genetic abnormalities in bronchial epithelial cells.

2. Lung Cancer Molecular Changes

Several allelotyping and comparative genomic hybridization (CGH) studies have revealed that multiple genetic changes (estimated at between 10 and 20) are found in clinically evident lung cancer involving known and putative recessive oncogenes and several dominant oncogenes [14, 15]. Examples of abnormal dominant oncogenes in lung cancer are the *ras* family members (K-*ras*, H-*ras* and N-*ras*), the *myc* family members (c-*myc*, N-*myc*, and L-*myc*) and the *Her-2/neu* gene [14]. *Ras* mutation occurs in approximately 20% of non-small cell lung carcinomas (NSCLC), mainly in adenocarcinomas. *Ras* mutations have however not been detected in any small cell lung carcinoma (SCLC) [16–18]. Another example of a dominant oncogene in lung cancer is overexpression of the *myc* family of genes, which occurs in nearly all SCLC and in many NSCLC [19–22].

The list of recessive oncogenes involved in lung cancer is likely to include as many 10 to 15 known and putatives genes [23]. These include changes in *p53* (17p13), *Rb*(13q14), *CDKN2* (9p21), 5q (*MCC*, *APC* region) and new candidate recessive oncogenes in the short arms of chromosome 8 (8p) and 3 (3p) at 3p12–14, 3p21 and 3p25 regions. Two key examples in lung cancer are the *p53* and the *Rb* genes. Mutations of *p53* are very common in lung cancer, occurring in over 90% of SCLC and approximately 50% of NSCLC [24]. Another well-documented genetic change that occurs frequently in lung cancer is that of the *Rb* gene. In more than 80% of SCLC and 20% to 30% of NSCLC, the protein has been mutated, so that it cannot fulfill its normal regulatory function [25–28].

Many recessive oncogenes remain to be identified, although in most instances their chromosomal locations are known from cytogenetic and molecular analysis. Loss of heterozygosity (LOH) analysis using polymorphic microsatellite markers is frequently used to identify allelic losses at specific chromosomal regions. The most common of these changes in both SCLC and NSCLC is loss of genetic material on chromosome 3p, which involves at least three distinct regions at 3p12–14, 3p21 and 3p25 [23]. Presumably, these regions are sites of undiscovered recessive oncogenes, inactivation of which is critical for the development of lung cancer. At 3p21 several groups have found large homozygous deletions in lung cancers, indicating the presence of one or more recessive oncogenes in this area [29, 30]. Recent attention has focused on *FHIT*, a candidate tumor suppressor gene at 3p14.2 which spans FRA3B, the most fragile of the common fragile sites [31]. Molecular abnormalities of the *FHIT* gene and the FRA3B region are frequent in lung cancer [32]. Analyses of microsatellite markers within *FHIT* have shown that LOH is found in 70% of both major types of lung cancer [33]. However, the frequent deletions involving *FHIT* may only reflect the fragility of the fragile site in which this gene is located.

Another relevant recessive oncogene area for lung cancer is the interferon gene cluster in chromosome region 9p21–22 [34, 35]. A putative tumor suppressor gene in 9p has been identified [36, 37]. The gene, *CDKN2* (also known as *MTS1* or *p16^{INK4}*) encodes a previously identified inhibitor (*p16*) of cyclin-dependent kinase 4. A second related cyclin/cdk inhibitor, *p15*, was also found in chromosome 9p adjacent to the gene coding for *p16^{INK4}* [38], and homozygous loss in lung cancer at chromosome 9p frequently encompasses both *p15* and *p16* [39, 40]. LOH at 9p21–22 locus has been reported to be 33% in NSCLC, with a much higher frequency in squamous cell carcinomas (55 to 59%) than adenocarcinomas (21% to 36%) [41, 42].

3. Tumor Type Specific Molecular Changes are Found in Lung Cancers

Studies of large numbers of lung cancers have shown different patterns of involvement between the two major groups of lung carcinomas (SCLC and NSCLC), with mutations in *Rb*, *p53*, and 3p21 allele loss found in >90% of SCLC but only uncommon mutations of *CDKN2*, whereas *p53*, 3p21, and *CDKN2* mutations/deletions occur frequently in NSCLC [23]. Our results of allelotyping lung tumor cell lines and microdissected invasive primary tumors indicate that SCLC also demonstrated more frequent losses at 5q (*MCC/APC* region) and 10q loci, while losses at 9p are more frequent in NSCLC. Our unpublished data and those of others [42] have found different patterns of LOH involving the two major types of NSCLC (squamous carcinoma and adenocarcinoma), with higher incidence of LOH at *p53*(17p), *Rb* (13q), 9p21 and 3p regions in squamous cell carcinomas.

4. Molecular Changes Found in Preneoplastic Lung Lesions

Although or knowledge of the molecular events in invasive lung cancer is relatively extensive, until recently our knowledge about the sequence of events in preneoplastic lesions was limited. A few studies have provided suggestions that molecular lesions can be identified at early stages of the pathogenesis of lung cancer [23, 43–45]. Mutant K-*ras* has been detected in the sputum up to several months prior to diagnosis [46] and K-*ras* mutation has been detected in bronchoalveolar lavage fluid in a high proportion of patients with adenocarcinoma (56%), but not in patients with squamous cell carcinoma or with another diagnosis [47]. Although *p53* mutations have been demonstrated in nonmalignant epithelium of lung specimens resected for lung cancer [43, 45, 48], little information is available on the chronology of *p53* mutation in preneoplastic epithelium. Whether or when *Rb* genetic abnormalities occur prior to the occurrence of invasive tumor is not known.

4.1 Sequential Molecular Changes in Lung Preneoplastic Changes

To understand the sequential molecular changes involved in lung cancer pathogenesis, we have developed a scheme to search systematically for mutations in preneoplastic lesions and normal epithelium using archival paraffin-embedded materials. Microsection from lung cancer resections and bronchoscopy biopsies containing preneoplastic lesions and normal respiratory epithelium are examined for the presence of genetic changes. Using a precise microdissection technique under direct microscopic observation a variable number of cells form these areas are precisely isolated along with invasive primary tumor and stromal lymphocytes (as a source of normal constitutional DNA). Using PCR-based techniques, these different specimens are typed for *ras* and *p53* mutations, for allele loss for 3p (at different chromosomal regions such as 3p12, 3p14.2 *FHIT* gene, 3p14, 3p21 and 3p24–25), 5q, 9p21, 13q (*Rb* gene) and 17p (*p53*).

Our published [49–51] and unpublished data have demonstrated that in lung cancer the developmental sequence is not random, with LOH at one or more 3p regions and 9p21, and to a lesser extent at 13q (*Rb*) and 17p (*p53*), being detected quite frequently at the early stage of hyperplasia in most of the major types of lung carcinoma (SCLC and NSCLC). By contrast, LOH at 5q and K-*ras* mutations were only detected at the carcinoma *in situ* (CIS) stage, and *p53* mutations appear at variables times. Our preliminary data also indicate that different patterns of sequential mutations (either LOH and point mutations) are detected in the pathogenesis of the different histological types of lung cancers. Overall, more cumulative and earlier molecular changes (LOH and point mutations) are found in centrally arising SCLC and squamous cell carcinomas than in peripheral adenocarcinomas (our unpublished data).

We have detected some of these early allelic losses in normal-appearing respiratory epithelium accompanying invasive carcinoma in a subset of cases. It is believed that the developmental of epithelial cancer requires multiple mutations [52], the stepwise accumulation of which may represent a mutator phenotype [53, 54]. Thus, it is possible that those preneoplastic lesions that have accumulated multiple mutations are at highest risk for progression to invasive carcinoma. As some of these lowgrade preneoplastic lesions and normal-appearing epithelia have demonstrated multiple genetic changes, we postulated that CIS and invasive tumors may arise directly either from normal or abnormal epithelium, without passing through the entire histological sequence (parallel theory of cancer development) [55]. A similar process may be involved in the pathogenesis of breast cancer [56].

4.2 Similar Molecular Changes are Found in Invasive Lung Cancer and Accompanying Preneoplastic Lesions

We and others have noted that the precise molecular changes (specific base substitution or allele loss) found in primary cancer were also found in the preneoplastic changes [45, 49, 51, 57] and normal appearing epithelium (our unpublished data), even at a distance from the primary cancer. We have referred to this phenomenon as allele specific loss. We have proposed two possibilities for allele specific loss: a) a single cell or small clone of cells develops loss or point mutation at a specific allele at one or more loci, migrates widely throughout the respiratory epithelium of both lungs and eventually gives rise to a tumor; or b) in individuals, one of any pair of alleles has a greater tendency to be lost, perhaps as a result of some form of genomic imprinting or the presence of fragile sites. Whatever its mechanisms, allele specific loss is likely to be a phenomenon of major biological significance. Our more recent observations confirm that allele specific loss is a widespread phenomenon involving several tumor types and involving genes on multiple chromosomes.

4.3 Microsatellite Alterations

In addition to the specific genetic changes discusses above, other evidence indicates that genomic instability occurs in lung cancer and its preneo-plastic lesions.

This evidence includes our finding of widespread aneuploidy throughout the respiratory epithelium of lung cancer patients [58]. Another molecular change frequently present in a wide variety of cancer types is microsatellite alterations (MAs), also known as genomic alterations. MAs represent changes in the size of polymorphic microsatellite markers compared to the normal germline in individual persons. They have been described in human lung cancers at frequencies ranging from 0 to 45% [59–62]. While lesions in mismatch repair genes account for the more generalized microsatellite instability seen for example in cancers in hereditary nonpolyposis coli patient [63], the mechanism underlying the less frequent MAs in lung and other cancers is currently unknown. However, it is believed that MAs reflect a form of genomic instability [64]. Nevertheless, MAs are attractive candi-dates for the early molecular detection of cancer [59, 65]. Our preliminary results demonstrated the presence of MAs in a subset of lung carcinomas (either SCLC and NSCLC), as well in their accompanying preneoplastic lesions and normal appearing epithelium.

4.4 Smoking-Related Damage

Of great interest, we have recently identified multiple molecular changes (LOH and MAs) in bronchial biopsies form current and former smokers. These changes, present in about 50% of biopsies, are present both in preneoplastic and normal appearing epithelium. The changes are similar in those detected in preneoplastic lesions accompanying invasive lung cancers [66, 67].

5. Conclusions

In summary, lung cancer cells appear to require many mutations in both dominant and recessive oncogenes to become clinically evident. The identification of the specific genes undergoing such mutations and the sequence of cumulative changes that lead to the neoplastic changes is still in progress. Our recent findings suggest that identifying biopsies with extensive or certain patterns of mutations may provide new methods for assessing the risk in smokes of developing invasive lung cancer and for monitoring response to chemoprevention. However, many un-answered questions regarding premalignant changes and early malignant lesions in respiratory mucosa must be addressed before advances in their clinical application to individuals at high risk can be achieved.

Acknowledgment

Supported by contract N01-CN-45580-01 from the Early Detection Research Network, and Specialized Program of Research Excellence grant 1-P50-CA70907-01 from the National Cancer Institute, Bethesda, MD, USA.

References

1. Parker SL, Tong T, Bolden S, Wingo PA (1996) Cancer statistics, 1996. *CA Cancer J Clin* 46: 5–27.
2. Garfinkel L, Stellman SD (1988) Smoking and lung cancer in women: findings in a prospective study. *Cancer Res* 48: 6951–6955.
3. Parkin DM, Pisani P, Lopez AD, Masuyer E (1994) At least one in seven cases of cancer is caused by smoking. Global estimates for 1985. *Int J Cancer* 5904: 494–504.
4. Saccomanno G, Archer VE, Auerbach O, Saunders RP, Brennan LM (1974) Development of carcinoma of the lung as reflected in exfoliated cells. *Cancer* 33: 256–270.
5. Weng S, Tsuchiya E, Satoh Y, Kitagawa T, Nakagawa K, Sugano H (1990) Multiple atypical adenomatous hyperplasia of type II pneumonocytes and bronchiolo-alveolar carcinoma. *Histopahology* 16: 101–103.
6. Nakanishi K (1990) Alveolar epithelial hyperplasia and adenocarcinoma of the lung. *Arch Pathol Lab Med* 114: 363–368.
7. Weng SY, Tsuchiya E, Kasuga T, Sugano H (1992) Incidence of atypical bronchioloalveolar cell hyperplasia of the lung: relation to histological subtypes of lung cancer. *Virchows Arch A Pathol Anat Histopathol* 420: 463–471.
8. Strong MS, Incze J, Vaughan CW (1984) Field cancerization in the aerodigestive tract – its etiology, manifestation, and significance. *J Otolaryng* 13: 1–6.
9. Slaughter DP, Southwick HW, Smejkal W (1954) "Field cancerization" in oral stratified squamous epithelium: Clinical implications of multicentric origin. *Cancer* 6: 963–968.
10. Auerbach O, Stout AP, Hammond EC, Garfinkel L (1961) Changes in bronchial epithelium in relation to smoking and cancer of the lung. *New Engl Med* 265: 253–267.
11. Auerbach O, Hammonad EC, Garfinkel K (1979) Changes in bronchial epithelium in relation to cigarette smoking, 1955–1960 vs 1970–1977. *N Engl J Med* 300: 381–385.
12. Bertram JF, Rogers AW (1981) Recover of bronchial epithelium on stopping smoking. *Br Med J (Clin Res Ed)* 283: 157–1569.
13. US Department of Health and Human Service (1990) The health benefits of smoking cessation. US Department of Health and Human Services, Public Health Service, Centers for Disease Control, Center for Chronic Disease Prevention and Health Promotion, Office on Smoking and Health.
14. Gazdar AF, Bader S, Hung J, Kishimoto Y, Sekido Y, Sugio K, Virmani A, Carbone DP, Minna JD (1995) Molecular genetic changes found in human lung cancer and its precursor lesions. *In:* Harlow E (eds.): *Molecular genetic changes found in human lung cancer and its precursor lesions*. Cold Spring Harbor Laboratory, Cold Spring Harbor, NY, pp 656–572.
15. Minna JD, Sekido Y, Fong K, Gazdar AF (1997) Molecular biology of lung cancer. *In:* DeVita VT Jr, Hellman S, Rosenberg SA (eds): *Molecular biology of lung cancer*. Lippincott, Philadelphia, Chapter 30.1.
16. Sugio K, Ishida T, Yokoyama H, Inoue T, Sugimachi K, Sasazuki T (1992) ras gene mutations as a prognostic marker in adenocarcinoma of the human lung without lymph node metastasis. *Cancer Res* 52: 2903–2905.
17. Mitsudomi T, Viallet J, Mulshine JL, Linnoila RI, Minna JD, Gazdar AF (1991) Mutations of *ras* genes distinguish a subset of non-small-cell lung cancer cell lines from small-cell lung cancer cell lines. *Oncogene* 6: 1353–1362.
18. Bos JL (1989) ras oncogenes in human cancer: a review. *Cancer Res* 49: 4682–2689.
19. Little CD, Nau MM, Carney DN, Gazdar AF, Minna JD (1983) Amplification and expression of the c-*myc* oncogene in human lung cancer cell lines. *Nature* 306: 194–196.
20. Nau MM, Carney DN, Battey J, Johnson B, Little C, Gazdar A, Minna JD (1984) Amplification, expression and rearrangement of c-*myc* and N-*myc* oncogenes in human lung cancer. *Curr Topics Microbiol Immunol* 113: 172–177.

21. Nau MM, Brooks BJ, Carney DN, Gazdar AF, Battey JF, Sausville EA, Minna JD (1986) Human small cell lung cancers show amplification and expression of the N-*myc* gene. *Proc Natl Acad Sci USA* 83:1092–1096.

22. Nau MM, Brooks BJ, Battey J, Sausville EA, Gazdar AF, Minna JD (1985) L-*myc*: A new *myc*-related gene amplified and expressed in human small cell lung cancer. *Nature* 318: 69–73.

23. Gazdar AF, Bader S, Hung J, Kishimoto Y, Sekido Y, Sugio K, Virmani A, Carbone DP, Minna JD (1995) Molecular genetic changes found in human lung cancer and its precursor lesions. *In*: (eds): *Molecular genetic changes found in human lung cancer and its precursor lesions,* Cold Spring Harbor Laboratory, Cold Spring Harbor, NY, pp 565–572.

24. Greenblatt MS, Bennett WP, Hollatein M, Harris CC (1994) Mutations in the p53 tumor supressor gene: clue to cancer etiology and molecular pathogenesis. *Cancer Res* 54: 4855–4878.

25. Horowitz JM, Park SH, Bogenmann E, Cheng JC, Yandell DW, Kaye FJ, Minna JD, Dryja TP, Weinberg RA (1990) Frequent inactivation of the retinoblastoma anti-oncogene is restricted to a subset of human tumor cells. Proceedings of the National Academy of Sciences of the United States of America, 87: 2775–2779.

26. Harbour JW, Sali SL, Whang-Peng J, Gazdar AF, Minna JD, Kaye FJ (1988) Abnormalities in structure and expression of the human retinoblastoma gene in SCLC. *Science* 241: 353–357.

27. Mori N, Yokota J, Akiyama T, Sameshima Y, Okamoto A, Mizoguchi H, Toyoshima K, Sugimura T, Terada M (1990) Variable mutations of the RB gene in small-cell lung carcinoma. *Oncogene* 5: 1713–1717.

28. Hensel CH, Hsieh CL, Gazdar AF, Johnson BE, Sakaguchi AY, Naylor SL, Lee WH, Lee EY (1990) Altered structure and expression of the human retinoblastoma susceptibility gene in small cell lung cancer. *Cancer Res* 50: 3067–3072.

29. Daly MC, Xiang RH, Buchhagen D, Hensel CH, Garcia DK, Killary AM, Minna JD, Naylor SL (1993) A homozygous deletion on chromosome 3 in a small cell lung cancer cell line correlates with a region of tumor suppressor activity. *Oncogene* 8:1721–1792.

30. Yamakawa K, Takahashi T, Horio Y, Murata Y, Takahashi E, Hibi K, Yokoyama S, Ueda R, Takahashi T, Nakamura Y (1993) Frequent homozygous deletions in lung cancer cell lines detected by a DNA marker located at 3p21.3-p22. *Oncogene* 8: 327–330.

31. Ohta M, Inoue H, Cotticelli MG, Kastury K, Baffa R, Palazzo J, Siprashivili Z, Mori M, McCue P, Druck T, Croce CM, Huebner K (1996) The *FHIT* gene, spanning the chromosome 3p14.2 fragile site and renal carcinoma-associated t(3;8) breakpoint, is abnormal in digestive tract cancers. *Cell* 84:587–597.

32. Sozzi G, Veronese ML, Negrini M, Baffa R, Corticelli MG, Inoue H, Tornielli S, Pilotti S, Ohta M, Huebner K, Croce CM (1996) The FHIT gene at 3p14.2 is abnormal in lung cancer. *Cell* 85:17–26.

33. Kastury K, Baffa R, Druck T, Ohta M, Cotticelli MG, Inoue H, Negrini M, Rugge M, Huang D, Croce CM, Palazzo J, Huebner K (1996) Potential gastrointestinal tumor suppressor locus at the 3p14.2 FRA3B site identified by homozygous deletions in tumor cell lines. *Cancer Res* 56: 978–983.

34. Olopade OI, Buchhagen DL, Minna JD, Gazdar AF, Malik KC, Rowley JD, Diaz MO (1991) Deletions of the short arm of chromosome 9 that include the alpha and beta interferon genes are associated with lung cancers (meeting abstract). *Proc Annu Meet Am Assoc Cancer Res* 32: A1814.

35. Olopade OI, Buchhagen DL, Malik K, Sherman J, Nobori T, Bader S, Nau MM, Gazdar AF, Minna JD, Diaz MO (1993) Homozygous loss of the interferon genes defines the critical region on 9p that is deleted in lung cancers. *Cancer Res* 53(10 Suppl): 2410–2415.

36. Kamb A, Gruis NA, Weaver-Feldhaus J, Liu Q, Harshman K, Tavtigian SV, Stockert E, Day RS, Johnson BE, and Skolnick MH (1994) A cell cycle regulator potentially involved in genesis of many tumor types. *Science* 264: 436–440.

37. Hayashi N, Sugimoto Y, Tsuchiya E, Ogawa M, Nakamura Y (1994) Somatic mutations of the MTS (multiple tumor suppressor) 1/CDK41 (cyclin-dependent kinase-4 inhibitor) gene in human primary non-small cell lung carcinomas. Biochem. *Biophys. Res. Commun* 202: 1426–1430.

38. Hannon GJ, Beach D (1994) p15INK4B is a potential effector of TGF-beta-induced cell cycle arrest. *Nature* 371: 257–261.

39. Washimi O, Nagatake M, Osada H, Ueda R, Koshikawa T, Seki T, Takahashi T, Takahashi T (1995) In vivo occurrence of p16 (MTS1) and p15 (MTS2) alterations preferentially in non-small cell lung cancers. *Cancer Res* 55: 514–517.

40. Xiao S, Li D, Corson JM, Vijg J, Fletcher JA (1995) Codeletion of p15 and p16 genes in primary non-small cell lung carcinoma. *Cancer Res* 55: 2968–2971.

41. Kishimoto Y, Sugio K, Mitsudomi T, Oyama T, Virmani A, McIntire DD, Gazdar AF (1995) Frequent loss of the short arm of chromosome 9 in resected non-small cell lung cancers from Japanese patients and its association with squamous cell carcinoma. *J Cancer Res Clin Oncol* 121: 291–296.

42. Sato S, Nakamura Y, Tsuchiya E (1994) Difference of allelotype between squamous cell carcinoma and adenocarcinoma of the lung. *Cancer Res* 54: 5652–5655.

43. Sozzi G, Miozzo M, Donghi R, Pilotti S, Cariani CT, Pastorino U, Della-Porta G, Pierotti MA (1992) Deletions of 17p and p53 mutations in preneoplastic lesions of the lung. *Cancer Res* 52: 6079–6082.

44. Sozzi G, Miozzo M, Tagliabue E, Calderone C, Lombardi L, Pilotti S, Pastorino U, Pierotti MA, Della Porta G (1991) Cytogenetic abnormalities and overexpression of receptors for growth factors in normal bronchial epithelium and tumor samples of lung cancer patients. *Cancer Res* 51: 400–404.

45. Sundaresan V, Ganly P, Hasleton P, Rudd R, Sinha G, Bleehen NM, Rabbitts P (1992) p 53 and chromosome 3 abnormalities, characteristic of malignant lung tumours, are detectable in preinvasive lesions of the bronchus. *Oncogene* 7: 1989–1997.

46. Mao L, Hruban RH, Boyle JO, Tockman M, Sidransky D (1994) Detection of oncogene mutations in sputum precedes diagnosis of lung cancer. *Cancer Res* 54:1634–1637.

47. Mills NE, Fishman CL, Scholes J, Anderson SE, Rom WN, Jacobson DR (1995) Detection of K-ras oncogene mutations in bronchoalveolar lavage fluid for lung cancer diagnosis. *J Natl Cancer Inst* 87: 1056–1060.

48. Sozzi G, Miozzo M, Pastorino U, Pilotti S, Donghi R, Giarola M, De Gregorio L, Manenti, G Radice P, Minoletti F et al. (1995) Genetic evidence for an independent origin of multiple preneoplastic and neoplastic lung lesions. *Cancer Res* 55: 135–2140.

49. Hung J, Kishimoto Y, Sugio K, Virmani A, McIntire DD, Minna JD, Gazdar AF (1995) Allele-specific chromosome 3p deletions occur at an early stage in the pathogenesis of lung carcinoma. *JAMA* 273: 558–563.

50. Sugio K, Kishimoto Y, Virmani A, Hung JY, Gazdar AF (1994) K-*ras* mutations are a relatively late event in the pathogenesis of lung carcinomas. *Cancer Res* 54: 5811–5815.

51. Kishimoto Y, Sugio K, Mitsudomi T, Oyama T, Virmani A, McIntire DD, Gazdar AF (1958) Allele specific loss of chromosome 9p in preneoplastic lesions accompanying non-small cell lung cancers. *J Natl Cancer Inst* 87: 1224–1229.

52. Fisher JC (1958) Multiple mutation theory of carcinogenesis. *Nature* 181: 651–652.

53. Loeb LA (1991) Mutator phenotype may be required for multistage carcinogenesis. *Cancer Res* 51: 3075–3079.

54. Loeb LA (1994) Microsatellite instability: marker of a mutator phenotype in cancer. *Cancer Res* 54: 5059–5063.

55. O'Connell P, Pekkel V, Fuqua S, Osborne CK, Allred DC (1994) Molecular genetic studies of early breast cancer evolution. *Breast Cancer Res Treat* 32: 5–12.

56. Deng G, Lu Y, Zlotnikov G, Thor AD, Smith HS (1996) Loss of heterozygosity in normal tissue adjacent to breast carcinomas. *Science* 274: 2057–2059.

57. Chung GT, Sundaresan V, Hasleton P, Rudd R, Taylor R, Rabbitts PH (1995) Sequential molecular genetic changes in lung cancer development. *Oncogene* 11: 2591–2598.

58. Smith AL, Hung J, Walker L, Rogers TE, Vuitch F, Lee E and Gazdar AF (1996) Extensive areas of aneuploidy are present in the respiratory epithelium of lung cancer patients. *Br J Cancer* 73: 203–209.

59. Mao L, Lee DJ, Tockman MS, Erozan YS, Askin F, Sidransky D (1994) Microsatellite alterations as clonal markers for the detection of human cancer. *Proc Natl Acad Sci USA* 91: 9871–9875.

60. Fong KM, Zimmerman PV, Smith PJ (1995) Microsatellite instability and other molecular abnormalities in non-small cell lung cancer. *Cancer Res* 55: 28–30.

61. Merlo A, Mabry M, Gabrielson E, Vollmer R, Baylin SB, Sidransky D (1994) Frequent microsatellite instability in primary small cell lung cancer. *Cancer Res* 54: 2098–2101.

62. Adachi J-I, Shiseki M, Okazaki T, Ishimuru G, Noguchi M, Hirohashi S, Yokota Y (1995) Microsatellite instability in primary and metastatic lung carcinomas. *Genes Chrom Cancer* 14: 301–306.
63. Fishel R, Lescoe, MK, Rao MR, Copeland NG, Jenkins NA, Garber J, Kane M, Kolodner R (1993) The human mutator gene homolog MSH2 and its association with hereditary nonpolyposis colon cancer. *Cell* 75: 1027–1038.
64. Fishel R (1996) Genomic instability, mutators, and the development of cancer: Is there a role for p53? *J Natl Cancer Inst* 88: 1608–1609.
65. Miozzo M, Sozzi G, Musso K, Pilotti (1996) Incarbone M, Pastorino U, Pierotti MA (1996) Microsatellite alterations in bronchial and sputum specimens of lung cancer patients. *Cancer Res* 56: 2285–2288.
66. Wistuba II, Lam S, Behrens C, Virmani AK, Fong KM, LeRiche J, Samet JM, Srivastava S, Minna JD, Gazdar AF (1997) Molecular damage in the bronchial epithelium of current and former smokers. *J Natl Cancer Inst* (in press)
67. Mao L, Lee JS, Kurie JM, Fan YH, Lippman SM, Lee JJ, Ro JY, Broxson A, Yu R, Morice RC, Kemp BL, Khuri FR, Walsh CG, Hittelman WN, Hong WK (1997) Clonal genetic alterations in the lungs of current and former smokers. *J Natl Cancer Inst* 89: 857–862.

Clinical and Biological Basis of Lung Cancer Prevention
ed. by Y. Martinet, F.R. Hirsch, N. Martinet, J.-M. Vignaud
and J.L. Mulshine
© 1998 Birkhäuser Verlag Basel/Switzerland

CHAPTER 6
Application of *In Situ* PCR and *In Situ* Hybridization to the Characterization of Lung Cancers

Alfredo Martínez

Cell and Cancer Biology Department, National Cancer Institute, National Institutes of Health, Rockville, Maryland, USA

1   Introduction
2   In Situ Hybridization
3   In Situ Gene Amplification
3.1   Protocol
3.2   Additional Comments
3.2.1   DNase or no DNase?
3.2.2   Designing Primers
3.2.3   Double Labelling
References

1. Introduction

Lung cancer is the result of chronic exposure of a range of normal respiratory epithelial cells to carcinogens. This exposure produces a complicated biology which is reflected by the numerous histologies of lung cancer [1]. Currently, the precise sequence of genetic events leading to an invasive cancer is speculative, but the development of new techniques offers possibilities of understanding this process. In addition, these techniques could be instrumental in identifying early markers for the detection of lung tumors before they metastasize [2].

We have applied in situ methods for the detection of particularly relevant nucleic acids and their protein products in tissue sections, in an attempt to characterize the involvement of these molecules in lung carcinogenesis. Our approach involves in situ hybridization for mRNA when the expression of the specific gene is abundant enough [3, 4] or in situ RT-PCR, which involves amplification of the template nucleic acid, for the detection of mRNA from low-expression genes [5–7]. The colocalization of the nucleic acids with the protein for which they code in the same cells can be achieved by a combination of the previous techniques with immunohistochemistry, further strengthening the initial observations [4]. Another important application of in situ gene amplification techniques could be the detection of single point mutations in tissue sections, as we have recently reported [8].

In the following pages we summarize the techniques used in our laboratory, paying special attention to in situ gene amplification.

2. In Situ Hybridization

In situ hybridization has become an important tool for the detection of specific nucleic acid sequences (both DNA and RNA) in chromosome preparations, cytospins and tissue sections. Since the first procedures were published [9], continuous improvements have been made in the different steps that are essential for successful hybridization of the target nucleic acid, which lies buried in the tissue section (for reviews, see [10, 11].

Preparation of cells and tissue sections for in situ hybridization usually involves fixation with a crosslinking fixative (10% formalin or 4% paraformaldehyde) and attachment to a glass slide, followed by proteolytic digestion to allow penetration of the probes. This requires a delicate balance between preservation of cell morphology and the efficiency of the hybridization procedure. Usually a series of slides is required to establish the optimal digestion.

Different probes can be used for in situ hybridization including double-stranded DNA, single-stranded RNA and oligonucleotides. Each of them has its advantages and disadvantages and the decision to use one or the other depends on the abundance and nature of the target. Another factor to consider is how to label the probe. Although the first protocols made use of radioisotopes, the introduction of stable, nonradioactive labels has become the method of choice, and since many hapten-labelling protocols are available [12], the possibilities for combination with other techniques are also numerous. On top of that, the nonradioactive methods have the added bonus of a better localization of the signal.

Special care has to be taken when attempting the detection of mRNA since the ubiquitous, rather efficient and very stable RNases can easily contaminate the tissue section and render our efforts unfruitful.

3. In Situ Gene Amplification

The possibility of performing DNA or mRNA amplification in tissue sections has been proposed since the beginning of the polymerase chain reaction (PCR) era. Unfortunately, the technique has proved to be more elusive than a quick glance at various protocols [13, 14] suggests. Nevertheless, the reward to those able to master the technique is high: unlimited sensitivity in the detection of specific nucleic acids expressed in subpopulations of cells. A single "available" molecule is enough to produce a detectable signal. This promise has persuaded a great number of investigators dealing with low levels of expression (growth factors, receptors, developmental signals, etc.), with newly acquired DNA (viral infections, point mutations, transpositions, deletions, etc.), or trying to follow vectors after gene therapies, to pursue in situ PCR technology.

The advent of specific thermocyclers for tissue sections has solved many of the technical problems and our laboratory has recently developed a protocol for the direct detection of DNA and mRNA in archival material using one such instrument [15]. In the past, one of the bigger problems accompanying this technique was the lack of reproducible results, which arose from: (1) difficulties in performing synchronized "hot Start" applications; (2) limitations in the number of slides that can be processed at the same time; (3) heterogeneous heating of the slides (they were usually placed on top of a regular thermocycler block, with holes for the tubes, and even if a small aluminium foil boat was used great variations in temperature between different areas of the section occurred). We overcame the first obstacle using a monoclonal antibody that blocks the Taq polymerase until the temperature reaches 70 °C and the denatured antibody liberates an active enzyme to the PCR solution [16], and the other two difficulties were resolved by performing the reaction in a specifically designed thermocycler (OmniSlide System, Hybaid, UK).

The conceptual protocol is simple: if we want do detect DNA, after dewaxing and rehydrating the sections three steps must be performed: (1) protein digestion to facilitate reagent penetration, (2) PCR reaction with simultaneous labelling of the PCR products, and (3) visualization of the labelled products by immunocytochemical methods. The detection of mRNA incorporates a reverse transcription step, to generate cDNA, before amplification.

Fixation is critical for obtaining positive results. It has been reported that in samples treated with alcohol – or acetone – based fixatives the PCR products ended up in the supernatant. Conversely, crosslinking fixatives like paraformaldehyde or formalin were able to retain the labelled products in the tissue, possibly because of the lattice they created among the proteins [17].

In situ amplification combines all the advantages of histological and PCR technologies but, unfortunately, it also suffers from the possible artefacts of both of them. This is why attention to appropriate controls is of paramount importance for successful interpretation of the results.

These are some of the controls we use: (1) positive control, which includes a section of a tissue or cell line known to have high expression of the target nucleic acid as determined by other techniques (Northern blotting, regular PCR, in situ hybridization); (2) negative control, where substitution of the primers by water in the PCR mixture will reveal nonspecific endogenous priming (necrosis, apoptosis, repair processes); (3) negative control when looking for mRNA, by RNase pretreatment or omission of the reverse transcriptase; (4) colocalization of the signals for the mRNA (in situ RT-PCR) and its translated protein (immunocytochemistry); (5) extraction of the DNA from the tissue section after amplification and analysis by electrophoresis and Southern blot; (6) in situ hybridization with a labelled nested probe after amplification. This last procedure is routinely used in the indirect method of in situ PCR.

3.1. Protocol

In situ amplification can be done on cytospin preparations, or on sections from paraffin-embedded and frozen tissues. Here we present a protocol for the detection of mRNA in paraffin sections, because of the importance of archival material. For the detection of DNA step No. 4 is omitted.

1. Take the usual precautions for working with RNA, even when cutting the sections: wear gloves, bake the glassware, use DEPC-treated water, etc.
2. Sections are deparaffinized by immersion in xylene (20 min) and rehydrated in decreasing concentrations of ethanol in DEPC-treated water. Always use new solutions for in situ RT-PCR: you can reuse them for regular histological procedures.
3. Permeabilization of the tissue is achieved by incubation with protein-ase K. We found that a concentration of 10 µg/ml proteinase K at 37 °C for 15 min is appropriate for most archival material, but variations of concentration or exposure time are recommended to optimize the results.
4. Reverse transcription. The reverse transcriptase needs to be primed and it is possible to use either specific primers designed to target the requir-ed message or an oligo (dT) that binds to the polyA tail of the mRNAs. For this step we use the SuperScript Preamplification System (Gibco BRL, Gaithersburg, MD): a drop (60 µl) containing the primers is placed on top of the section and covered with parafilm and the sections are incubated for 10 min at 70 °C in the thermocycler. After removing the coverslips, another solution containing the enzyme (100 U/section) is added and covered with a new piece of parafilm. The slides are then maintained at room temperature for 10 min, at 45 °C for 45 min, and at 70 °C for 10 min.

    Alternatively, a single reaction mixture for RT and PCR can be per-formed when using the rTth DNA polymerase. In the presence of Mn salts this enzyme has an efficient enough RT activity [18]. Whether it acts as RT or DNA polymerase depends on the temperature profile as established by the thermocycler [19].
5. PCR. All the parameters for the PCR reaction must be optimized by regular PCR before attempting in situ amplification.
    a) In a sterile microcentrifuge tube mix 0.5 µl of Taq polymerase (Perkin-Elmer Cetus, Norwalk, CT) and 0.5 µl of TaqStart antibody (Clontech, Palo Alto, CA) per slide and incubate for 5 min at room temperature to block the enzyme.

b) Add the rest of the components of the PCR mixture to obtain the following composition: 2.5 mM $MgCl_2$ (has to be tested for each set of primers), 200 µM dNTPs, 100 µM digoxigenin-11-dUTP (Boehringer Mannheim, Indianapolis, IN), 1 ng/µl primers, 50 mM KCl, 10 mM Tris-HCl.

c) An 80 µl aliquot of solution is applied to each slide, the section is covered by a glass coverslip which is sealed with rubber cement to prevent evaporation and placed in the thermocycler. Recently, efficient coverslipping systems, able to survive thermocycling, have been developed.

d) The number of cycles and the annealing temperature have to be optimized for each tissue and target nucleic acid. A standard run could be like this: begin with 2 min at 72 °C; 15 cycles of 94 °C for 15 sec, 55 °C for 15 sec, 72 °C for 60 sec; finish with 5 min at 72 °C.

e) Remove coverslips and wash the sections twice in $0.1 \times SSC$ at 45 °C, 20 min each.

6. Detection of digoxigenin-tagged DNA. We use the Digoxigenin Detection kit (Boehringer Mannheim): it involves a 2-hour incubation with an antidigoxigenin antibody bound to alkaline phosphatase at a dilution of 1:500, thorough washes and incubation with the appropriate substrates (nitroblue tetrazolium and a complex phosphate) to produce a dark blue precipitate.

7. Check under the microscope until the proper color intensity is reached. Stop the reaction before the background in the negative controls begins to increase. Mount the slides in a water-soluble mounting medium because the blue precipitate is soluble in organic solvents.

8. Compare the test slides with the controls.

3.2 Additional Comments

3.2.1. DNase or no DNase? In some protocols for in situ RT-PCR the authors recommend a digestion with RNase-free DNase before the reverse transcription step. This treatment is intended to remove nuclear and mitochondrial DNA to avoid genomic amplification during PCR. We repeatedly observed, using a variety of DNases, that this digestion step resulted in nonspecific nuclear staining [15]. This problem seems to be due to the behaviour of the DNase enzyme which cuts the DNA into oligonucleotides but does not reduce it to mononucleotides. The remaining oligonucleotides are used as primers by the DNA polymerase and nonspecific staining occurs. Therefore we strongly recommend the omission of this step. A careful choice of the primers and a reduced number of cycles (15 to 20) is useful to avoid nonspecific nuclear staining.

3.2.2. Designing primers: When choosing primers consider the following: (a) A good size range for the PCR product is 100 to 500 bp. If the product is too small it could leak out of the fixative-induced lattice and be washed away from the tissue. On the other hand products which are too long could be hard to amplify in the tissue sections and, especially when looking at archival material, the probability of finding nicks (that will prevent amplification) in the nucleic acid template increases with size. (b) If the primers bridge an intron it is easier to eliminate the possibility of genomic amplification. (c) Take the usual precautions with palindromic sequences and hairpin formation.

3.2.3. Double labelling: It is possible to combine in situ amplification with immunocytochemistry or in situ hybridization. In the first case, we suggest performing the immunological detection first because the thermal cycles could destroy most of the antigens present in the tissue. If trying to do mRNA localization, remember to use RNase-free reagents during the whole process by using DEPC-treated water in all the solutions and adding RNase inhibitors to the antisera.

References

1. Linnoila RI, Aisner SC (1995) Pathology of lung cancer: an exercise in classification. *In:* Johnson BE, Johnson DH (eds): *Lung cancer*, Wiley-Liss, New York, pp 73–95.
2. Mulshine JL, Scott F, Zhou J, Avis I, Vos M, Miller MJ, Szabo E, Martínez A, Treston AM, Cuttitta F, et al. (1996) Development of molecular approaches to early lung cancer detection. *Seminars in Radiation Oncology* 6: 72–75.
3. Saldise I, Martínez A, Montuenga LM, Treston A, Springall RD, Polak JM, Vásquez JJ (1996) Distribution of peptidyl-glycine α-amidating mono-oxygenase (PAM) enzymes in normal human lung and in lung epithelial tumors. *J Histochem Cytochem* 44: 3–12.
4. Martínez A, Treston AM, Saldise L, Montuenga LM, Linnoila RI (1996) Expression of peptidyl-glycine α-amidating mono-oxygenase (PAM) enzymes in morphological abnormalities adjacent to pulmonary tumors. *Am J Pathol* 149: 707–716.
5. Martínez A, Miller MJ, Unsworth EJ, Siegfried JM, Cuttitta F (1995) Expression of adrenomedullin in normal human lung and in pulmonary tumors. *Endocrinology* 136: 4099–4105.
6. Avis I, Jett M, Boyle T, Vos MD, Moody T, Treston AM, Martínez A, Mulshine JL (1996) Growth control of lung cancer by interruption of 5-lipoxygenase-mediated growth factor signaling. *J Clin Invest* 97: 806–813.
7. Miller MJ, Martínez A, Unsworth EJ, Thiele CJ, Moody TW, Elsasser T, Cuttitta F (1996) Adrenomedullin expression in human tumor cell lines, its potential role as an autocrine growth factor. *J Biol Chem* 271: 23345–23351.
8. Ebina M, Martínez A, Birrer MJ, Linnoila RI (1995) Topographic mapping of p53 mutations in non-small cell lung cancer, novel approach to carcinogenesis using in situ PCR. *Proc Am Assoc Cancer Res* 36: 578.
9. John HA, Birnstiel ML, Jones KW (1969) RN-DNA hybrids at the cytological level. *Nature* 223: 582–587.
10. Polak JM, McGee JO'D (eds) (1990): *In situ hybridization, principles and practice.* Oxford University Press, New York.
11. Terenghi G, Fallon RA (1990) Techniques and applications of in situ hybridization. In: Underwood JCE (ed) *Current topics in pathology.* 82: Pathology of the nucleus. Berlin, Springer-Verlag, 289–337.
12. Speel EJM, Ramaekers FCS, Hopman AHN (1995) Cytochemical detection systems for in situ hybridization, and the combination with immunocytochemistry: "Who is still afraid of red, green and blue?". *Histochem J* 27: 833–858.

13. Nuovo GJ (ed) (1992) *PCR in situ hybridization; protocols and applications.* New York: Raven Press.
14. Corcoran M, Levin M, Jacobson S, Liotta L (1994) From hot starts and false starts to smart starts: in situ PCR. *NIH Catalyst* (May): 12–14.
15. Martínez A, Miller MJ, Quinn K, Unsworth EJ, Ebina M, Cuttitta F (1995) Non-radioactive localization of nucleic acids by direct in situ PCR and in situ RT-PCR in paraffin-embedded sections. *J Histochem Cytochem* 43: 739–747.
16. Kellogg DE, Rybalkin I, Chen S, Mukhamedova N, Vlasik T, Siebert PD, Chenchik A (1994) TaqStart antibody; "hot start" PCR facilitated by a neutralizing monoclonal antibody directed against Taq DNA polymerase. *BioTechniques* 6: 1134–1137.
17. O'Leary JJ, Browne G, Landers RJ, Crowley M, Bailey Healy I, Street JT, Pollock AM, Murphy J, Johnson MI, Lewis FA, et al. (1994) The importance of fixation procedures on DNA template and its suitability for solution-phase polymerase chain reaction and PCR in situ hybridization. *Histochem J* 26: 337–346.
18. Myers TW, Gelfand DH (1991) Reverse transcription and DNA amplification by a *Thermus thermophilus* DNA polymerase. *Biochemistry* 30: 7661–7663.
19. Macri CJ, Martínez A, Moody TW, Gray KD, Miller MJ, Gallagher M, Cuttitta F (1996) Detection of adrenomedullin, a hypotensive peptide, in amniotic fluid and fetal membranes. *Am J Obstet Gynecol* 175: 906–911.

Clinical and Biological Basis of Lung Cancer Prevention
ed. by Y. Martinet, F.R. Hirsch, N. Martinet, J.-M. Vignaud
and J.L. Mulshine
© 1998 Birkhäuser Verlag Basel/Switzerland

CHAPTER 7
Tumor Stroma Formation in Lung Cancer

Jean-Michel Vignaud *,[1,3], Béatrice Marie[1], Evelyne Picard[1], Karim Nabil[3],
Jöelle Siat[2], Francoise Galateau-Salle[4], Jacques Borrelly[2], Yves Martinet[2,3]
and Nadine Martinet[3]

[1] *Laboratoire d'Anatomie Pathologique, Université de Nancy, Nancy, France*
[2] *Clinique Pneumologique Médico-Chirugicale, Université de Nancy, Nancy, France*
[3] *INSERM U14, Université de Nancy, Nancy, France*
[4] *Laboratoire d'Anatomie Pathologique, Université de Caen, Caen, France*

1. Introduction

Lung carcinomas are heterogeneous in composition. The malignant cells
are surrounded by a specialized connective tissue called stroma, consisting
of an extracellular matrix (ECM) and a cellular compartment made of
fibroblasts, inflammatory cells and endothelial cells. The ability of carcinoma cells to induce a stroma is a phenotypic trait that is maintained at
metastatic sites. Stromal tissue is qualitatively distinct from the connective
tissue which develops in inflammatory conditions: for instance, stromal
inflammatory and mesenchymal cells have distinct phenotypic characteristics, and specific spliced variants of ECM components, such as fibronectin and tenascin, have been reported in carcinomas. Blood vessels are
another essential component of the stroma. A vascular supply is necessary
for tumor growth over 2 mm³. This is achieved by the complex multistep

---

* Autor for correspondence.

process of angiogenesis (see chapter by Castronovo et al., this volume). Moreover, the stroma, as opposed to normal connective tissue, is an unstable structure, remodelled throughout tumor development. This plasticity, controlled in part by the neoplastic cells themselves, is the result of a spatially and temporally changing imbalance between the agonist and antagonist stromal mechanisms that control tumor progression.

It is now currently accepted that stroma acts for tumor cells as: (1) a mechanical support, (2) a feeding support and pathway for metabolic wasteproducts, (3) a participant in the control of differentiation, proliferation, adhesion, and migration via a complex network of extracellular signals, and (4) ultimately promotes the tumor invasive phenotype and the metastatic process, although a number of histochemical studies have demonstrated the presence of infiltrating immune cells within carcinomas. Understanding the complex relationships established between neoplastic cells and cellular and non-cellular stroma components may lead, in the near future, to the design of new anticancer treatments targeted against tumor stroma constituents.

2. Extracellular Matrix Components of Lung Carcinomas

2.1. Carcinoma Cell-ECM Interactions are Mediated by Surface Receptors: Integrins, Non-integrins and Cell Surface Proteoglycans

The most extensively studied of ECM receptors is the integrin family, a group of transmembrane α and β subunit glycoprotein heterodimers [1, 2]. Integrins play an important role in both tumor cell-ECM and carcinoma cell-stromal cell interactions, especially with endothelial cells and leukocytes. Integrins and the mechanisms coupled to them undergo extensive changes during malignant transformations and tumor progression. For instance, in normal lung tissue $\alpha 6\ \beta 4$ integrin was found at a low level, but its expression increased significantly in epidermoid carcinomas and adenocarcinomas, mostly at carcinoma/stroma interfaces [3]. In small cell lung carcinoma (SCLC) cell lines, $\beta 1$ expression is predominantly associated with the $\alpha 3$ subunit (and to a lesser extent, with αM and $\alpha 1$ [4]. This $\alpha 3\ \beta 1$ integrin is involved in laminin adhesion of SCLC cells.

Among non-integrins, the laminin/elastin receptors and the collagen receptors-cell surface proteoglycans (including CD44) play a central role. The latter are less specified elements, but provide an important support for cell-ECM interactions.

2.2 Extracellular Matrix Components

The ECM is composed of four major classes of component (collagens, elastin, proteoglycans and hyaluronic acid, and glycoproteins), a wide range of molecules that constitute a very complex network. During the last decade, the presence of homologous sequences repeated in different proteins of the ECM has been extensively demonstrated. Motifs that share a common structure are called modules, and the great diversity of ECM proteins can be reduced to a relatively small number of distinct modules such as epidermal growth factor (EGF), fibronectin (FN) type III and proteoglycan tandem repeat. The modules from which a particular protein is built up can play both a structural and a functional role. The resulting interactions account for the integrity of the ECM, and a mutation affecting a single module can induce a loss of function of the protein.

2.2.1. Collagen and elastin fibers: Each tumor builds a specific stroma, using different quantities of ECM and cellular components. A wide range of ECM stroma patterns has been described, each of them broadly related to a histological type: for instance, while abundant in non-small cell lung cancer (NSCLC) the stroma is sparse in neuroendocrine carcinomas, especially SCLC, and in bronchioalveolar carcinomas. These distinct ECM patterns are mainly supported by qualitative and quantitative differences in collagen and elastic fiber content as shown in Table 1 [5, 6]. Concerning the nature of the cells that constitute the ECM, experimental studies have clearly demonstrated that, in accordance with their embryological origin, sarcoma cells produce the ECM that surrounds them, but carcinoma cells subcontract their ECM production to the surrounding fibroblasts [7]. Elastin, collagens (particularly type I and III) and basement membrane type IV, the major constituents of the ECM, may act as a barrier for tumor cell invasion, but can also favor the migration of tumor cells. When carcinoma cells move through the stroma, their cytoplasmic membrane interacts with both elastin and collagen fibers. The interaction between carcinoma cells and elastin fibers [8] is mediated, in sarcomas and in some carcinomas [9], by both insoluble and soluble elastin binding receptors (IEBR, SEBR). IEBRs bind the tumor cells to elastic fibers and allow surface elastase to release elastin peptides. SEBR binding of the elastin peptides may stimulate cells to increase levels of the membrane-bound protein phosphokinase C, which is thought to correlate with an increase in migratory activity [10].

Table 1. Extracellular matrix profile in lung cancer (adapted from [5])

	NSCLC	SCLC	BAC
Collagen type III	+++	++	+
Pro collagen III	+++	–	+/–
Collagen type VI	–	+++	–
Oxytalan fibers	–	++	+++
Elastic fibers	+	+++	++

NSCLC: non-small cell lung carcinoma; SCLC: small-cell lung carcinoma; BAC: bronchioloalveolar cell carcinoma.

2.2.2. Proteoglycans: Proteoglycans (PGs) are macromolecules consisting of a core protein covalently linked to one or more glycosaminoglycans (GAG) side chains that are sulfated or non-sulfated repeating dissacharide units. GAGs have a strongly negative charge that makes them able to bind growth factors and proteins specific to them. For instance, hyaluronic acid, a free GAG that lacks sulfate, is the ligand for CD44, a lymphocyte-homing receptor [11]. Many PGs are constituents of the ECM (e.g. aggrecan, decorin, fibromodulin and perlecan) [12]. PGs act as modulators of growth factor activity [12]. Decorin, associated with type I collagen, binds transforming growth factor-β (TGF-β) in an inactive form through its core protein [13]. The binding of TGF-β to decorin is reversible; as a consequence, decorin may form a reservoir of this growth factor. In colonic carcinoma stroma, the amount of decorin is markedly increased and the glycosylation pattern is modified and identical to that found in embryonic tissues [14]. These changes correlate with an increase in decorin mRNA and the hypomethylation of the decorin gene [15] in stromal cells. In the same way, perlecan, a basement membrane PG, interacts with basic- and acid-fibroblast growth factors (FGFs) [16] and granulocyte-macrophage-colony stimulating factor (GM-CSF) [17], regulating the corresponding growth factor activities. Furthermore, perlecan, by promoting the binding of bFGF to its receptor, is a potent inducer of angiogenesis [18], and PGs, such as versican, have EGF-like domains [19]. It has also been suggested that the accumulation of hyaluronic acid in tumors, providing a well-hydrated matrix, may favor the growth and migration of carcinoma cells [20] by creating a loose hydrated extracellular pathway which is conducive to cell migration, in addition to a direct interaction via carcinoma cell surface hyaluranan specific receptors [21]. Although data on the GAG profile of different tumors are very variable, there is a consistent tendency to produce more hyaluronic acid than sulfated GAG [22]. Lung carcinomas and mesotheliomas are highly enriched in hyaluranan [23, 24], although in lung adenocarcinoma, staining for hyaluranan is confined to the remnants of the infiltrated connective tissue stroma [25]. Furthermore, it has been suggested that tumor cells stimulate stromal mesenchymal cells to synthesize PGs rather than producing PG themselves. Thus an increased content of PGs in stroma could (1) favor tumor cell migration in a highly hydrated tissue, (2) promote tumor cell growth through reservoir-bound growth factors and (3) participate in the process of angiogenesis.

2.2.3. Stromal glycoproteins: Fibronectin might be considered as the prototype of stromal glycoproteins. FNs are glycoproteins present in the ECM, which play a crucial role in cell adhesion, spreading and migration. A single pre-mRNA is transcribed from the FN gene, which undergoes alternative splicing in three regions referred to as EDB, EDA and III CS. The expression of FN isoforms can vary in an oncodevelopmental manner, and in general, EDB+, EDA+ and III CS+FN mRNAs are expressed in foetal and tumor tissue rather than adult or normal tissue [26]. Carcinoma cells do not express FN, but stromal fibroblasts surrounding the tumor are positive for FN. In well-differentiated laryngeal and cervical carcinomas, the level of FN mRNAs is increased 7- to 13-fold in stromal fibroblasts versus fibroblasts of healthy tissues [27]. This decreases in corresponding poorly differentiated tumors. The induction of FN mRNAs is associated with the release of growth factors by carcinoma cells into the peritumoral stroma. It has been reported that TGF-β, and its extracellular deposition, could stimulate the synthesis of FN, especially the isoforms containing EDB$^+$, EDA$^+$ and the III CS variant 2, encoding FNs that initiate the fibrillogenesis of the ECM [28, 29]. Since FN participates in the maintenance of normal cell phenotype, the FN produced by fibroblasts and deposited around carcinoma cells may antagonize tumor cell growth and invasion. However, tumor cells and stromal fibroblasts release proteases leading to the degradation of FN (and other matrix proteins), with the generation of FN fragments. These fragments exhibit proteolytic activities for FNs and collagens [30, 31], and probably other ECM proteins, and could favor tumor invasion. The imbalance between the antagonistic function of fibroblasts producing FNs and tumor cells leading to FN fragment release may contribute to the regulation of mechanisms that control the dormancy or growth and invasion of carcinoma cells.

The functions of many glycoprotein molecules remain unclear. Tenascin, a good example, is expressed at the embryonic stage, but no expression is found in adult lung. In benign tumors and cancer, tenascin reappears in the stroma [32], but there is no fixed level of expression: some lung carcinomas show an increased expression of tenascin mRNA, while others have a low expression [33]. Tenascin shows various, and sometimes opposite, effects: cell adhesion/anti-adhesion, promotion/inhibition of cell growth according to assay conditions used. The multidomain structure of the molecule, and the different isoforms regulated by alternative splicing, allow us to speculate that cells can produce different types of tenascin, depending on the tissue environment, which may explain the various actions of this molecule in cancer development. Indeed, only the high molecular weight variant, containing a type II fibronectin repeat, supports mitogenic activity [33] and the ability to downregulate focal adhesion [34]. This isoform has been suggested as a marker of stromal proliferation and tumor invasion [35]. Furthermore, in some adenocarcinomas, large cell carcinomas and many squamous cell carcinomas, a significant increase of the tenascin/ fibronectin mRNA ratio has been shown [36, 37]. The value of such a high ratio, in prognostic terms, has not yet been investigated.

In summary, the ECM, as a result of the cooperation between host stromal mesenchymal cells and tumor cells, strongly influences the histological characteristics and behavior of lung carcinoma cells (cell adhesion, migration and differentiation). If tumor cells can modify their extracellular environment, the ECM in turn may also control tumor cell behavior by modulating the activity of growth factors/cytokines.

3. Stromal Cell Populations

3.1. Fibroblasts

Tumor associated fibroblasts (TAF) are an important subpopulation of stromal cells in NSCLC, synthesizing collagen and elastic fibers and other ECM components. TAF are phenotypically distinct from their counterparts in healthy tissues. They display characteristics similar to those of foetal cells: in particular they have an extended *in vitro* lifespan [38, 39], and express foetal-specific cell surface antigens [40]. They also synthesize tumor-specific isoforms of ECM components such as EDB fibronectin. Furthermore, they can produce proteases (particularly stromelysin-3, gelatinase-A and -B) and growth factors such as interleukin (IL)-6, and so participate in ECM remodelling, angiogenesis and tumor progression [41, 42]. However, these fetal-like TAFs are not tumor-specific. They are observed in noncancerous tissues in diverse pathological conditions such as wound healing. They also represent a phenotypically heterogeneous population, with respect to their distribution inside the tumor [43]. The factors that allow the persistence of foetal cell phenotypic characteristics by TAFs have yet to be specified, but probably involve the complex interactions of cytokines and matrix molecules. For instance, in NSCLC tumor associated macrophages (TAM), and to a lesser extent tumor cells, strongly express platelet-derived growth factor (PDGF) A and B proteins and TAF constantly express PDGF receptor α and β subunits. There is also a superposition of the sites where PDGF-producing TAM are present in high concentration and the sites where TAF are replicating, which strongly suggests the role of PDGF in TAF growth [44]. Other growth factors such as TGF-β [45] increase collagen and fibronectin synthesis and secretion in several fibroblast cell lines [46, 47]. Thus TAF, by interacting with inflammatory cells and carcinoma cells, favor carcinoma cell progression through the ECM, angiogenesis and ultimately the metastatic process.

3.2. Tumor Stroma Inflammatory Cells

Lymphocytes and macrophages are the main inflammatory cells infiltrating lung carcinomas, but we should not underestimate the role of other cell populations such as Langerhans cells, polymorphonuclear leukocytes and mastocytes.

3.2.1. Tumor-infiltrating lymphocytes (TIL): TIL, in lung carcinomas, are a heterogeneous population consisting of mainly CD3$^+$ T lymphocytes, a minority of B lymphocytes, and a few natural killer (NK) cells. These represent, in NSCLC (independently of histological type), an average of 80%, 20% and 1% respectively of TIL population (personal data). TIL are mainly CD8+, with a low (5% to 20%) CD4/CD8 ratio [48]. When compared to peripheral blood lymphocytes (PBL), TIL show an increased expression of several activation markers (CD45 Ro, HLA-DR, CD25, CD69), indicating that they have been activated, possibly by encountering specific tumor antigens. CD8+ TIL may kill carcinoma cells that express peptides derived from mutant cellular proteins and presented in association with class I MHC (major histocompatibility complex) molecules. The lytic capacity of CD56+ NK cells is MHC-unrestricted. NK cells can be targeted to antibody-coated cells because they express low affinity Fc receptors (CD16) for IgG molecules. Their lytic capacity can be increased by interferon-γ (IFN-γ), tumor necrosis factor-α (TNF-α), IL-2 and IL-12. Therefore, their cytotoxic potential may depend on the simultaneous activation of CD4+ TIL, tumor cells and TAM producing these cytokines. Although CD4+ T-cells are not generally cytotoxic for tumor cells, they are necessary for a successful antitumor immune response mediated via the cytokines secreted by the Th1 subset (IL-2, IFN-γ, TNF-β) and the Th2 subset (IL-4, IL-5, IL-10, IL-13) [49], that regulate the induction of immune cells. TNF-α and IFN-γ can increase tumor cell class I MHC expression and sensitivity to lysis by CD8+ TIL. A minority of tumors that express class II MHC molecules may directly activate tumor-specific CD4+ T cells.

However: (1) class I MHC molecule expression *in vivo* is strongly downregulated on epidermoid and lung adenocarcinoma cells (personal data), as well as in SCLC [50], so that efficient complexes of processed tumor antigen peptides and MHC molecules required for CD8+ Tcell recognition cannot be formed; (2) using RT-PCR a decreased expression of mRNA has been shown for IL-2, IL-4, IL-6, GM-CSF and IFN-γ in TIL freshly isolated form lung cancer [51] versus PBL; (3) using iododeoxuridine (IdU) technique to follow TIL kinetics *in vivo* [44], we observed a low rate of replication of these cells (2%). These three observations suggest that TIL are relatively functionally deficient in their capacity to mediate a strong antitumor cytotoxicity, to release cytokines, and to proliferate. However, the extension of the T helper 1 and 2 paradigm of functional CD4 subsets into the CD8 lineage suggests that complex subsets of functionally distinct CD8+ T cells may be present within tumors. One or several of them, although few in number, could display significant cytotoxic capacity using the perforin-dependent induction of membrane lysis, and/or the Fas-induced DNA fragmentation and apoptosis [52]. Furthermore, through the complex network of cytokines they produce, CD4+ T cells can interfere with the mechanisms regulating ECM production, and the functions of tumor cells and other inflammatory cells. In contrast, carcinoma cell products such as TGF-β may decrease the antitumor immune response [45]. It has also been shown that NSCLC carcinoma cells express a type 2 lymphocyte-like cytokine pattern [53] that can facilitate the immune response. Thus, although the interactions between TIL and cancer cells are not fully understood, clinical observations and experimental studies may lead to clinical trials of adoptive immunotherapy.

3.2.2. Tumor-associated macrophages (TAM): TAM are a major component of the stroma in NSCLC, with many sometimes contradictory functions [54]. These pleiotropic cells have the capacity (1) to affect production and remodelling of the ECM, (2) to exert a cytotoxic influence but also promote carcinoma cell growth and (3) to favor the process of angiogenesis. Currently some evidence suggests that the protumor functions of TAM prevail over their cytotoxic functions.

Macrophage infiltration of tumors is mainly relevant to a superfamily of cytokines called chemokines, which are produced by tumor cells, but also by mesenchymal cells, endothelial cells and mononuclear phagocytes. A kinetic study showed that TAM replicate weakly in NSCLC ($1 \pm 0.5\%$) [44] but are mainly recruited at a tumor site [55]. Monocyte chemotactic protein 1 (MCP-1), a chemoattractant active on monocytes (but inactive on lymphocytes and neutrophils) is the major chemokine, a family which includes other members such as MCP-2, -3, MIP-1α, -1β and gro-α. It has been shown that local inoculation of MCP-1 determines monocyte infiltration in rats [56], and MCP-1 gene transfer into murine melanoma cells results in an increased infiltration by blood monocytes in nude mice [57]. Factors other than chemokines, such as M-CSF and GM-CSF, are also involved in TAM recruitment, as demonstrated by gene transfer experiments in mice [58]. TIL produce GM-CSF [59] and participate in monocyte recruitment. Anti-inflammatory cytokines such as TGF-β and IL-10 may counterbalance the action of these chemokines.

The activation of macrophages is a prerequisite for cellular cytotoxicity. Many factors produced by carcinoma cells and stromal cells, especially by inflammatory cells, are potent activators of TAM (e.g. IFN-γ, TNF-α, -β, and GM-CSF) [60]. Appropriately activated macrophages can kill cancer cells via different mediators, including cytokines (IL-12, TNF-α, IL-6) and reactive intermediates of oxygen or nitrogen. The cytolytic process is dependent upon cell-cell contact, mediated by specific cell-surface receptors present on macrophages. Adhesion molecules, particularly of the β-integrin family, are clearly involved in several forms of TAM-tumor cell interaction, antibody-independent as well as dependent forms. 64% of TAM from NSCLC express low affinity Fc receptor III (CD16) [61], which makes them potent effectors for killing antibody-sensitized carcinoma cells. However, this cytolytic potential may be modulated by the fact that TAM, in lung cancer, are relatively poor producers of IL-1 and TNF-α [51]. Furthermore, carcinoma cells produce IL-10 [62] which demonstrates various immunosuppressive bioactivities, including alteration of monocyte cytotoxicity, downregulation of class II MHC molecule expression and inhibition of proinflammatory cytokine production [63].

TAM interactions with carcinoma cell growth and ECM production take place through growth factor synthesis, and interact within the intratumoral cytokine network. Mononuclear phagocytes are capable of producing high amounts of growth factors (such as EGF, GM-CSF, IL-1, IL-6, IL-12, PDGF, TGF-α, TNF-α, VEGF), and can respond to effectors (such as GM-CSF, IFN-γ, IL-3, IL-4, IL-7, IL-10, MCP-1, PDGF, TGF-β, TNF-α and VEGF). It is therefore not surprising that these cells, in association with cytokines produced by other stromal cells and by carcinoma cells themselves [64], can promote *in vitro* growth of tumor cells, favor ECM production and participate in angiogenesis. However, in this tightly meshed network, the key cytokines to control stroma development are not known. But it can be hypothesized that growth factors directly involved in ECM production and angiogenesis play a central role. PDGF and TGF-β are thus serious candidates for the control of ECM regulation, since NSCLC cell lines expressing these genes induce a significant tumor stroma when injected into nude mice [65].

A potent chemotactic and growth factor for mesenchymal cells and endothelial cells is PDGF. It is composed of two chains, A and B, the B chain being coded for by the c-*sis* proto-oncogene. PDGF interacts on target cells with a receptor composed of two subunits, α and β. Besides being involved, in a paracrine fashion, in different human fibrotic disorders (especially lung fibrosis) [66, 67], PDGF has been suggested to participate, in an autocrine and paracrine fashion, in both the production of ECM and the replication of endothelial cells and cancer cells in NSCLC [44]. In this process, TAM may play a central role. In 92% of lung cancers, TAM express PDGF A and B chain genes and produce PDGF proteins. These PDGF-producing TAM are found mainly in the peripheral part of the tumor, in close connection with the surrounding normal lung tissue. In this area 10%−25% of PDGF-positive TAM are observed. TAM also express both PDGF receptor α and β subunits. Furthermore, stromal mesenchymal cells, as well as endothelial cells, strongly express PDGF receptors. In addition, 30% of NSCLC express PDGF genes and proteins at carcinoma cell level, with frequent co-expression of receptors. We propose a sequence of events contributing to stroma formation [44]: (1) recruitment of TAM from blood monocytes by the release of chemotactic factors such as MCP-1 by tumor cells, and then (2) recruitment and local proliferation of mesenchymal and endothelial cells due to the release of PDGF by TAM and to a lesser extent by tumor cells. This concept is further supported by the fact that the higher levels of PDGF-producing TAM and of replicating endothelial and mesenchymal cells are observed in the same area.

TGF-β proteins belong to a superfamily of structurally related regulatory proteins. TGF-β1, the most abundant isoform, is a multifunctional cytokine, acting in both autocrine and paracrine ways, producing a wide range of frequently opposing effects on different cells and human tissues. TGF-β1, both a stimulator and inhibitor of cell replication, may control the production of many components of the ECM, and modulate cell differentiation, angiogenesis and cellular migration [68, 69]. In most cells, TGF-β1 is secreted as a latent complex (LTGF-β1). TGF-β1 is activated when cleaved from the LTGF-β1 complex by acidification or proteolysis [70], catalyzed by different proteolytic enzymes, such as plasmin and cathepsin D. The active form of TGF-β1 binds to TGF-β receptors (I, II and III) present on virtually all cells. In NSCLC, the major sources of TGF-β1 are tumor cells, ECM components and TAM. It has been demonstrated that the rapid release of TGF-β1 induced by treatment with plasmin was due to TGF-β1 release from ECM [71].

TGF-β1 stimulates the expression of a wide range of ECM proteins, including FN, laminin, elastin, thrombospondin and various collagens [72]. TGF-β1 modulates the expression of these proteins at transcriptional or post-transcriptional levels. ECM synthesis and deposition, in turn, regulate TGF-β1 expression, leading to a negative feedback mechanism [73]. It has been shown that the appearance of central fibrosis in lung adenocarcinoma is significantly related to positive staining for TGF-β1, which suggests that TGF-β1 plays some role in central fibrosis formation [74]. In addition to the induction of ECM proteins, TGF-β1 also increases the amount of ECM by inhibiting ECM degradation (inhibition of preteolysis), especially by inducing the release of protease inhibitors [75]. Furthermore, TGF-β1 stimulates the adhesiveness of both normal and malignant cells, in part by modulating the integrin-mediated adhesion.

Most knowledge of TGF-β and cell proliferation in lung cancer comes from investigations carried out in cell cultures. These have clearly demonstrated the growth inhibitory effect of TGF-β for cells of ectodermal origin, and conversely, its ability to stimulate the growth of most cells of mesodermal origin such as fibroblast cell lines. Little is known about the intracellular signaling cascade which mediates the growth inhibitory effect of TGF-β, but its growth stimulatory action is thought to be due to the induction of PDGF synthesis [76]. Thus PDGF, in addition to an ability to induce carcinoma cell proliferation, may counterbalance the inhibitory effect of TGF-β1 on carcinoma cells. This hypothesis correlates with the observation that in NSCLC, TGF-β1 and PDGF A and B chains are strongly expressed, both by tumor cells and TAM. In addition to the strong expression of PDGF by TAM (and to a lesser extent by tumor cells themselves), two immunohistochemical studies of tissue sections have shown that half of lung adenocarcinomas strongly express TGF-β1 [77, 78]. Similarly, a variety of TGF-β1 effects has been shown in NSCLC cell lines, including growth inhibition [79], increased *in vitro* invasion, and cell attachment [80].

TGF-β stimulates angiogenesis [81], although TGF-β1 exerts a pronounced anti-proliferative effect on endothelial cells *in vitro* by increasing production of thrombospondin, an ECM associated anti-angiogenic protein [82]. *In vivo* studies have revealed that the angiogenic effect of TGF-β is operative in tumorigenesis and metastasis. TGF-β1-transfected rodent cells inoculated into nude mice were found to induce a marked angiogenesis, which was completely abolished by TGF-β1 neutralizing antibodies [83].

TAM may be important for intratumoral fibrin formation and the fibrinolytic process. Extensive studies have provided evidence that intratumoral fibrin plays an important role in tumor growth, invasion and metastasis formation [84]. It may have a barrier function, interfere with antitumoral immunity, and favor angiogenesis. ECM macromolecules are embedded in fibrin deposits, in most if not all lung cancers, although the extent of fibrin deposition varies from one tumor to another. TAM, from NSCLC, show increased amounts of procoagulant activity [85], as do intra-alveolar macrophages collected from areas close to the tumor [86]. Fibrinogen extravased from leaky blood vessels is quickly clotted. The clotting cascade is activated, either by tumor cells themselves producing coagulation activators, and/or by TAM, triggered by carcinoma cells to express procoagulant activity. TAM can provide all the clotting factors (factors II, V, VII and X) necessary for in situ thrombin generation [87] and the stabilization of the fibrin network (factor XIII) [88]. TAM can also produce two main components of the fibrinolytic mechanism: the urokinase-plasminogen activator (u-PA) [89] and the plasminogen inhibitor type 2 [90]. They also express surface receptors for u-PA and plasminogen. Upon binding to its receptor, u-PA is converted into an active form that catalyses plasmin formation from plasminogen on the cell surface. Plasmin is a serine protease with a broad substrate specificity, able to degrade the majority of ECM components. Part of its activity is due to the induction of a proteolytic cascade that activates other proteases, such as metalloproteases (MMPs) and latent growth factors as FGFs, TGF-β and insulin-like growth factor-1.

4. Extracellular Matrix Remodelling

The stroma is a continuously expanding and remodelling structure, characterized by both active degradation and synthesis of ECM components. These tightly regulated processes are the consequence of complex relationships. Degradation of basement membranes containing type IV collagen and other ECM components is required as cancer cells locally invade, enter vessels, and exit vasculature into metastatic sites. Matrix degradation is controlled by proteases grouped into four main classes: serine-proteases (such as plasmin, elastase), cysteine-proteases (e.g. cathepsin B and L), aspartyl proteases (cathepsin D) and MMPs. MMPs are a family of zinc atom-dependent endopeptidases (14 have so far been described) with specific and selective activities against many classical components of the ECM including growth factor/cytokine domains [91, 92].

They are secreted as proenzymes, extracellularly activated and classified into three subgroups: gelatinases, stromelysins, and interstitial and neutrophil collagenases. The functions of MMPs in the ECM can be regulated at many stages from gene activation to proenzyme activation and inactivation by inhibitors. Gelatinase-A excepted production of MMPs is induced by IL-1β, TNF-α, PDGF, TGF-α, EGF and b-FGF. However, most of these reagents stimulate only one or two MMPs, and many are repressed by TGF-β [91]. Most MMPs may be activated by the plasmin cascade. All the MMPs are inhibited by a group of inhibitors known as tissue inhibitors of metalloproteases (TIMPs). MMPs, except stromelysin-3, are secreted in inactive forms, and bound to their natural inhibitors (TIMPs). Several TIMPs have been identified: TIMP-1, that preferentially forms complexes with interstitial collagenase, stromelysin-1 and gelatinase-B; TIMP-2, that presents a high affinity for progelatinase-A; and TIMP-3, with a preferential binding to ECM components. The activation of MMP-2 takes place after binding of the proenzyme, or its complex with TIMP-2, to the cytoplasmic membrane of tumor cells. Activation is due to a tumor cell membrane type-matrix metalloproteinase (MT-MMP). A strong correlation between the existence of the activated form of MMP-2 and the expression of MT-MMP is observed in lung carcinomas [93]. The imbalance of MMP/TIMP ratios and other local determinants in the tumor determines net MMP activity. In NSCLC [42], stromelysin-3 transcripts and protein are constantly expressed in stromal mesenchymal cells, but not in carcinoma cells. Gelatinase-A (MMP-2) and -B (MMP-9) mRNAs are present in both tumor and stromal cells, but proteins are mainly observed in tumor cells. One study has localized MMP-2 mRNAs exclusively to stromal cells [94]. Discrepancies between the cellular localization of transcripts and protein could be due either to the transfer of the enzyme from fibroblasts to the tumor cell surface, or to the methodological procedure used for immunohistochemistry. TIMP-1 and -2 mRNAs are mainly localized to the stroma. The observation of a strong expression of MMP-2, MMP-9 and stromelysin-3 in fibroblasts (rather than in tumor cells themselves), suggests that peritumoral fibroblasts are induced to produce MMPs by factors derived from tumor cells, such as the tumor cell-derived collagenase-stimulating factor that can increase the expression of MMP-1, -2, -3 in breast cancer [95]. Numerous studies correlate low TIMP expression with enhanced invasive and metastatic properties [96, 97]. Therefore, TIMP-1 and -2 may function as natural suppressors of cellular invasion. There is also evidence for the role of MMPs and TIMPs in angiogenesis [98, 99]. Early stages of endothelial tube formation are dependent on a critical balance of active gelatinase-A versus TIMP-2. It has also been shown that TIMP-2 can block b-FGF-stimulated endothelial cell growth [100].

In summary, it appears that peritumoral fibroblasts are the major source of MMPs. MMPs, in association with other proteinases produced by inflammatory cells (especially macrophages) and tumor cells themselves, (1) contribute to the control of ECM turnover, (2) allow the progression of carcinoma cells through the ECM, (3) favor angiogenesis and (4) finally the metastatic process. However, it is currently accepted that an adequate level of MMP-inhibitors in situ counterbalances these effects, at least temporarily.

5. Submucosal Modifications in Preneoplastic Lesions of the Bronchial Tree

The literature provides extensive studies concerning the premalignant lesions of the bronchi. Most focus on the events occurring in the epithelial compartment [101–103], but a few investigate submucosal modifications occurring beneath the precancerous lesions. In situ carcinoma (CIS) and severe dysplasia obviously show submucosal modifications, consisting of an increased number of vessels and strong infiltration by inflammatory cells, that may account for a stroma. However, in the earlier steps of the preneoplastic process, from basal cell hyperplasia to mild dysplasia, presence of stroma components is less obvious. There is no specific accumulation of inflammatory cells underneath the epithelial lesions, and when present, these cells are generally part of a nonspecific bronchitis observed in smokers.

One study of ECM modification in preneoplastic lesions [104] noticed a progressive decrease of basement membrane thickness from mild dysplasia (5.3 µm) to CIS (1 µm), an accumulation of type I and III collagens and in the more advanced lesions an increased number of capillary vessels stained for laminin. In a recent paper on the frequency of matrix protease mRNA expression in epithelial cells and submucosa cells [105], the authors concluded that (1) matrilysin and stromelysin-3 are expressed, in the epithelial compartment, very early in the carcinogenesis process and (2) stromelysin-1, -3, matrilysin, and collagenase-1 in stromal cells from the stage of dysplasia. This clearly demonstrates that myofibroblasts of the submucosa present a tumor-like phenotype, at least in the dysplasia stage.

Neovascularization was also recently investigated in preneoplastic lesions by evaluation of microvessel density [106]. For this purpose, microvessels were counted in selected areas of highest neovascularization underneath the basement membrane in the tunica propria. This microvessel count showed, in parallel with a more severe dysplasia, an increasing neovascularization close to the basement membrane: 33 vessels/0.6 mm^2 were found associated with squamous cell metaplasia, 50 vessels with squamous cell metaplasia with different degrees of dysplasia, and 61 vessels with CIS. These results are in agreement with our data: we investigated preneoplastic lesions for endothelial cell density and IdU labelling index of endothelial cells present underneath the basement membrane of preneoplastic lesions. These parameters were counted all along the epithelial lesion in a 1 mm thick band of submucosa, compared to the same surface in the surrounding normal looking mucosa. Samples with inflammatory cell infiltration were rejected, to eliminate angiogenesis due to a nonspecific inflammatory process. This study showed a progressive increase in the density of endothelial cells from the slight dysplasia stage, and an IdU labelling index of endothelial cells gradually increasing from the squamous metaplasia, to the more advance dysplastic lesions (7-fold increase of IdU labelling index associated with severe dysplasia versus normal mucosa). The angiogenic factors controlling the neovascularization process have yet to be investigated.

Thus, in the preneoplastic lesions that develop in the bronchial tree, the basis of stromal construction is already present, consisting of phenotypic modifications of fibroblasts, production of matrix proteases, and angiogenesis, followed in the more advanced stages by the recruitment of inflammatory cells.

Acknowledgement

This work was supported in part by grants from the Programme Hospitalier de Recherche Clinique 95 from Ministère des Affaires Sociales, de la Santé et de la Ville, France and from the Ligue Nationale contre le Cancer (Comités de Meurthe et Moselle, Moselle et Meuse).

References

1. Albelda SM (1993) Role of integrins and other cell adhesion molecules in tumor progression and metastasis. *Lab Invest* 68: 4–17.
2. Damjanovich L, Albelda SM, Mette SA, Buck CA (1992) The distribution of integrin cell adhesion receptors in normal and malignant lung tissue. *Am J Resp Cell Mol Biol* 6: 197–206.
3. Costantini RM, Falconi R, Battista P, Zupi G, Kennel SJ, Colasante A, Venturo I, Curcio CG, Sacchi A (1990) Integrin ($\alpha 6 \beta 4$) expression in human lung cancer as monitored by specific monoclonal antibodies. *Cancer Res* 50: 6107–6112.
4. Feldman IE, Shin KC, Natale RB, Todd RF (1991) $\beta 1$ integrin expression on human small cell lung cancer cells. *Cancer Res* 51: 1065–1070.
5. Galateau-Salle F, Peyrol S, Grimaud JA (1993) Stroma réaction des cancers bronchopulmonaires. *Ann Pathol* 13: 381–389.
6. Ohori NP, Yousem SA, Griffin J, Stanis K, Stetler-Stevenson WG, Colby TV, Sonmez-Alpan E (1992) Comparison of extracellular matrix antigens in subtypes of bronchioloalveolar carcinoma and conventional pulmonary adenocarcinoma. An immunohistochemical study. *Am J Surg Pathol* 16: 675–686.
7. Duprez A, Guerret S, Vignaud JM, Plénat F, Hartmann D, Grimaud JA (1987) Interstitial matrix of human carcinomas and sarcomas transplanted to the nude mouse: immunolocalization of some human and murine components. *Cell Mol Biol* 83: 647–654.
8. Parsons DF (1993) Tumor cell interactions with stromal elastin and type I collagen: the consequences of specific adhesion and proteolysis. *Tumor Biol* 14: 137–143.
9. Timar J, Lapis K, Fulop T, Varga ZS, Tixier JM, Robert L, Hornebeck W (1991) Interaction between elastin and tumor cell lines of different metastatic potential: in-vitro and in-vivo studies. *J Clin Res Clin Oncol* 117: 232–238.
10. Gopalakrishna R, Barsky SH (1988) Tumor promoter-induced membrane-bound protein kinase C regulates hematogenous metastasis. *Proc Natl Acad Sci USA* 85: 612–616.
11. Ruoslahti E, Yamaguchi Y (1991) Proteoglycans as modulators of growth factor activities. *Cell* 64: 867–869.
12. Ruoslahti E, Yamaguchi Y, Hildebrand A, Border WA (1992) *Extracellular matrix/growth factor interactions. Cold Spring Harbor Symposia on Quantitative Biology; Volume LVII,* Cold Spring Harbor Laboratory Press.

13. Yamaguchi Y, Mann DM, Ruoslahti E (1990) Negative regulation of transforming growth factor-β by the proteoglycan decorin. *Nature* 346: 281–284.
14. Iozzo RV (1995) Tumor stroma as a regulator of neoplastic behavior. *Lab Invest* 73:157–160.
15. Adany R, Iozzo RV (1991) Hypomethylation of the decorin proteoglycan gene in human colon cancer. *Biochem J* 276: 301–306.
16. Burgess WH, Maciag T (1989) The heparin-binding (fibroblast) growth factor family of proteins. *Annu Rev Biochem* 58: 575–606.
17. Roberts R, Gallagher J, Spooncer E, Allen TD, Bloomfield F, Dexter TM (1988) Heparan sulphate bound growth factor: a mechanism for stromal cell mediated haemopoiesis. *Nature* 332: 376–378.
18. Aviezer D, Hecht D, Safran M, Eisinger M, David G, Yayon A (1994) Perlecan, basal lamina proteoglycan, promotes basic fibroblast growth factor-receptor binding, mitogenesis, and angiogenesis. *Cell* 79: 1005–1013.
19. Krusius T, Gehlsen KR, Ruoslahti E (1987) A fibroblast chondroitin sulfate proteoglycan core protein contains lectin-like and growth factor-like sequences. *J Biol Chem* 262: 13120–13125.
20. Turley EA, Tretiak M (1985) Glycosaminoglycan production by murine melanoma variants in vivo and in vitro. *Cancer Res* 45: 5098–5105.
21. Underhill CB (1992) CD44: the hyaluronan receptor. *J Cell Sci* 103: 293–298.
22. Iozzo RV (1985) Neoplastic modulation of extracellular matrix colon carcinoma cells release polypeptides that alter proteoglycan metabolism in colon fibroblasts. *J Biol Chem* 260: 7464–7473.
23. Horai T, Nakamura N, Tateishi R, Hattori S (1981) Glycosaminoglycans in human lung cancer. *Cancer* 48: 2016–2021.
24. Li XQ, Thonar EJMA, Knudson W (1989) Accumulation of hyaluronate in human lung carcinoma as measured by a new hyaluronate ELISA. *Connective Tissue Res* 19: 243–253.
25. Knudson W, Knudson CB (1995): Overproduction of hyaluronan in the tumor stroma. *In:* Adany R (ed.): *Tumor matrix biology.* CRC Press, New York, pp 55–79.
26. Oyama F, Hirohashi S, Shimosato Y, Titani K, Sekiguchi K (1990) Oncodevelopmental regulation of the alternative splicing of fibronectin premessenger RNA in human lung tissues. *Cancer Res* 50: 1075–1078.
27. Barlati S, Colombi M, De Petro G (1995) Differential expression of fibronectin and its degradation products in malignant tumors. *In:* Adany R (ed.): *Tumor matrix biology.* CRC Press, New York, pp 81–100.
28. Magnuson VL, Young M, Schattenberg DG, Mancini MA, Chen D, Steffensen B, Klebe RJ (1991) The alternative splicing of fibronectin pre-mRNA is altered during aging and in response to growth factors. *J Biol Chem* 266: 14654–14662.
29. Balza E, Borsi L, Allemanni G, Zardi L (1988) Transforming growth factor-β regulates the levels of different fibronectin isoforms in normal human cultured fibroblasts. *FEBS Lett* 228: 42–44.
30. Emod I, Lafaye P, Planchenault T, Lambert-Vidmar S, Imhoff JM, Keil-Dlouha V (1990) Potential proteolytic activity of fibronectin: fibronectin laminase and its substrate specificity. *Biol Chem Hoppe Seyler* 371: 129–135.
31. Planchenault T, Lambert-Vidmar S, Imhoff JM, Blondeau X, Emod I, Lottspeich F, Keil-Dlouha V (1990) Potential proteolytic activity of human plasma fibronectin: fibronectin gelatinase. *Biol Chem Hoppe Seyler* 371: 117–128.
32. Natali PG, Nicotra MR, Bigotti A, Botti C, Castellani P, Risso AM, Zardi I (1991) Comparative analysis of the expression of the extracellular matrix protein tenascin in normal human fetal, adult and tumor tissues. *Int J Cancer* 47: 811–816.
33. End P, Panayotou G, Entwistle A, Waterfield MD, Chiquet M (1992) Tenascin: a modulator of cell growth. *Eur J Biochem* 209: 1041–1051.
34. Murphy-Ullrich JE, Lightner VA, Aukhil I, Yan YZ, Erickson HP, Höök M (1991) Focal adhesion integrity is downregulated by the alternatively spliced domain of human tenascin. *J Cell Biol* 115: 1127–1136.
35. Borsi L, Carnemolla B, Nicolo G, Spina B, Tanara G, Zardi L (1992) Expression of different tenascin isoforms in normal, hyperplastic and neoplastic human breast tissues. *Int J Cancer* 52: 688–692.

36. Oyama F, Hirohashi S, Shimosato Y, Titani K, Sekiguchi K (1991) Qualitative and quantitative changes of human tenascin expression in transformed lung fibroblast and lung tissues: comparison with fibronectin. *Cancer Res* 51: 4876–4881.
37. Sakakura T (1995) Role of tenascin in cancer development. *In:* Adany R (ed.): *Tumor matrix biology.* CRC Press, New York, pp. 101–129.
38. Azzarone B, Marell M, Billard C, Scemana P, Chaponnier C, Marciera-Coelho M (1984) Abnormal properties of skin fibroblasts from patients with breast cancer. *Int J Cancer* 33:759–764.
39. Wynford-Thomas D, Smith P, Williams ED (1986) Prolongation of fibroblast life-span associated with epithelial rat tumor development. *Cancer Res* 46: 3125–3127.
40. Bartal AH, Lichtig C, Cardo CC, Feit C, Robinson E, Hirshaut Y (1986) Monoclonal antibody defining fibroblasts appearing in fetal and neoplastic tissue. *J Natl Cancer Inst* 76: 415–419.
41. Basset P, Bellocq JP, Wolf C (1990) A novel metalloproteinase gene specifically expressed in stromal cells of breast carcinoma. *Nature* 348: 699–704.
42. Urbanski SJ, Edwards DR, Maitland A, Leco KJ, Watson A, Kossakowska AE (1992) Expression of metalloproteinases and their inhibitors in primary pulmonary carcinomas. *Br J Cancer* 66: 1188–1194.
43. Schor SL (1995) Fibroblast subpopulations as accelerators of tumor progression: the role of migration stimulating factor. *In:* Goldberg ID, Rosen EM, (eds.) *Epithelial mesenchymal interactions in cancer.* Birkhäuser Verlag, Basel, pp 273–296.
44. Vignaud JM, Marie B, Klein N, Plénat F, Pech M, Borrelly J, Martinet N, Duprez A, Martinet Y (1994) The role of platelet-derived growth factor production by tumor-associated macrophages in tumor stroma formation in lung cancer. *Cancer Res* 54: 5455–5463.
45. Norgaard P, Hougaard S, Poulsen HS, Spang-Thomsen M (1995) Transforming growth factor-β and cancer. *Cancer Treat Rev* 21: 367–403.
46. Ignotz RA, Massagué J (1986) Transforming growth factor-beta stimulates the expression of fibronectin and collagen and their incorporation in the extracellular matrix. *J Biol Chem* 261: 4337–4345.
47. Ignotz RA, Endo T, Massagué J (1987) Regulation of fibronectin and type I collagen mRNA levels by transforming growth factor-β. *J Biol Chem* 262: 6443–6446.
48. Rabinowich H, Cohen R, Bruderman L (1987) Functional analysis of mononuclear cells infiltrating into tumours: lysis of autologous human tumour cells by cultured infiltrating lymphocytes. *Cancer Res* 47: 173–177.
49. Yoong KF, Adams DH (1996) Tumour infiltrating lymphocytes: insights into tumour immunology and potential therapeutic implications. *J Clin Pathol Mol Pathol* 49: M256–267.
50. Doyle A, Martin WJ, Funa K, Gazdar A, Carney D, Martin SE, Linnoila I, Cuttitta F, Mulshine J, Bunn P, Minna J (1985) Markedly decreased expression of class I histocompatibility antigens, protein, and mRNA in human small-cell lung cancer. *J Exp Med* 161: 1135–1151.
51. Gingras MC, Roussel E, Roth JA (1995) Little expression of cytokine mRNA by fresh tumour-infiltrating mononuclear leucocytes from glioma and lung adenocarcinoma. *Cytokine* 7:580–588.
52. Kagi D, Vignaux F, Ledermann B (1994) Fas and perforin pathways as major mechanisms of T cell-mediated cytotoxicity. *Science* 265: 528–530.
53. Huang M, Wang J, Lee P, Sharma S, Mao JT, Meissner H, Uyemura K, Modlin R, Wollman J, Dubinett SM (1995) Human non-small cell lung cancer cells express a type 2 cytokine pattern. *Cancer Res* 55: 3847–3853.
54. Mantovani A (1994) Tumor-associated macrophages in neoplastic progression: a paradigm for the in vivo function of chemokines. *Lab Invest* 71: 5–16.
55. Martinet N, Beck G, Bernard V, Plénat F, Vaillant P, Schooneman F, Vignaud JM, Martinet Y (1992) Mechanism for the recruitment of macrophages to cancer site: in vivo concentration gradient of monocyte chemotactic activity. *Cancer* 70: 854–860.
56. Zachariae CO, Anderson AO, Thompson HL, Appella E, Mantovani A, Oppenheim JJ, Matsushima K (1990) Properties of monocyte chemotactic and activating factor (MCAF) purified from a human fibrosarcoma cell line. *J Exp Med* 171: 2177–2182.
57. Bottazzi B, Walter S, Govoni D, Colotta F, Mantovani A (1992) Monocyte chemotactic cytokine gene transfer modulates macrophage infiltration, growth, and susceptibility to IL-2 therapy of a murine melanoma. *J Immunol* 148: 1280–1285.

58. Dorsch M, Hock H, Kunzendorf U, Diamantstein T, Blankenstein T (1993) Macrophage colony-stimulating factor gene transfer into tumor cells induces macrophage infiltration but not tumor suppression. *Eur J Immunol* 23: 186–190.

59. Tazi A, Bouchonnet F, Grandsaigne M, Boumsell L, Lance AJ, Soler P (1993) Evidence that granulocyte macrophage-colony-stimulating factor regulates the distribution and differentiated state of dendritic cells/langerhans cells in human lung and lung cancers. *J Clin Invest* 91: 566–576.

60. Adams DO, Hamilton TA (1992) Macrophages as destructive cells in host defense. *In:* Galin JI, Goldstein IM, Snyderman R (eds): *Inflammation: basic principles and clinical correlates.* Raven Press, New York, *pp* 637–661.

61. Van Ravenswaay Claasen, HH, Kluin PM, Fleuren GT (1992) Tumor infiltrating cells in human cancer. On the possible role of CD16+ macrophages in antitumor cytotoxicity. *Lab Invest* 67: 166–174.

62. Smith DR, Kunkel SL, Burdick MD, Wilke CA, Orringer MB, Whyte RI, Strieter RM (1994) Production of interleukin-10 by human bronchogenic carcinoma. *Am J Pathol* 145: 18–25.

63. Fiorentino DF, Ziotnik A, Mosmann TR, Howard M, Ogarra A (1991) Il-10 inhibits cytokine production by activated macrophages. *J Immunol* 147: 3815–3822.

64. Betsholtz C, Berg J, Bywater M, Petterson M, Johnsson A, Heldin CH, Ohlsson R, Knott TJ, Scott J, Bell GI, Westermark B (1987) Expression of multiple growth factors in a human lung cancer cell line. *Int J Cancer* 39: 502–507.

65. Berg J (1988) The expression of the platelet-derived and transforming growth factor genes in human non-small lung cancer lines is related to tumor stroma formation in nude mice tumors. *Am J Pathol* 133: 434–439.

66. Martinet Y, Rom W, Grotendorst GR, Martin GR, Crystal RG (1987) Exaggerated spontaneous release of platelet-derived growth factor by alveolar macrophages of patients with idiopathic pulmonary fibrosis. *N Engl J Med* 317: 202–209.

67. Vignaud JM, Allam M, Martinet N, Pech M, Plénat F, Martinet Y (1991) Presence of platelet-derived growth factor in normal and fibrotic lung is specifically associated with interstitial macrophages while both interstitial macrophages and alveolar epithelial cells express the c-sis proto-oncogene. *Am J Resp Cell Mol Biol* 5: 531–538.

68. Mooradian DDL, McCarthy JB, Komandduri KV, Furcht LT (1992) Effects of transforming growth factor-beta 1 on human pulmonary adenocarcinoma cell adhesion, motility, and invasion in vitro. *J Natl Cancer Inst* 84:523–527.

69. Pertovaara L, Kaipainen A, Mustonen T, Orpana A, Ferrara N, Saksela O, Alitalo K (1994) Vascular endothelial growth factor is induced in response to transforming growth factor-beta in fibroblastic and epithelial cells. *J Biol Chem* 269: 6271–6274.

70. Lyons R, Keski-Oja J, Moses HL (1988) Proteolytic activation of latent transforming growth factor-β from fibroblast-conditioned medium. *J Cell Biol* 106: 1659–1665.

71. Taipale J, Miyazono K, Heldin CH, Keski-Oja J (1994) Latent transforming growth factor-β1 associates to fibroblast extracellular matrix via latent TGF-β binding protein. *J Cell Biol* 124: 171–181.

72. Roberts AB, McCune BK, Sporn MB (1992) TGF-β: regulation of extracellular matrix. *Kidney* Int 41: 557–559.

73. Streuli CH, Schmidhauser C, Kobrin M, Bissell MJ, Derynck R (1993) Extracellular matrix regulates expression of the TGF-β1 gene. *J Cell Biol* 120: 253–260.

74. Asakura S, Kato H, Fujino S, Konishi T, Asada Y, Tezuka N, Mori A (1995) Immunohistochemical study of transforming growth factor-beta and central fibrosis in T1 adenocarcinoma of the lung. *Nippon Kyobu Geka Gakkai Zasshi* 43: 1924–1928.

75. Roberts AB, Sporn MB (1990) Peptide growth factors and their receptors. Handbook of experimental pharmacology. 95th ed. Heidelberg/FRG: Springer Verlag. The transforming growth factor-βs: 419–472.

76. Moses HL, Yang EY, Pientenpol JA (1990) TGF-β stimulation and inhibition of cell proliferation: new mechanistic insights. *Cell* 63: 245–247.

77. Takanami I, Imamura T, Hashizume T, Kikuchi K, Yamamoto Y, Kodaira S (1994) Transforming growth factor-beta 1 as a prognostic factor in pulmonary adenocarcinoma. *J Clin Pathol* 47: 1098–1100.

78. Inoue T, Ishida T, Takenoyama M, Sugio K, Sugimachi K (1995) The relationship between the immunodetection of transforming growth factor-beta in lung adenocarcinoma and longer survival rates. *Surg Oncol* 4: 51–57.

79. Newman MJ (1993) Inhibition of carcinoma and melanoma cell growth by type 1 trans-forming growth factor-β is dependent on the presence of polyunsaturated fatty acids. *Proc Natl Acad Sci USA* 87: 5543–5547.
80. Mooradian DL, McCarthy JB, Komanduri KV, Furcht LT (1992) Effects of transforming growth factor-β1 on human pulmonary adenocarcinoma cell adhesion motility and inva-sion in vitro. *J Natl Cancer Inst* 84: 523–527.
81. Yang EY, Moses HL (1990) Transforming growth factor-β1-induced changes in cell migration, proliferation, and angiogenesis in the chicken chorioallantoic membrane. *J Cell Biol* 111: 731–741.
82. RayChaudhury A, Frazier WA, D'Amore PA (1994) Comparison of normal and tumori-genetic endothelial cells: differences in thrombospondin production and responses to transforming growth factor-beta. *J Cell Sci* 107: 39–46.
83. Ueki N, Nakazato M, Okhawa T, Ikeda T, Amuro Y, Hada T, Higashino K (1992) Excessive production of transforming growth-factor β1 can play an important role in the develop-ment of tumorigenesis by its action for angiogenesis: validity of neutralizing antibodies to block tumor growth. *Biochem Biophys Acta* 1137: 189–196.
84. Nagy JA, Brown IF, Senger DR, Lanir N, VanDeWater I, Dvorak AM, Dvorak HF (1988) Pathogenesis of tumour stroma generation: a critical role for leaky blood vessels and fibrin deposits. *Biochim Biophys Acta* 948: 305–326.
85. Ornstein DL, Zacharski LR, Memoli VA, Kisiel W, Kudryk BJ, Hunt J, Rousseau SM, Stump DC (1991) Coexisting macrophage-associated fibrin formation and tumor cell urokinase in squamous cell and adenocarcinoma of the lung tissues. *Cancer* 68: 1061–1067.
86. Semeraro N, DeLucia O, Lattanzio A, Montemurro P, Giordano D, Loizzi M, Carpagnano F (1986) Procoagulant activity of human alveolar macrophages: different expression in patients with lung cancer. *Int. J Cancer* 37: 525–529.
87. Adany R, Kappelmayer J, Berényi E, Szegedi A, Fabian E, Muszbek L (1989) Factors of the extrinsic pathway of blood coagulation in tumour associated macrophages. *Thromb Haemost* 62: 850–855.
88. Adany R, Nemes Z, Muszbek L (1987) Characterization of factor XIII containing-macro-phages in lymph nodes with Hodgkin's disease. *Br J Cancer* 55: 421–426.
89. Falcone DJ, McCaffrey TA, Haimovitz-Friedman A, Garcia M (1993) Transforming growth factor-β1 stimulates macrophage urokinase expression and release of matrix-bound basic fibroblast growth factor. *J Cell Physiol* 155: 595–605.
90. Wohlwend A, Belin D, Vassalli JD (1987) Plasminogen activator-specific inhibitors pro-duced by human monocytes/macrophages. *J Exp Med* 165: 320–339.
91. Birkedal-Hansen H, Moore WGI, Bodden MK (1993) Matrix metalloproteinases: a review. *Crit Rev Oral Biol Med* 4: 197–250.
92. Ray JM, Stetler-Stevenson WG (1994) The role of matrix metalloproteases and their inhibitors in tumour invasion, metastasis and angiogenesis. *Eur Respir J* 7: 2062–2072.
93. Shi YE, Liu Y (1995) Stroma-epithelial interaction in type IV collagenase expression and activation: the role in cancer metastasis. *In:* Goldberg ID, Rosen EM (eds): *Epithelial mesenchymal interactions in cancer.* Birkhäuser Verlag, Basel, *pp* 215–234.
94. Soini Y, Paakko P, Autio-Harmainen H (1993) Genes of lamnin B1 chain, alpha 1 (IV) chain of type IV collagen and 72 kDa type IV collagenase are mainly expressed by the stroma cells of lung carcinomas. *Am J Pathol* 142: 1622–1630.
95. Kataoka H, DeCastro R, Zucker S, Biswas C (1993) Tumor cell-derived collagenase-stimulatory factor increase expression of interstitial collagenase, stromelysin, and 72-kDa gelatinase. *Cancer Res* 53: 3154–3158.
96. DeClerck YA, Perez N, Shimada H, Boone TC, Langley KE, Taylor SM (1992) Inhibition of invasion and metastasis in cells transfected with an inhibitor of metalloproteinases. *Cancer Res* 52: 701–708.
97. Schultz RM, Silberman S, Persky B, Bajkowski AS, Carmichael DF (1988) Inhibition by human recombinant tissue inhibitor of metalloproteinases of human amnion invasion and lung colonization by murine B-16F10 melanoma cells. *Cancer Res* 48: 5539–5545.
98. Takigawa M, Nishida Y, Suzuki F, Kishi J, Yamashita K, Hayakawa T (1990) Induction of angiogenesis in chick yolk-sac membrane by polyamines and its inhibition by tissue in-hibitors of metalloproteinases (TIMP and TIMP2). *Biochem Biophys Res Commun* 171: 1264–1271.

 99. Schnapper HW, Grant DS, Stetler-Stevenson WG (1993) Type IV collagenase(s) and TIMPs modulate endothelial cell morphogenesis in vitro. *J Cell Physiol* 156: 235–246.
100. Murphy AN, Unsworth EJ, Stetler-Stevenson WG (1993) Tissue inhibitor of metalloproteinases-2 inhibits bFGF-induced human microvascular endothelial cell proliferation. *J Cell Physiol* 157: 351–358.
101. Klein N, Vignaud JM, Sadmi M, Plénat F, Borrelly J, Duprez A, Martinet Y, Martinet N (1993) Squamous metaplasia expression of proto-oncogenes and P53 in lung cancer patients. *Lab Invest* 68: 26–32.
102. Boers JE, Ten Velde GPM, Thunnissen FBJM (1996) P53 in squamous metaplasia: a marker for risk of respiratory tract carcinoma. *Am J Respir Crit Care Med* 153: 411–416.
103. Thiberville L, Payne P, Vielkinds J, LeRiche J, Horsman D, Nouvet G, Palcic B, Lam S (1995) Evidence of cumulative gene losses with progression of premalignant epithelial lesions to carcinoma of the bronchus. *Cancer Res* 55: 5133–5139.
104. Fisseler-Eckhoff A, Prebeg M, Voss B, Müller KM (1990) Extracellular matrix in preneoplastic lesions and early cancer of the lung. *Pathol Res Pract* 186: 95–101.
105. Bolon I, Brambilla E, Vandenbunder B, Robert C, Lantuejoul S, Brambilla C (1996) Changes in the expression of matrix proteases and of the transcription factor c-Ets-1 during progression of precancerous bronchial lesions. *Lab Invest* 75: 1–13.
106. Fisseler-Eckhoff A, Rothstein D, Müller KM (1996) Neovascularization in hyperplastic, metaplastic and potentially preneoplastic lesions of the bronchial mucosa. *Virchow Arch* 429: 95–100.

Clinical and Biological Basis of Lung Cancer Prevention
ed. by Y. Martinet, F. R. Hirsch, N. Martinet, J.-M. Vignaud
and J. L. Mulshine
© 1998 Birkhäuser Verlag Basel/Switzerland

CHAPTER 8
Tumor Angiogenesis: Basis for New Prognostic Factors and New Anticancer Therapies

Dorina Belotti and Vincent Castronovo*

Metastasis Research Laboratory, University of Liège, 4000 Sart Tilman via Liège, Belgium

1. Summary

There is now abundant experimental and clinical evidence that angiogenesis is an essential phenomenon for tumor growth and dissemination. Major progress has been achieved this last decade in both the understanding of the molecular bases for the change to an angiogenic phenotype, and the development of natural and synthetic angiogenesis inhibitors. Some of these have already reached clinical trials and are likely to improve cancer treatment profoundly in the very near future. Evaluation of the angiogenic phenotype of a patient's individual tumor by microvessel density count, or by serum angiogenic factor titration, appears to be of great independent prognostic value. In this chapter, we present an overview of some of the more interesting new developments in prognostic evaluation and cancer treatment following recent tumor angiogenesis research.

2. Introduction

Formation of new blood vessels is essential for embryogenesis, growth, reproduction and wound repair. During embryogenesis two processes, vasculogenesis and angiogenesis, generate blood vessels. During vasculogenesis, blood vessels derive directly from endothelial cell progenitors

---

* Author for correspondence.

while angiogenesis capillaries derive from pre-existing blood vessels [1]. In adult new blood vessels are formed only through angiogenesis. Under physiological conditions, angiogenesis is highly spatiotemporally regulated and is mainly activated during ovulation, menstruation, implantation and pregnancy. Angiogenesis is also activated during wound healing [2].

Persistent angiogenesis is involved in several diseases. Among them are some of the most frequent ocular diseases: diabetic retinopathy, retrolental fibroplasia, trachoma, glaucoma and corneal graft neovascularizations. Persistent vascularization is one of the most common causes of blindness worldwide [3]. Abnormal vascularization is also present in joint diseases such as rheumatoid arthritis, where newly proliferating capillaries penetrate the cartilage of a joint, eventually leading to its destruction [4]. Psoriasis, a skin disease, appears to depend on abnormal capillary proliferation in the dermis [5]. A malignant tumor is dependent upon angiogenesis for its growth and dissemination. Cancer cells continuously stimulate the formation of new capillaries which, in turn, support tumor growth and provide a gateway for tumor cells to enter the circulation and metastasize to distant sites [6, 7]. There is now a body of experimental and clinical evidence to support the hypothesis that angiogenesis is a key event in the complex process leading to tumor progression. It is considered that any cancer cell more than 200 μm distant from a blood vessel is a dead cell. Modulation of angiogenesis could therefore represent a potential therapeutic approach in the treatment of diseases implicating abnormal vascularization. In particular, angiogenesis is an interesting target for the development of new anticancer therapies. It has been postulated that inhibition of tumor angiogenesis will restrain the growth of the primary tumor as well as the metastasis. Angiogenesis inhibitors could potentially be inducers of tumor dormancy.

3. Switching to the Angiogenic Phenotype

Like other morphogenic events, angiogenesis is a complex process, during which endothelial cells are subjected to important changes which include proliferation, motility, production of matrix degrading enzymes and selective interactions with other cells and the extracellular matrix [2]. In response to an appropriate stimulus, quiescent endothelial cells (with turnover time exceeding 1000 days) are induced to proliferate with a turnover time of around five days [8]. This proliferation of endothelial cells is accompanied by degradation of the basement membrane surrounding the blood vessels, invasion of the underlying stroma, cell migration and reorganization into tube-like structures. The switching on or off of the angiogenic phenotype depends on the relative balance of angiogenic inducers and inhibitors [8]. Low concentrations of angiogenesis inducers or the presence of angiogenesis inhibitors keep the switch off, while either reduction of angioinhibin concentrations or increase of angiogenic factor

Table 1. Endogenous stimulating factors of angiogenesis

Stimulating factors	Reference
Acidic fibroblast growth factor	[2] [9]
Angiogenin	[10]
Basic fibroblast growth factor	[2] [9]
Hepatocyte growth factor	[11]
Interleukin-8	[12]
Platelet-derived endothelial cell growth factor	[13]
Transforming growth factor α	[14]
Transforming growth factor β	[15]
Tumor necrosis factor α	[16]
Vascular endothelial growth/factor/Vascular permeability factor	[17–19]

Table 2. Endogenous inhibitors of angiogenesis

Inhibitory factors	Reference
Angiostatin	[20]
Cartilage-derived inhibitor	[21]
Interferon α	[22]
Platelet factor 4	[23]
Prolactin 16k fragment	[24]
Placental proliferin-related protein	[25]
Thrombospondin-1	[26]
Tissue inhibitors of metalloproteinases (TIMP)	[27]

unbalance this dynamic equilibrium and turn on the angiogenic phenotype. Table 1 and Table 2 list the more important angiogenic factors and angio-inhibins respectively.

Some angiogenesis inducers, like basic fibroblast growth factor (bFGF) and vascular endothelial growth factor (VEGF) are polypeptide growth factors that have a direct mitogenic effect on endothelial cells, induce endothelial cell migration and capillary-like structure formation *in vitro*. Others like tumor growth factor-β (TGF-β) and tumor necrosis factor-α (TNF-α) inhibit endothelial cells growth *in vitro*, and their angiogenic effect is probably partly mediated by angiogenic factors released from chemoattracted inflammatory cells. VEGF and bFGF have been demonstrated to have a synergistic effect in the induction of angiogenesis *in vitro* [28].

4. Tumor Angiogenesis

Tumor growth and metastasis require the development of new blood vessels. Without angiogenesis, a tumor cannot expand to a volume larger than 2 to 3 mm^3. Tumor cells become necrotic and/or apoptotic and their rate of proliferation reaches equilibrium with their rate of dying. A tumor becomes vascularized and begins to grow rapidly when a clone of tumor cells "switches" to an angiogenic phenotype and the equilibrium between positive and negative regulators of tumor growth is disrupted [8]. The model of the endothelial cell and the tumor cell compartment in a tumor, described by Judah Folkman [2], is important for understanding how tumor and endothelial cells can stimulate each other to grow. Tumor cells can stimulate endothelial cell proliferation and migration by production of bFGF, VEGF, platelet-derived endothelial cell growth factor (PD-ECGF) and other angiogenic factors. Endothelial cells can stimulate, in a paracrine fashion, the growth of tumor cells by production of platelet-derived growth factor (PDGF), insulin-like growth factor 1 (IGF-1), bFGF, heparin binding-epithelial growth factor (HB-EGF), granulocyte-colony stimulating factor (G-CSF) and interleukin-6 (IL6). In addition, a vascularized tumor is perfused by nutrients and oxygen and the catabolites can be easily removed from it. All these together permit tumor and metastasis expansion.

5. Evaluation of the Angiogenic Phenotypes as a Means of Tumor Prognosis and Diagnosis

Quantification of angiogenesis in cancer specimens can help to predict the risk of metastasis or recurrence [29]. The number of vessels, visualized by immunostaining of endothelial cells, provides reproducible prognostic information. The prognostic significance of microvessel density was found to be a marker independent of traditional prognostic markers [30]. Many studies performed on different types of tumors show an association between increasing intratumor microvessel density and tumor aggressiveness, incidence of metastases and/or decreased patient survival. This association was found in breast [31–33], lung [34–36], prostate [37–39], squamous head and neck [40, 41], ovarian [42], rectal [43], testicular [44] and bladder carcinoma [45], malignant melanoma [46, 47], soft tissue [48], central nervous system tumors [49], and multiple myeloma [50]. In other studies, no relationship was found between intratumor microvessel density and prognosis in breast carcinoma [51, 52]. No relationship was found either between intratumor microvessel density and prognosis in patients with malignant melanoma and lymph nodal metastases [53], or in patients with squamous carcinoma of the tongue [54]. Discrepancies in these results probably derive from methodological differences. Another method which has been proposed to quantify angiogenesis in patients with solid cancers is to measure the level of bFGF in the urine or serum [55] or, for the patients with brain tumors, in the cerebrospinal fluid [50]. Measuring bFGF does give an indirect indication of angiogenic activity and can be used as a predictor of outcome once a cancer has been diagnosed [60]. The third model of multistage tumorigenesis is epidermal carcinogenesis. The development of squamous cell carcinoma begins as hyperplasia of kerationocytes, with a mild increase in vessel density which progresses to dysplasia, marked by morphologically aberrant kerationocytes with a high proliferation index and by abundant neovascularization; finally two classes of squamous carcinoma arise, both showing extensive angiogenesis [58]. A similar pattern of angiogenesis activation has been described for several premalignant lesions that precede several human cancers, including dysplastic melanocytic lesions (naevi) thought to precede malignant melanoma [61], mammary ductal carcinoma *in situ* (CIS) seen in association with invasive breast carcinomas, and moderate to high-grade cervical dysplasias implicated as progenitors of uterine cervical carcinomas [8]. These human cancers and their murine models suggest that premalignant activation of angiogenesis is a general parameter of tumor development and predict early activation of the angigenic switch as a distinct, potentially rate limiting step in the pathway of cancer. Following these observations, there are now experimental studies on the mechanism of activation of the angiogenic switch, and on new preclinical and clinical tests of compounds that interfere with angiogenesis.

6. Angiogenic Inhibitors and Cancer Therapy

In the last few years, the importance of endogenous or exogenous angiogenic inhibitors for cancer therapy has become evident. These compounds have been found to inhibit endothelial cell functions like secretion of proteases, chemotaxis and proliferation, inhibiting production of angiogenic factors by tumors, or antagonizing the action of angiogenic factors. Some of these angiogenesis inhibitors are already used in clinical trials or have been used to synthesize analogs with characteristics more useful for therapy (solubility, yield of synthesis, less degradability, less toxicity and so on). Anti-angiogenic therapy can be used to potentiate conventional chemotherapy and radiotherapy, and to maintain metastases and tumors in a "dormant" state.

One of the most promising angiogenic inhibitors seems to be angiostatin, a 38 kD fragment of plasminogen secreted by tumor cells and purified from urine of mice with primary tumors [20]. Anigostatin has been shown to inhibit neovascularization and growth of metastases and to increase tumor cell apoptosis. No resistance to this compound seems to develop even after prolonged treatment. Another endogenous inhibitor of angiogenesis with considerable therapeutic potential for cancer treatment is the 16 kD fragment of prolactin. Like angiostatin and plasminogen, the intact molecule does not appear to have any anti-angiogenic effect but the 16 kD fragment inhibits proliferation of endothelial cells [62], organization into capillary-like structures in type I collagen gels [24] *in vitro*, and capillary formation in the chick embryo chorioallantoic membrane assay [24]. Other endogenous inhibitors of angiogenesis are α-interferon [22], platelet factor 4 [23], thrombospondin-1, a p53-regulated glycoprotein [26], the 29 kD fragment of fibronectin [63], tissue inhibitor of metalloproteases (TIMP) [27], and cartilage extracts [21]. Cartilage was the first reported biological inhibitor of neovascularization. It was shown to inhibit blood vessel development in the chick chorioallantoic membrane and in the rabbit cornea, and proliferation and migration of endothelial cells. A liquid extract of shark cartilage has been developed by a Canadian company and given as a food supplement to cancer patients who have not responded to any conventional therapy. Because of several anecdotal reports of tumor stabilization or regression, this product is being developed as a anticancer drug.

Several synthetic inhibitors of angiogenesis have been also developed, characterized and used in clinical trials. Among these, Batimastat [64] (an inhibitor of metalloproteases), and TNP-470 (AGM-1470 (a derivative of fumagillin), an antibiotic produced by the fungus *Aspergillus fumigatuss serenius*, (reviewed in [65]) are the most promising.

7. Conclusions

The importance of angiogenesis for tumor growth and metastasis development is well recognized, but the mechanism by which tumor cells develop the ability to stimulate new capillary formation is not yet fully elucidated. Evaluation of the angiogenic potential of a malignant tumor is seen as one of the most potent predictors of disease progression. Furthermore, the use of angiogenesis inhibitors offers a new and promising concept for anticancer therapy. Rather than directly attacking the cancer cells, anti-angiogenesis therapy aims to stop the energy supplies that cancer cells need in order to expand. These new approaches could therefore turn the deadly disease cancer into a chronic one. Long-term treatment will therefore probably be necessary. Because most anti-angiogenic factors under evaluation do not have any major side effects, and no resistance to angiogenesis inhibitors has been reported to date, it is very likely that this new anticancer treatment will soon be available to cancer patients.

References

1. Risau W (1995) Differentiation of endothelium. *FASEB J* 9: 926–933.
2. Folkman J, Shing YJ (1992) Angiogenesis. *J Biol Chem* 267: 10931–10934.
3. Pat A (1980) Studies on retinal neovascularization. Friedenwald Lecture. *Invest Ophthalmol Vis Sci* 19: 1133–1138.
4. Colville-Nash PR (1992) Angiogenesis and rheumatoid arthritis: pathogenic and therapeutic implications. *Ann Rheum Dis* 51: 919–925.
5. Wolf JEJ (1989) Angiogenesis in normal and psoriatic skin. *Lab Invest* 61: 139–142.
6. Folkman J (1995) Clinical application of research in angiogenesis. *J Nature Med* 1: 27–31.
7. Dvorak HF, Nagy JA, Dvorak AM (1991) Structure of solid tumors and their vasculature: implications for therapy with monoclonal antibodies. *Cancer Cell* 3: 77–85.

8. Hanahan D, Folkman J (1996) Patterns and emerging mechanisms of the angiogenic switch during tumorigenesis. *Cell* 86: 353–364.

9. Friesel RE, Maciag T (1995) Molecular mechanisms of angiogenesis fibroblast growth factor signal. *FASEB J* 9: 919–925.

10. Fett JW, Strydom DJ, Lobb RR, Alderman EM, Bethune JL, Riordan JF, Riordan BL (1985) V. Isolation and characterization of angiogenin, an angiogenic protein from human carcinoma cells. *Biochemistry* 24: 5480–5486.

11. Grant DS, Kleinman HK, Goldberg ID, Bhargava MM, Nickloloff BJ, Kinsella JL, Polverini P, Rosen EM (1993) Scatter factor induces blood vessel formation in vivo. *Proc Natl Acad Sci USA* 90: 1937–1941.

12. Koch AE, Polverini PJ, Kunkel SL, Harlow LA, DiPietro LA, Elner VM, Elner SG, Strieter RM (1992) Interleukin-8 as a macrophage-derived mediator of angiogenesis. *Science* 258: 1798–1801.

13. Risau W, Drexler H, Mironov V, Smits A, Siegbahn A, Funa K, Heldin CH (1992) Platelet derived growth factor is angiogenic in vivo. *Growth Factors* 7: 261–266.

14. Yamamoto T, Terada N, Nishizawa Y, Petrow V (1994) Angiostatic activities of medroxyprogesterone acetate and its analogues. *Int J of Cancer* 56: 393–399.

15. Schott RJ, Morrow LA (1993) Growth factors and angiogenesis. *Cardiovascular Res* 27: 1155–1161.

16. Frater-Schroder M, Risau W, Hallmann R, Gautschi P, Bohlen P (1987) Tumor necrosis factor type alpha, a potent inhibitor of endothelial cell growth in vitro, is angiogenic in vivo. *Proc Natl Acad Sci USA* 84: 5277–5281.

17. Kolch W, Martiny-Baron G, Kieser A, Marmé (1995) Regulation of the expression of the VEGF/VPS and its receptors: role in tumor angiogenesis. *Breast Cancer Res and Treat* 36: 139–155.

18. Joukov V, Pajusola K, Kaipanen A, Chilov D, Lahtinen I, Kukk E, Saksela O, Kalkkinen N, Alitalo KA (1996) A novel vascular endothelial growth factor, VEGF-C, is a ligand for the Flt-4(VEGFR-3) and KDR (VEGFR-2) receptor tyrosine kinases. *EMBO J* 15: 290–298.

19. Olofsson B, Pajusola K, Kaipanen A, von Euler G, Joukov V, Saksela O, Orpana A, Pettersson RF, Alitalo K, Eriksson U (1996) Vascular endothelial growth factor B, a novel growth factor for endothelial cells. *Proc Natl Acad Sci USA* 93: 2576–2581.

20. O'Reilly MS, Holmgren L, Shing Y, Chen C, Rosenthal RA, Moses M, Lane WS, Cao Y, Sage EH, Folkman J (1994) Angiostatin: a novel angiogenesis inhibitor that mediates the suppression of metastases by a Lewis lung carcinoma. *Cell* 79: 315–328.

21. Brem H, Folkman J (1975) Inhibition of tumor angiogenesis mediated by cartilage. *J Exp Med* 141: 427–439.

22. Sydky YA, Borden EC (1987) Inhibition of angiogenesis by interferons: effects on tumor- and lymphocyte-induced vascular responses. *Cancer Res* 47: 5155–5161.

23. Gupta SK, Hassel T, Singh JPA (1995) A potent inhibitor of endothelial cell proliferation is generated by proteolytic cleavage of the chemokine platelet factor-4. *Proc Natl Acad Sci USA* 92: 7799–7803.

24. Clapp C, Martial JA, Guzman RC, Rentier-Delrue F, Weiner RI (1993) The 16-kilodalton N-terminal fragment of human prolactin is a potent inhibitor of angiogenesis. *Endocrinology* 133: 1292–1299.

25. Jackson D, Volpert OV, Bouck N, Linzer DIH (1994) Stimulation and inhibition of angiogenesis by placental proliferin and proliferin-related protein. *Science* 266: 1581–1584.

26. Dameron KM, Volpert OV, Tainsky MA, Bouck N (1994) Control of angiogenesis in fibroblasts by p53 regulation of thrombospondin-1. *Science* 265: 1582–1584.

27. Takigawa M, Nishida Y, Suzuki F, Kishi J, Yamashita K, Hayakawa T (1990) Induction of angiogenesis in chick yolk-sack membrane by polyamines and its inhibition by tissue inhibitors of metalloproteinases (TIMP and TIMP-2). *Biochem Biophys Res Commun* 171: 1264–1271.

28. Pepper MS, Ferrara N, Orci L, Montesano R (1992) Potent synergism between vascular endothelial growth factor and basic fibroblast growth factor in the induction of angiogenesis in vitro. *Biochem Biophys Res Commun* 165: 1198–1206.

29. Weidner N (1995) Intratumor microvessel density as a prognostic factor in cancer. *Am J Pathol* 147: 9–19.

30. Craft PS, Harris AL (1994) Clinical prognostic significance of tumour angiogenesis. *Annals of Oncol* 5: 305–311.
31. Weidner N, Folkman J, Pozza F, Bevilacqua P, Allred EN, Moore DH, Meli S, Gasparini G (1992) Tumor angiogenesis: a new significant and independent prognostic indicator in early-stage breast carcinoma. *J Natl Cancer Inst* 84: 1875–1887.
32. Bosari S, Lee AKC, DeLellis RA, Wiley BD, Heatley GJ, Silverman MC (1992) Microvessel quantitation and prognosis in invasive breast carcinoma. *Hum Pathol* 23: 755–761.
33. Gasparini G, Weidner N, Bevilacqua P, Maluta S, Dalla Palma P, Caffo O, Barbareschi M, Boracchi P, Marubini E, Pozza F (1994)Tumor microvessel density, p53 expression, tumor size, and peritumoral lymphatic vessel invasion are relevant prognostic markers in node-negative breast carcinoma. *J Clin Oncol* 12: 454–466.
34. Macchiarini P, Fontanini G, Hardin MJ, Squartini F, Angeletti CA (1992) Relation of neovasculature to metastasis of non-small-cell lung cancer. *Lancet* 340: 145–146.
35. Macchiarini P, Fontanini G, Dulmet E, de Montpreville V, Chapelier AR, Cerrin J, Le Roy Ladurie F, Dartevelle PG (1994) Angiogenesis: an indicator of metastasis in non-small-cell lung cancer invading the thoracic inlet. *Ann Thorac Surg* 57:1534–1539.
36. Yamazaki K, Abe S, Takekawa H, Sukoh N, Watanabe N, Ogura S, Nakajima I, Isobe H, Inoue K, Kawakami Y (1994) Tumor angiogenesis in human lung adenocarcinoma. *Cancer* 74: 2245–2250.
37. Wakui S, Furusato M, Itoh T, Sasaki H, Akiyama A, Kinoshita I, Asano K, Tokuda T, Aizawa S, Ushigome S (1992) Tumor angiogenesis in prostatic carcinoma with and without bone marrow metastasis: a morphometric study. *J Pathol* 68: 257–262.
38. Weidner N, Carroll PR, Flax J, Blumenfeld W, Folkman J (1993) Tumor angiogenesis correlates with metastasis in invasive prostate carcinoma. *Am J Pathol* 43: 401–409.
39. Fregene TA, Khanuja PS, Noto AC, Gehani SK, Van Egmont EM, Luz DA, Pienta KJ (1993) Tumor-associated angiogenesis in prostate cancer. *Anticancer Res* 1993: 2377–2381.
40. Gasparini G, Weidner N, Bevilacqua P, Maluta S, Boracchi P, Testolin A, Pozza F, Folkman J (1993) Intratumoral microvessel density and p53 protein: correlation with metastasis in head- and -neck squamous-cell carcinoma. *Int J Cancer* 55: 739–744.
41. Albo D, Granick MS, Jhala N, Atkinson B, Solomon MP (1994) The relationship of angiogenesis to biological activity in human squamous cell carcinomas of the head and neck. *Ann Plast Surg* 32: 588–594.
42. Hollingsworth HC, Kohn EC, Steinberg SM, Rothenberg ML, Merino MJ (1995) Tumor angiogenesis in advanced stage ovarian carcinoma. *Am J Pathol* 147: 33–41.
43. Saclarides TJ, Speziale NJ, Drab E, Szeluga DJ, Rubin DB (1994) Tumor angiogenesis and rectal carcinoma. *Dis Colon Rectum* 37: 921–926.
44. Olivarez D, Ulbright T, De Riese W, Foster R, Reister T, Einhorn L, Sledge GA (1994) A testicular germ cell tumor: prediction of metastatic disease. *Cancer Res* 54: 2800–2802.
45. Jaeger TM, Weidner N, Chew K, Moore DH, Kerschmann RL, Waldman FM, Carroll PR (1994) Tumor angiogenesis and lymph node metastases in invasive bladder carcinoma. *J Urol* 151: 348 (abstr).
46. Barnhill RL, Fandrey K, Levy MA, Mihm MC, Hyman B (1992) Angiogenesis and tumor progression of melanoma: quatitation of vascularity in melanocytic nevi and cutaneous melanoma. *Lab Invest* 67: 331–337.
47. Graham CH, Rivers J, Kerbel RS, Stankiewicz KS, White WL (1994) Extent of vascularization as a prognostic indicator in thin (0.76 mm) malignant melanoms. *Am J Pathol* 145: 510–514.
48. Ewaskov SP, Collins CA, Conrad EU, Gown AM, Schmidt RA (1993) Quantitative assessment of blood vessel density and size in soft-tissue tumors. *Mod Pathol* 6: 6A.
49. Li VW, Folkerth RD, Watanabe H, Yu C, Rupnick M, Barnes P, Scott RM, Black PM, Sallan SE, Folkman J (1994) Microvessel count and cerebrospinal fluid basic fibroblast growth factor in children with brain tumors. *Lancet* 334: 82–86.
50. Vacca A, Ribatti D, Roncali L, Ranieri G, Serio G, Silvestris F, Dammacco F (1994) Bone marrow angiogenesis and progression in multiple myeloma. *Br J Haematol* 87: 503–508.
51. Van Hoef MEHM, Knox WF, Dhesi SS, Howell A, Schor AM (1993) Assessment of tumor vascularity as a prognostic factor in lymph node negative invasive breast cancer. *Eur J Cancer* 29A: 1141–1145.

52. Hall NR, Fish DE, Hunt N, Goldin RD, Guillou PJ, Monson JRY (1992) Is the relationship between angiogenesis and metastasis in breast cancer real? *Surg Oncol* 1: 223–229.
53. Carnochan P, Briggs JC, Westbury G, Davies AJ (1991) The vascularity of cutaneous melanoma: a quantitative histologic study of lesions 0.85–1.25 mm in thickness. *Br J Cancer* 64: 102–107.
54. Leedy DA, Trune DR, Kronz JD, Weidner N, Cohen JI (1994) Tumor angiogenesis, the p53 antigen, and cervical metastasis in squamous carcinoma. *Ontolarygol Head and Neck Surg* 111: 417–422.
55. Nguyen M, Hiroyouki W, Budson AE, Richie JP, Folkman J (1994) Elevated levels of an angiogenic peptide, basic fibroblast growth factor, in the urine of patients with wide spectrum of cancers. *J Natl Cancer Inst* 86: 356–361.
56. Hanahan D (1985) Heritable formation of pancreatic β-cell tumors in transgenic mice expressing recombinant insulin/simian virus 40 oncogenes. *Nature* 315: 115–121.
57. Lacey M, Alpert S, Hanahan D (1986) The bovine papillomavirus genome elicits skin tumours in transgenic mice. *Nature* 322: 609–612.
58. Arbeit C, Munger K, Howley P, Hanahan D (1994) Progressive squamous epithelial neoplasia in K14-HPV16 transgenic mice. *J Virol* 68: 4358–4368.
59. Folkman J, Watson K, Ingber D, Hanahan D (1989) Induction of angiogenesis during the transition from hyperplasia to neoplasia. *Nature* 339: 58–61.
60. Kandel J, Bossy-Wetzel E, Radvany F, Klagsbrun M, Folkman J, Hanahan D (1991) Neovascularization is associated with a switch to the export of bFGF in the multistep development of fibrosarcoma. *Cell* 66: 1095–1104.
61. Rak JW, St Croix BD, SC, Kerbel RS (1995b) Consequences of angiogenesis for tumor progression, metastasis and cancer therapy. *Anticancer Drugs* 6: 3–18.
62. Ferrara N, Clapp C, Weiner R (1991) The 16 K fragment of prolactin specifically inhibits basal or fibroblast growth factor stimulated growth of capillary endothelial cells. *Endocrinology* 129: 896–900, 129.
63. Homandberg GA, Williams JE, Grant D, Schumacher B, Eisenstein R (1985) Heparin-binding fragments of fibronectin are potent inhibitors of endothelial cell growth. *Am J Pathol* 120: 327–332.
64. Beattie GJ, Young HA, Smyth JF (1994) Phase I study of intra-peritoneal metalloproteinase inhibitor BB94 in patients with malignant ascites. *Ann Oncol* 5: suppl 5: 72.
65. Castronovo V, Belotti D (1996) TNP-470 (AGM-1470) mechanism of action and early clinical development. *Europ J Cancer* 32A(14): 2520–2527.

Clinical and Biological Basis of Lung Cancer Prevention
ed. by Y. Martinet, F.R. Hirsch, N. Martinet, J.-M. Vignaud
and J.L. Mulshine

CHAPTER 9
Cell Cycle Regulators and Mechanisms of Growth Control Evasion in Lung Cancer

Irene E. Schauer and Robert A. Sclafani*

Department of Biochemistry, Biophysics, and Genetics, University of Colorado Health Sciences Center, Denver, Colorado, USA

1. Introduction

The last several years have seen an explosion in our understanding of the components and mechanisms involved in regulation of the eukaryotic cell cycle. The explosion began with the discovery of cyclins and the identification of *Xenopus* maturation promoting factor as a complex of cyclin B and a cdc2-related protein kinase [1]. Since then cyclins and the cyclin-dependent kinases (CDKs) have been identified as the key mediators of cell cycle progression, and the cast of known players has expanded to include cyclins A, B1, B2, C, D1–3, E, F, G, H, and I and CDKs 1–7, as well as inhibitors and mediators of CDK activity [2–5].

The most complicated array of proteins now appears to be involved in the regulation of progression through the G1 phase of the cell cycle [5], the stage at which virtually all mammalian growth regulation occurs. Cells in G1 face decisions regarding their environment (presence or absence of growth factors), their readiness to divide (e.g. DNA damage checkpoints), their age (senescence involves arrest in G0) and their developmental destinies (whether to divide, differentiate, or undergo apoptosis). The evi-

---

* Author for correspondence.

dence increasingly suggests that the cyclin-CDK pathway is involved in all of these decisions. Since one aspect of oncogenesis is the loss of normal growth controls, it is not surprising that the evidence also increasingly indicates that one of the molecular events required for tumor development is a perturbation of the cell cycle machinery involved in G1 regulation.

2. Cell Cycle Regulators

2.1. CDKs

The actual promoters of cell cycle progression are the cyclin-dependent kinases (CDKs, reviewed in [6]). These highly regulated serine/threonine-directed protein kinases are best understood in yeast, where a single CDK is responsible for both the G1/S and G2/M transitions. In mammalian cells at least seven different CDKs have been identified. At least four of these clearly have roles in cell cycle progression with different CDKs acting at different stages and on different substrates (Fig. 1).

2.2. Cyclins

The activity of the CDKs is regulated by several different post-translational mechanisms including phosphorylation, which will not be addressed further here, and subunit interactions [6]. The kinase subunit is typically present at a constant level throughout the cell cycle but is inactive as a monomer. The activating subunit, a cyclin, is an unstable protein that is synthesized only at a specific time in the cell cycle and then rapidly degraded. Different cyclins are synthesized at different stages, interact with specific CDKs, and may have distinct effects on a given CDK. Thus, CDK kinase activity is regulated throughout the cell cycle. The number of known cyclins now stands at twelve and continues to grow. In general, not all possible cyclin/CDK complexes form. Instead, specific CDKs interact only with certain cyclins, although the subsets do overlap. For instance, cyclin B interacts only with CDK1, but CDK1 can also interact with cyclin A, which can also interact with CDK2, and so on. Thus, the cyclin/CDK complexes form an interlocking network around the cell cycle with any specific point in the cycle being represented by a characteristic CDK/cyclin profile, and an orderly, regulated progression through the numerous events of the cell cycle is assured (Fig. 1).

The mid-G1 phase of the cell cycle, during which the decisions described earlier are made, is characterized by high levels of the D-type cyclins. The three different D-type cyclins, D1, D2 and D3, are closely related and appear to differ primarily in tissue specificity, although some evidence for functional differences also exists [7]. Cyclin D2 expression is limited to

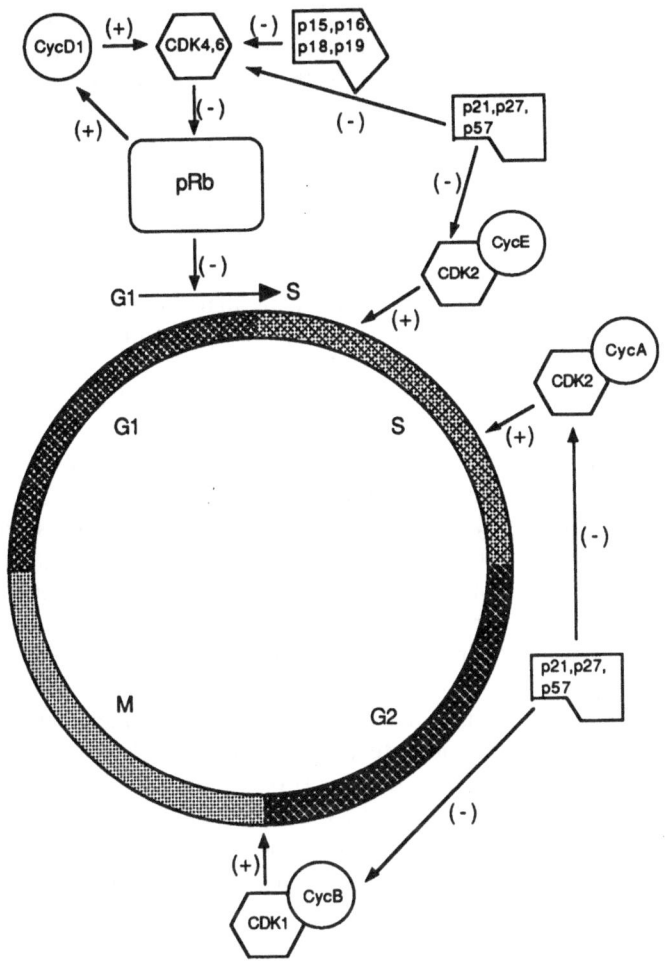

Figure 1. Cell cycle regulation by cyclins, CDKs, CKIs, and retinoblastoma protein. CDKs are regulated by a combination of cyclin activation (+) and CKI inhibition (–) through the cell cycle. Although several other CDKs and cyclins are involved in cell cycle progression, only those whose roles are best understood are illustrated here. Retinoblastoma protein, an inhibitor of the G1 to S phase transition that is inactivated by phosphorylation, is one of the important cyclin/CDK substrates. (+) = activation. (–) = inhibition.

hematopoietic lineages, while D3 appears to be ubiquitously expressed at very low levels. Cyclin D1, the best characterized of the three, is expressed at high levels in many cell types, including the frequently cultured fibroblasts, macrophages, and epithelial cells.

The D-type cyclins activate primarily CDK4 and CDK6 and are unusual in that their levels do not oscillate with the cell cycle as dramatically as those of other cyclins. That their role is in G1 is, however, clear. Injection of anti-cyclin D1 monoclonal antibodies into cells results in G1 arrest if the cells are injected during G1 [8–10]. Injection at other times does not interfere with cell cycle progression. Furthermore, cyclin D1 levels are also responsive to certain extracellular factors that affect G1 progression such as growth factors [11], cell-cell contacts, and anchorage to a solid medium [12]. This is consistent with a cell cycle regulatory role in G1 that monitors not only intrinsic readiness to divide, but also external influences.

Since mammalian cell growth is highly externally regulated, and the D-type cyclins appear to integrate extracellular signals into internal cell cycle regulation, it is perhaps not surprising that cyclin D1 has also recently been shown to act as an oncogene [13–15]. Cyclin D1 was originally identified as the product of the *bcl1* gene [16, 17]. In certain B cell lymphomas a translocation between chromosomes 11 and 14 places the *bcl1* gene under the control of the immunoglobulin heavy chain promoter, leading to dramatic and unregulated overexpression of cyclin D1. At the same time cyclin D1 was also identified as the product of the *PRAD1* gene [18, 19]. In this case cyclin D1 is unregulated and overexpressed in parathyroid adenomas due to a chromosomal inversion that places the *PRAD1* gene under the control of the parathyroid hormone promoter. Overexpression of cyclin D1 in cultured cells has been shown to shorten G1 and decrease growth dependence on mitogens, but it does not lead to a fully transformed phenotype [20–23]. However, further experiments have shown that the cyclin D1 gene can cooperate with other oncogenes including c-*myc*, activated Ha-*ras* and defective adenovirus E1A protein to give full transformation [24–26]. Thus, cyclin D1 overexpression is not sufficient for transformation, but can complement other partially transforming events and could constitute one step in a multistep oncogenic pathway.

Finally, herpes saimiri virus has recently been shown to encode a novel cyclin, v-cyclin, which is most closely related to the D-type cyclins and is a very strong activator of CDK6 [27]. Since this virus can cause malignant lymphomas, leukemias, and lymphosarcomas in new world primates, v-cyclin may also play a role in viral oncogenesis.

2.3. CDK inhibitors

The most recently discovered cell cycle regulators are the cyclin-dependent kinase inhibitors or CKIs [28, 29]. Like the cyclins, these proteins function as regulatory subunits of the CDKs. However, while the cyclins activate CDKs, the CKIs act to inhibit CDK kinase activity. Since unregulated kinase activity due to cyclin overexpression can be oncogenic, unregulated kinase activity due to CKI loss might also be expected to be oncogenic. Thus the genes for the CKIs would appear to be potential tumor suppressor genes. The known CKIs fall into two major groups, the p21 family and the p16 family.

2.3.1. The p21 family: Members of the p21 family including p21 (CIP1, WAF1), p27 (KIP1), and p57 (KIP2) act by forming higher order complexes with the CDK/cyclin complexes and are nonspecific, interacting with all CDK/cyclin complexes tested [28, 29]. Expression of the *p21* gene is regulated by p53, the product of a known tumor suppressor gene [30]. DNA damage induces *p53* gene expression and leads to G1 cell cycle arrest, during which cells assess the damage and either repair it or undergo apoptosis. It is likely that the p53-mediated cell cycle arrest is the result of p21 induction. However, while p53 is clearly a tumor suppressor that is lost in a large percentage of tumors, there is no direct evidence identifying *p21* as a tumor suppressor gene [31, 32]. It is likely, therefore, that p53's role as a tumor suppressor goes beyond its induction of p21. Thus far a role for loss of p21 protein or any of the p21 family members in oncogenesis remains to be established.

2.3.2. The p16 family: In contrast the gene for at least one member of the p16 family, *p16* itself, clearly does function as a tumor suppressor gene in several kinds of cancer [15, 28]. The p16 family of inhibitors consists of a number of related low molecular weight proteins including p15 (MTS2), p16 (MTS1), p18 and p19. These CKIs act as cyclin competitors, forming dimers with the CDKs and displacing or blocking the cyclin activator. They are more specific than the p21 family CKIs, interacting only with CDK4 and CDK6, the D-type cyclin specific kinases.

p16 was originally identified as the product of the melanoma tumor suppressor 1 (*MTS1*) gene, a gene that was localized by mapping the overlap of the regions of loss of heterozygosity on chromosome 9p21 among a large collection of melanomas [33]. Loss of heterozygosity at 9p21, implicating a tumor suppressor gene in the area, occurs in many cancers including non-small cell lung cancer (NSCLC). It is now clear that *MTS1* does function as a tumor suppressor gene for melanoma and certain other cancers, including T cell leukemias and gliomas [28]. However, although loss of heterozygosity analysis has clearly demonstrated a 9p21 tumor suppressor gene in many other cancer types, the lack of mutations in the remaining copy of *MTS1* has led to considerable controversy regarding the identification of *MTS1* as the relevant tumor suppressor gene. Most recently experiments have demonstrated that in many cancers, including NSCLC, the remaining *MTS1* gene, though unmutated, is hypermethylated and consequently not expressed [34]. Thus *MTS1* may function as a tumor suppressor gene that is inactivated by a completely novel mechanism in a variety of different cancers.

The p15 CKI is encoded by the *MTS2* gene which lies within about 20 kilobases of *MTS1*. An exon for an alternately spliced form of p16 is also located almost within the *MTS2* gene [35, 36]. This proximity to *MTS1* has made it very difficult to assess the role of *MTS2* in tumor suppression. Finally, very little is known regarding p18 and p19 cell cycle functions, and no direct evidence exists implicating their genes in tumor suppression.

2.4. Retinoblastoma protein

At the heart of G1 regulation is the retinoblastoma protein (pRb). Originally identified as the tumor suppressor gene involved in the retinal cancer retinoblastoma, the *Rb* gene is now known to function as a tumor suppressor gene for many cancers including small cell lung cancer (SCLC) [37]. In these cancers the *Rb* gene is usually deleted and/or mutated such that the tumor cells contain no detectable pRb. In addition a number of oncogenic viruses encode proteins such as SV40 T antigen, papilloma virus E7 protein, and adenovirus E1A protein that can bind to and inactivate pRb.

The product of the *Rb* gene, pRb, is a key regulator of G1 progression in many, if not all, cell types [37, 38]. Active pRb binds to and inhibits transcription factors required for transcription of genes essential for DNA replication and, therefore, for entry into S phase. Thus, active pRb acts as brake in the G1 phase of the cell cycle. pRb is active in an underphosphorylated form which can be inactivated by hyperphosphorylation, a reaction catalysed by cyclinD/CDK4,6 complexes. As was described earlier, injection of anti-cyclin D1 monoclonal antibodies into G1 phase cells can arrest cells in G1. This arrest can only be achieved in Rb$^+$ cells. In contrast injection of antibody into cells that are deficient for pRb has no effect on cell cycle progression [39]. These experiments suggest that cyclin D1/CDK complexes are essential for pRb inactivation *in vivo* and cannot be substituted by other normal cyclin/CDK complexes. They further suggest that this inactivation of pRb is the only essential cell cycle function of cyclin D1/CDK complexes.

3. Cell Cycle Regulators in Lung Cancer

When we began our studies on cell cycle regulators in lung cancer cell lines, one part of the story was already known. It was clear from a number of earlier studies that most SCLC tumors and cell lines lacked pRb [40–42]. However, the status of cell cycle regulators in NSCLC and the connection between pRb and other cell cycle regulators were not yet understood. Since then a much clearer picture of cell cycle regulation in lung cancer has emerged.

Our studies of levels of cell cycle proteins in SCLC, NSCLC, and primary culture normal human bronchioepithelial (NHBE) cells have revealed some significant differences between these cell types [43, 44]. A summary of the major differences is shown in Table 1. Of the cell lines tested all of the SCLC lines (11/11) produce no detectable pRb while all of the NSCLC lines contain normal levels of apparently wildtype pRb distributed between the hypo- and hyperphosphorylated forms. The p16 protein shows the exact opposite pattern, with all of the SCLC lines containing normal levels while all 17 of the NSCLC lines are completely

Table 1. Differences in cell cycle regulatory protein levels between SCLC and NSCLC

	pRb[a]	Cyclin D1	p16[a]	CDK4	CDK6
SCLC	–	low	+	high	low
NSCLC	+	high	–	low	high

[a] +, presence; –, absence.

deficient. Cyclin D1 also show tumor type specific differences in that all but one of the SCLC lines have little or no detectable cyclin D1, while the NSCLC lines contain variably elevated levels relative to normal bronchio-epithelial cells.

Further experiments with the NSCLC lines indicate that the elevation of cyclin D1 levels occurs at the transcriptional level (Schauer and Sclafani, unpublished results). We do not observe the cyclin D1 gene amplification or protein stabilization found in breast cancer cell lines (e.g. [45] and Daly, Langan, Schauer and Sclafani, unpublished results). Since the cyclin D1 level in the NHBE cells is intermediate to those seen in the two types of tumor cell lines, we conclude that the tumor cell line levels reflect both underexpression in SCLC lines and variable overexpression in NSCLC lines. Since active pRb is a positive regulator of cyclin D1 expression [46], at least some of the underexpression in SCLC lines is easily explained. Loss of pRb protein results in loss of some positive regulation of cyclin D1 expression and levels of the unstable cyclin D1 drop. We are currently investigating the mechanism of overexpression in NSCLC lines.

The NSCLC lines are also deficient for the CKI, p16. Analysis of gene copy number and mRNA levels indicate that this deficiency is the result of multiple mechanisms (Schauer and Sclafani, unpublished results). Nearly half the lines are deficient due to homozygous deletion of the MTS1 gene. A few of the remaining lines make apparently normal mRNA but fail to accumulate protein, suggesting that they contain p16 mutations. The rest of the lines contain no detectable p16 mRNA. Our preliminary experiments suggest that some of the NSCLC lines that fail to express p16 may also have inactivated their *MTS1* genes by hypermethylation. These results are consistent with results from other laboratories reporting multiple mechanisms of p16 loss, including hypermethylation, in NSCLC cell lines [47].

One problem with using cell lines to investigate oncogenesis is that cell lines consist of a selected population of cells that may not represent the tumor as a whole, or that changes may have occurred during the culturing of the cells. The lack of pRb seen in SCLC cell lines has also been observed by others by the immunohistochemical staining of tumor samples and is clearly not such an artefact of cell culture [40, 42, 48]. Analysis of cyclin D1 levels in breast and esophageal tumors by immunohistochemistry has indicated that overexpression of cyclin D1 also occurs in primary tumors [10, 49–52]. We are currently extending our studies to include immunohistochemical and RT-PCR determinations of pRb, cyclin D1, and p16 levels in primary lung tumor samples.

Taken together with the current understanding of G1 cell cycle regulation, our results are consistent with a model in which the two types of lung cancer typically bypass the pRb mediated G1 arrest by alternate mechanisms (Fig. 2). In normal cells (top panel) pRb brakes the cell cycle in G1.

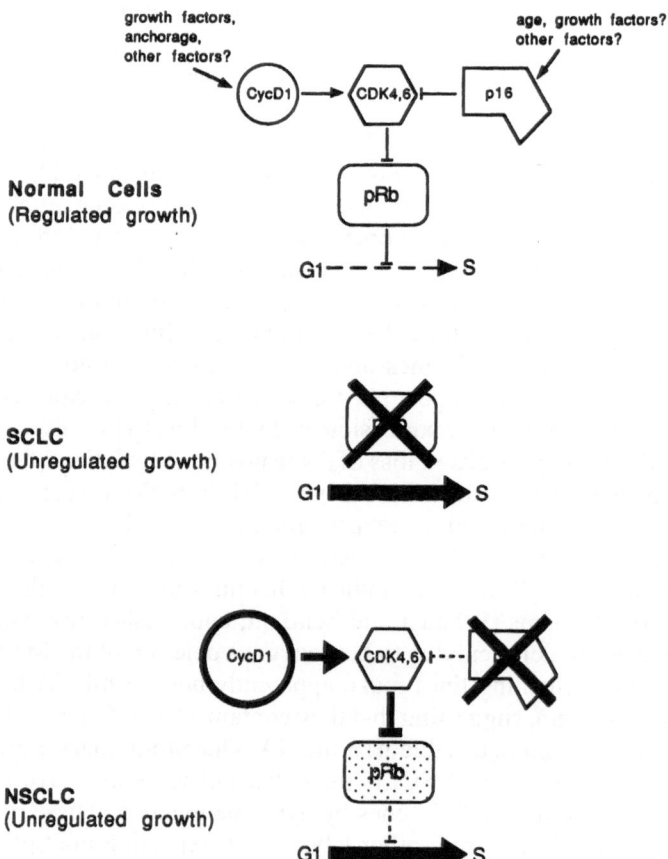

Figure 2. Model for the loss of cell cycle regulation in lung cancer. In normal cells growth is regulated at least in part by a pRb-mediated inhibition of the G1 to S transition (top panel). When conditions are appropriate, the balance of cyclin D1 and p16 shifts to allow CDK4,6 activation, pRb inactivation, and entry into a new round of cell division. Lung tumors cells typically are defective for this key regulatory event by one of two mechanisms. In most SCLC (middle panel) pRb is missing or mutant, leading to unregulated G1/S progression. This mechanism also occurs in retinoblastoma, osteosarcoma, extrapulmonary SC carcinomas, some esophageal cancers, glioblastoma, virally-mediated cancers, etc. In NSCLC (bottom panel) elevated cyclin D1 and/or a lack of the p16 CKI lead to inappropriate inactivation of pRb and the same loss of G1/S regulation. Other cancers that depend on this mechanism include melanoma, B-cell lymphoma, T-cell leukemias and lymphomas, glioblastoma, and some breast, colon, and esophageal carcinomas.

The balance of p16 and cyclin D1 levels maintains the G1 arrest until the appropriate conditions signal that cell division should occur. Increased cyclin D1 and, perhaps, decreased p16 levels then allow activated CDK4/CDK6 to inactivate pRb. This allows one round of cell division before the pRb brake is reset. In SCLC (as well as many other pRb⁻ and virally induced cancers) pRb is absent, effectively removing at least that brake on cell division (middle panel). In this case levels of cyclins, CDKs, and CKIs are irrelevant, and external control of the cell division is lost. In NSCLC (and other cancers such as melanoma) pRb is still present and active. However, the loss of p16 and artificial elevation of cyclin D1 levels have impaired the regulatory system. pRb is now inappropriately inactivated by the activated CDKs and regulation of cell division is lost or impaired (bottom panel). Studies of pRb expression in tumors have also found a high, but not perfect correlation between tumor type and pRb expression. That is, most, but not all, SCLC tumors lack pRb while most, but not all, NSCLC tumors express pRb [40–42, 53, 54]. The exceptions may indicate that in actual tumors a given tumor type shows a strong preference for a specific mechanism for overcoming the pRb cell cycle block but is not absolutely committed to that mechanism. Consequent selection during growth of cell lines may then enhance the apparent tumor type mechanism preference.

4. Implications for Diagnosis

One of the significant handicaps in lung cancer treatment today is the difficulty of early diagnosis. Mortality rates for cervical and breast carcinoma have decreased in recent years largely because the PAP smear and mammography have allowed for early diagnosis and early, premetastatic treatment of the disease. In lung cancer early lesions are difficult to detect and, once detected, are difficult to predict as many precancerous lesions do not appear to develop into metastatic disease. A clearer understanding of the early molecular changes involved in lung tumorigenesis could lead to new early detection methods. Since p16 and pRb are involved in growth regulation, their loss would be expected to lead to increased cell division, i.e. neoplasia, an early step in tumor progression. We are attempting to determine whether the pRb and p16 alterations are, in fact, present in precancerous lung lesions and might be good markers for early detection.

5. Implications for Gene Therapy

An understanding of the molecular changes involved in lung cancer would also present an opportunity for new treatment in the form of gene therapy. Experiments with tumor cell lines suggest that although multiple changes are involved in tumorigenesis, the reversal of any of these changes is sufficient to halt cell growth. Our results so far, as well as the results of others, indicate that p16 and antisense cyclin D1 expression in NSCLC tumor cell lines do effectively block cell growth ([9, 10] and Schauer, Siriwardana and Sclafani, unpublished results). We are currently developing systems for regulated p16 and antisense cyclin D1 expression which will be tested for efficacy in inhibiting the growth of NSCLC tumors in nude mice. If these experiments are successful, this area of research has the potential to translate into a gene therapy approach to the treatment of this most common form of lung cancer.

Acknowledgement

This work was supported by funds from the Public Health Service, National Institutes of Health/National Cancer Institute through a SPORE in lung cancer grant (1-P50-CA58187-01) awarded to Dr. Paul Bunn, Jr., M.D.

References

1. Minshull J (1993) Cyclin synthesis: who needs it? *BioEssays* 15: 149–155.
2. Graña X, Reddy EP (1995) Cell cycle control in mammalian cells: role of cyclins, cyclin dependent kinases (CDKs), growth suppressor genes and cyclin-dependent kinase inhibitors (CKIs). *Oncogene* 11: 211–219.
3. Nigg EA (1995) Cyclin-dependent protein kinases: key regulators of the eukaryotic cell cycle. *BioEssays* 17: 471–480.
4. Pines J (1993) Cyclins and cyclin-dependent kinases: take your partners. *Trends Biochem Sci* 18: 195–197.
5. Sherr CJ (1993) Mammalian G1 cyclins. *Cell* 73: 1059–1065.
6. Morgan DO (1995) Principles of CDK regulation. *Nature* 374: 131–134.
7. Kato JY, Sherr CJ (1993) Inhibition of granulocyte differentiation by G1 cyclins D2 and D3 but not D1. *Proc Natl Acad Sci USA* 90: 11513–11517.
8. Baldin V, Lukas J, Marcote MJ, Pagano M, Draetta G (1993) Cyclin D1 is a nuclear protein required for cell cycle progression in G1. *Genes and Dev* 7: 812–821.
9. Tam SW, Theodoras AM, Shay JW, Draetta GF, Pagano M (1994) Differential expression and regulation of Cyclin D1 protein in normal and tumor human cells: association with Cdk4 is required for Cyclin D1 function in G1 progression. *Oncogene* 9: 2663–2674.
10. Bartkova J, Lukas J, Müller H, Lützhoft D, Strauss M, Bartek J (1994) Cyclin D1 protein expression and function in human breast cancer. *Int J Cancer* 57: 353–361.
11. Sherr CJ (1994) G1 phase progression: cycling on cue. *Cell* 79: 551–555.
12. Bohmer R-M, Scharf E, Assoian RK (1996) Cytoskeletal Integrity is required throughout the mitogen stimulation phase of the cell cycle and mediates the anchorage-dependent expression of cyclin D1. *Molec Biol Cell* 7: 101–111.
13. Marx J (1994) How cells cycle towards cancer. *Science* 263: 319–321.
14. Motokura T, Arnold A (1993) Cyclin D and oncogenesis. *Curr Opin in Genet Devel* 3: 5–10.
15. Hunter T, Pines J (1994) Cyclins and cancer. II: Cyclin D and CDK inhibitors come of age. *Cell* 79: 573–82.
16. Lew DJ, Dulic V, Reed SI (1991) Isolation of three novel human cyclins by rescue of G1 cyclin (Cln) function in yeast. *Cell* 66: 1197–1206.
17. Xiong Y, Connolly T, Futcher B, Beach D (1991) Human D-type cyclin. *Cell* 65: 691–699.
18. Withers DA, Harvey RC, Faust JB, Melnyk O, Carey K, Meeker TC (1991) Characterization of a candidate *bcl-1* gene. *Molec Cell Biol* 11: 4846–4853.

19. Rosenberg CL, Wong E, Petty EM, Bale AE, Tsujimoto Y, Harris NL, Arnold A (1991) PRAD1, a candidate BCL1 oncogene: mapping and expression in centrocytic lymphoma. *Proc Natl Acad Sci USA* 88: 9638–9642.
20. Ando K, Ajchenbaum-Cymbalista F, Griffin JD (1993) Regulation of G1/S transition by cyclins D2 and D3 in hematopoietic cells. *Proc Natl Acad Sci USA* 90: 9571–9575.
21. Ohtsubo M, Roberts JM (1993) Cyclin-dependent regulation of G1 in mammalian fibroblasts. *Science* 259: 1908–1912.
22. Quelle DE, Ashmun RA, Shurtleff SA, Kato J-Y, Bar-Sagi D, Roussel MF, Sherr CJ (1993) Overexpression of mouse D-type cyclins accelerates G1 phase in rodent fibroblasts. *Genes and Dev* 7: 1559–1571.
23. Resnitzky D, Gossen M, Bujard H, Reed SI (1994) Acceleration of the G1/S phase transition by expression of cyclins D1 and E with an inducible system. *Molec Cell Biol* 14: 1669–1679.
24. Hinds PW, Dowdy SF, Eaton EN, Arnold A, Weinberg RA (1994) Function of a human cyclin gene as an oncogene. *Proc Natl Acad Sci USA* 91: 709–713.
25. Lovec H, Sewing A, Lucibello FC, Muller R, Moroy T (1994) Oncogenic activity of cyclin D1 revealed through cooperation with Ha-ras: link between cell cycle control and malignant transformation. *Oncogene* 9: 323–326.
26. Lovec H, Grzeschiczek A, Kowalski MB, Moroy T (1994) Cyclin D1/bcl-1 cooperates with myc genes in the generation of B-cell lymphoma in transgenic mice. *Embo J* 13:3487–3495.
27. Jung JU, Stager M, Desrosiers RC (1994) Virus-encoded cyclin. *Molec Cell Biol* 14: 7235–7244.
28. Harper JW, Elledge SJ (1996) Cdk inhibitors in development and cancer. *Curr Opin Genet Dev* 6: 56–64.
29. Sherr CJ, Roberts JM (1995) Inhibitors of mammalian G1 cyclin-dependent kinases. *Genes and Devel* 9: 1149–1163.
30. El-Deiry WS, Tokino T, Velculescu VE, Levy DB, Parsons R, Trent JM, Mercer WE, Kinzler KW, Vogelstein B (1993) WAF1, a potential mediator of p53 tumor suppression. *Cell* 75: 817–825.
31. Shiohara M, El-Diery WS, Wada M, Nakamaki T, Takeuchi S, Yang R, Chen DL, Vogelstein B, Koeffler HP (1994) Absence of WAF1 mutations in a variety of human malignancies. *Blood* 84: 3781–3784.
32. Deng C, Zhang P, Harper JW, Elledge SJ, Leder PJ (1995) Mice lacking p21[CIP1/WAF1] undergo normal development, but are defective in G1 checkpoint control. *Cell* 82: 675–684.
33. Kamb A, Gruis NA, Weaver-Feldhaus J, Liu Q, Harshman K, Tavtigian SV, Stockert E, Day RFI, Johnson BE, Skelnick MH (1994) A cell cycle regulator potentially involved in genesis of many tumor types. *Science* 264: 436–440.
34. Merlo A, Herman JG, Mao L, Lee DJ, Gabrielson E, Burger PC, Baylin SB, Sidransky D (1995) 5' CpG island methylation is associated with transcriptional silencing of the tumour suppressor p16/CDKN2/MTS1 in human cancers. *Nature Med* 1: 686–692.
35. Mao L, Merlo A, Bedi G, Shapiro GI, Edwards CD, Rollins BJ, Sidransky D (1995) A novel p16INK4a transcript. *Cancer Res* 55: 2995–2997.
36. Stone S, Jiang P, Dayanath P, Tavtigian SV, Katcher H, Parry D, Peters G, Kamb A (1995) Complex structure and regulation of the p16 (MTS1) locus. *Cancer Res* 55: 2988–2994.
37. Ewen ME (1994) The cell cycle and the retinoblastoma protein family. *Cancer Metastasis Rev* 13: 45–66.
38. Hollingsworth RE, Jr, Chen PL, Lee WH (1993) Integration of cell cycle control with transcriptional regulation by the retinoblastoma protein. *Curr Opin Cell Biol* 5: 194–200.
39. Lukas J, Bartkova J, Rohde M, Strauss M, Bartek J (1995) Cyclin D1 is dispensable for G1 control in retinoblastoma gene-deficient cells independently of cdk4 activity. *Molec Cell Biol* 15: 2600–2611.
40. Horowitz JM, Park S-H, Bogenmann E, Cheng J-C, Yandell DW, Kaye FJ, Minna JD, Dryja TP, Weinberg RA (1990) Frequent inactivation of the retinoblastoma anti-oncogene is restricted to a subset of human tumor cells. *Proc Natl Acad Sci USA* 87: 2775–2779.
41. Hensel CH, Hsieh C-L, Gazdar AF, Johnson BE, Sakaguchi AY, Naylor SL, Lee W-H, Lee EY-HP (1990) Altered structure and expression of the human retinoblastoma susceptibility gene in small cell lung cancer. *Cancer Res* 50: 3067–3072.

42. Harbour JW, Lai S-L, Whang-Penn J, Gazdar AF, Minna JD, Kaye FJ (1988) Abnormalities in structure and expression of the human retinoblastoma gene in SCLC. *Science* 241: 353–357.
43. Sclafani RA, Schauer IE (1996) Cell cycle control and cancer: lessons from lung cancer. *J Invest Dermatol* 106: 1S–5S.
44. Schauer IE, Siriwardana S, Langan TA, Sclafani RA (1994) Cyclin D1 overexpression vs. Rb inactivation: Alternate mechanisms of growth control evasion in non-small cell and small cell lung cancer. *Proc Natl Acad Sci USA* 91: 7827–7831.
45. Buckley MF, Sweeney KJE, Hamilton JA, Sini RL, Manning DL, Nicholson RI, deFazio A, Watts CKW, Musgrove EA, Sutherland RL (1993) Expression and amplification of cyclin genes in human breast cancer. *Oncogene* 8: 2127–2133.
46. Müller H, Lukas J, Schneider A, Warthoe P, Bartek J, Eilers M, Strauss M (1994) Cyclin D1 expression is regulated by the retinoblastoma protein. *Proc Natl Acad Sci USA* 91: 2945–2949.
47. Shapiro GI, Park JE, Edwards CD, Mao L, Merlo A, Sidransky D, Ewen ME, Rollins BJ (1995) Multiple mechanism of p16INK4A inactivation in non-small cell lung cancer cell lines. *Cancer Res* 55: 6200–6209.
48. Linardopoulos S, Gonos ES, Spandidos DA (1993) Abnormalities of retinoblastoma gene structure in human lung tumors. *Cancer Lett* 71: 67–74.
49. Bartkova J, Lukas J, Muller H, Strauss M, Gusterson B, Bartek J (1995) Abnormal patterns of D-type cyclin expression and G1 regulation in human head and neck cancer. *Cancer Res* 55: 949–56.
50. Bartkova J, Lukas J, Strauss M, Bartek J (1995) Cyclin D1 oncoprotein aberrantly accumulates in malignancies of diverse histogenesis. *Oncogene* 10: 775–778.
51. Gillett C, Fantl V, Smith R, Fisher C, Bartek J, Dickson C, Barnes D, Peters G (1994) Amplification and overexpression of cyclin D1 in breast cancer detected by immunohistochemical staining. *Cancer Res* 54: 1812–1817.
52. Jiang W, Zhang Y-J, Kahn SM, Hollstein MC, Santella RM, Lu S-H, Harris C, Montesano R, Weinstein IB (1993) Altered expression of the cyclin D1 and retinoblastoma genes in human esophageal cancer. *Proc Natl Acad Sci USA* 90: 9026–9030.
53. Reissmann PT, Koga H, Takahashi R, Figlin RA, Holmes EC, Piantadosi S, Cordan-Cardo C, Slamon DJ, Group LCS (1993) Inactivation of the retinoblastoma susceptibility gene in non small cell lung cancer. *Oncogene* 8: 1913–1919.
54. Yokota J, Akiyama T, Fung Y-KT, Benedict WF, Namba Y, Hanaoka M, Wada M, Terasaki T, Shimosato Y, Sugimura T, Terada M (1988) Altered expression of the retinoblastoma (RB) gene in small-cell carcinoma of the lung. *Oncogene* 3: 471–475.

Clinical and Biological Basis of Lung Cancer Prevention
ed. by Y. Martinet, F.R. Hirsch, N. Martinet, J.-M. Vignaud
and J.L. Mulshine
© 1998 Birkhäuser Verlag Basel/Switzerland

CHAPTER 10
Molecular Genetics of Lung Cancer

Xin W. Wang[1], Marc S. Greenblatt[2] and Curtis C. Harris[1]

[1] *Laboratory of Human Carcinogenesis, National Cancer Institute, National Institutes of Health, Bethesda, Maryland, USA*
[2] *Hematology/Oncology Unit, Fletcher Allen Health Care, MCHV Campus-Patrick 534, Burlington, Vermont, USA*

1. Genetic Changes in Multistep Lung Carcinogenesis

The specific genetic and epigenetic events leading to neoplastic transformation differ among tumor types, but several cellular pathways and important regulatory genes are known to be frequently involved. In lung cancer they include G protein signal transduction (*ras* genes and gastrin releasing peptides [GRPs]); epidermal growth factor (EGF), transforming growth factor alpha (TGF-α) and their family of receptors (EGFR and the products of the *erbB-1* and *erbB-2* proto-oncogenes); cell cycle regulation (involving the RB gene product, cyclins, cyclin-dependent kinases (cdk) and cdk inhibitors); and the *p53* tumor suppressor gene, which integrates functions of DNA repair, genomic stability, transcription control and programmed cell death (apoptosis). Studies have also demonstrated or implied abnormal regulation and mutation of other genes and proteins, including c-*myc*, *bcl-2*, unidentified tumor suppressor genes on chromosomes 3p and 9p, and transforming growth factor-beta (TGF-β) [1, 2]. The biological and clinical significance of most of these alterations, and the nature of differences between small cell (SCLC) and non-small cell lung cancers (NSCLC), remain to be determined.

2. Functional Implications of Molecular Changes in Lung Cancer

Mutations in K-*ras* are thought to have important consequences for bronchial cell growth deregulation. Activating K-*ras* mutations are found in 25%–30% of adenocarcinomas and 15% of large cell carcinomas, but

squamous cell carcinomas and never in SCLC [3]. Transfected
uses neoplastic transformation of immortalized human bronchial
l cells; the transformed cells produce adenocarcinomas when
ted into athymic nude mice [4]. Transfection of activated K-*ras*
CLC line induces features of NSCLC differentiation [5, 6]. Other
1 pathway events are implicated in SCLC, despite the absence of
tions. Gastrin-releasing peptides (GRP, including bombesin) are
it autocrine growth factors for SCLC [7], and also stimulate
f normal human bronchial epithelial (NHBE) cells [8].
otein encoded by the *p53* tumor suppressor gene performs many
ellular functions, including cell cycle arrest, regulation of DNA
response to DNA damage, transcriptional activation and suppres-
l triggering of apoptosis [9–11]. Mutations of *p53* can both ab-
s normal tumor suppressor functions and produce gain of new
;, which stimulate cell growth and neoplastic transformation [12,
:ations have been found in 72% of SCLC and 47% of NSCLC,
erences among histological types (see section 2.c.) [2]. Because of
e in the maintenance of genomic stability, loss of its function is
. to produce progressive genetic abnormalities, some of which
ntribute to tumor progression. Other p53 pathway events may
ut so far genes modulated by p53 (e.g. *mdm2*, *WAF1*, and
5) have not been found to be altered in lung cancer.
il other known tumor suppressor genes have been shown to be
or deleted in lung cancers (Table 1). The best characterized is the
.stoma gene *Rb*, which is abnormal (loss of expression, mutation,
f heterozygosity) in over 90% of SCLC and 20%–30% of NSCLC
nd lines [3, 14, 15]. Analysis in the same tumors of the expression
ational status of *Rb* and two other cell cycle proteins, p16^{INK4}
and cyclin D1, supports the hypothesis that a single abnormality
athway is sufficient for dysregulation of the cell cycle G1 check-

---

lasses of oncogenes and tumor suppressor genes, with examples of genes found to
n lung cancer

:tors: PDGF-B

isduction Proteins:

 Factor Receptor Tyrosine Kinases: EGFR, erbB-1, erbB-2 [Her2/neu]
:eptor Membrane-Associated Kinases: fms, fes
ismic Kinases: raf
ins: ras, GRP

oteins:

iption Factors, DNA Binding Proteins: p53, myc, fos, jun
cle Regulators: p53, Rb, p16, cyclin D1

Regulators: p53, bcl-2

Itability Regulators: p53

---

point. Okamoto et al. [16] found that loss of either *Rb* expression (3/9) or p16 expression (6/9), but not both, occurred in NSCLC lines. Schauer et al. [17] found that 11/12 NSCLC lines overexpressed cyclin D1 but did not lose *Rb* protein, whereas 9/9 SCLC lines had lost *Rb* protein but only one overexpressed cyclin D1. These results are analogous to the differences in G protein pathway abnormalities seen between SCLC and NSCLC (GRP expression in SCLC, *ras* mutation in NSCLC), implying separate pathogenesis for these tumor types.

Studies demonstrating consistent chromosomal deletions or loss of heterozygosity suggest that other tumor suppressor genes contribute to lung carcinogenesis. Strong evidence exists that unidentified tumor suppressor genes critical in SCLC and often NSCLC development reside on chromosome 3p21 and 3p14 [3, 18, 19]. Candidate genes at these loci include the beta-retinoic acid receptor (*β-RAR*) and protein-tyrosine phosphatase-gamma (*PTP-γ*) [20, 21]. A tumor suppressor gene on chromosome 5 important in colon carcinogenesis, *APC*, also shows frequent loss of heterozygosity in SCLC, without mutations in the remaning allele [22], which suggests the involvement of an adjacent tumor suppressor gene. Cytogenetic analyses frequently demonstrate losses of chromosome 9p21 in NSCLC; a tumor suppressor gene may reside in the interferon gene cluster in this region [1, 23–25]. *p16^{INK4}* (*MTS1*) and *p15^{INK4}* (*MTS2*) are candidate tumor suppressor genes at this locus [26] which are infrequently involved in primary lung cancers [16]. Other chromosomes frequently deleted in lung cancers (e.g. chromosome 11) also may contain tumor suppressor genes [27–29].

The *bcl-2* gene, identified at the breakpoint of the t (14;18) translocation in lymphomas, is one of many factors in the programmed cell death pathway. When complexed with Bax, another protein in this family, Bcl-2 inhibits apoptosis; Bax homodimers accelerate apoptosis. Study of the interactions of these and other families of genes in the apoptosis pathway promise to yield an improved paradigm of cell death [30]. Bcl-2 is expressed in some NSCLC [31], but the balance between Bax homodimers and Bax-Bcl-2 heterodimers, and its relationship to apoptosis in lung cancers, remains to be determined.

The *myc* gene, whose product binds DNA and regulate gene transcription, is overexpressed in 10%–15% of primary lung cancers, more often in SCLC than NSCLC [3], and activated c-*myc* may correlate positively with poor prognosis [28, 32]. Other DNA binding oncogene products such as *fos* and *jun* also are overexpressed in lung cancer [33, 34]. The downstream genes in these pathways which might be relevant to lung carcinogenesis are unknown.

As cells age, normal cellular senescence is partially regulated by the progressive shortening of chromosomal telomeres, the repetitive DNA sequences at chromosomal ends. The enzyme telomerase can elongate telomeres by replicating these sequences. Telomerase activity generally is not present in normal somatic cells, but is reactivated in immortalized cells [35]. Dysregulation of the telomerase pathway is thought to be a major event in cellular immortalization, and has been described in some lung cancers [36]. The first gene in this pathway, *TLC1*, has recently been discovered [37]; rapid advances in this area of carcinogenesis research are anticipated.

Growth factor pathways, autocrine and paracrine, are important in lung carcinogenesis. EGF and TGF-α both act by binding to the EGF receptor [38]. They stimulate proliferation, and may be important autocrine and paracrine agents in lung regulation as they are produced by a variety of lung cells [39]. Evidence to suggest the importance of these growth factors in lung carcinogenesis is the frequent overexpression and amplification of EGF and other genes in the EGF receptor family. These include the products of the *erbB-1* and *erbB-2* (*Her2/neu*) oncogenes, whose native ligands are unknown [28]. EGFR, erbB-1, and erbB-2 have tyrosine kinase activity and can neoplastically transform cells when overexpressed; transfection of c-*erbB-2* into nontumorigenic bronchial cells can contribute to but is not sufficient for malignant transformation [40]. Overexpression of EGFR, erbB-1, and erbB-2 is common in NSCLC [3, 33, 38, 41].

Retinoids are important regulators of bronchial epithelia, inhibiting squamous and promoting mucociliary differentiation [39], and inhibiting NHBE squamous differentiation *in vitro* [42]. The recent identification of retinoid receptors as transcription factors [39] suggests that regulation of the genes involved in the pathways of growth arrest and squamous differentiation, (such as cell cycle proteins Rb and cdc2-kinase, and transcription factors c-myc and E2F-1) [43], may be the mechanism of action.

Other growth factors important in lung carcinogenesis include TGF-β, a cytokine produced by various normal and malignant cells that inhibit proliferation and induce terminal squamous differentiation of NHBE cells [44]. Receptors for TGF-β are present on lung and many other cells, but its signal transduction pathways are still being defined. Several members downstream from TGF-β receptors (including *DPC4* and *SMAD2*) have been implicated the tumor suppressor genes that are important in lung carcinogenesis [45,46]. TGF-β exposure reduces phosphorylation of the retinoblastoma protein, which may account for the growth arresting activity of TGF-β [39]. Insulin and insulin-like growth factors (IGFs) also stimulate bronchial epithelial cells *in vitro*; production of IGFs by pulmonary macrophages may play a role in lung neoplasia *in vivo* [39]. Platelet derived growth factor (PDGF-B) is not a common autocrine growth factor in lung cancers, but may participate in paracrine growth loops between lung epithelial and mesenchymal cells [47]. Dopamine pathways have also been implicated in SCLC growth control [48].

3. Timing and Sequence of Genetic Abnormalities

Knowledge of the sequence of genetic and epigenetic changes in multi-stage lung carcinogenesis is still sparse [1]. Correlation of genetic events with detectable phenotypes might define patients who can benefit from chemoprevention, resection, or molecularly targeted therapy to halt or reverse progression of premalignant lesions. Squamous cell carcinomas (25% of lung cancers) usually progress through multiple, histologically recognizable stages of dysplasia (usually subdivided as mild, moderate, and severe), carcinoma in situ (CIS) and invasive cancer, marked by transgression of the basement membrane. The phenotypes of premalignant lesions of other histological types of lung cancer are unclear. Some studies of genetic and biochemical markers, including allelic deletion, sequence analysis, and immunohistochemistry (IHC) have been carried out on premalignant mucosae.

Molecular and cytogenetic analyses of bronchial dysplasia have shown that *p53* mutations and 3p deletion can occur in dysplastic lesions, and *ras* mutations usually occur at the development of CIS [49–53]. Composite data from IHC studies show a progressive increase in the frequency of p53 protein accumulation from 0% of normal bronchial mucosae to two thirds of severe dysplasias, CIS and microinvasive carcinomas [49–51, 54–56], although one study has found that staining did not occur in early dysplasias and was rare in high grade dysplasias [57]. Most of these studies support a multistage model for squamous lung carcinoma in which *p53* mutation occurs in 25% of the earliest neoplastic lesions, and most mutations occur before invasion develops. The sequence of events may or may not be identical in all cancers; study of carefully characterized premalignant lesions may clarify this. The accumulation of a critical amount of damage, or of abnormalities in a threshold number of key cellular pathways, may be more important than the precise sequence of events. In addition, the rate and probability of progression of a dysplastic lesion to carcinoma may depend on the genetic changes present in the lesion. For example, a mild dysplasia containing cells with mutant p53 may progress to malignancy at a faster rate than one containing only normal p53.

The genetic events associated with tumor progression are unclear. Study of primary tumors and lymph nodes suggests that some changes, such as expression of oncogenes c-*jun* and c-*myc*, occur more frequently in metastases than in primary tumors. *Ras* mutations usually precede metastasis, whereas other changes such as c-*fos*, c-*erbB-1*, and c-*erbB-2* may or may not precede metastasis [34]. The use of these markers as prognostic indicators is discussed below. Tumor angiogenesis is thought to be critical to metastatic potential *in vitro* and *in vivo* [58]. In preliminary studies, expression of the extracellular matrix molecule thrombospondin, which is regulated by p53 [59], has been shown to correlate inversely with tumor progression in cell lines derived from lung and other cancers [60].

4. Therapeutic Implications

Molecular targets promise future cancer therapy. Potential avenues include gene therapy, antisense DNA, monoclonal antibodies carrying toxins, and combinations of cytotoxic and biological agents to enhance programmed cell death.

Surprisingly, correction of one molecular abnormality can reverse a malignant phenotype *in vitro*, even in a cancer cell with multiple genetic anomalies [61–64]. *In vitro* and animal studies have demonstrated that antisense inhibition of mutated K-*ras* or introduction of wildtype *p53* gene via a retroviral vector can suppress growth and tumorigenicity of NSCLC cell lines [61, 62, 64]. The use of cell type-specific promoters may allow the introduction of toxic genes with specificity for cell types, including lung cancers [65]. Cytotoxicity is seen in nontransduced cells adjacent to cells incorporating the new gene; this "bystander effect" may make gene therapies more effective [66]. The identification of other molecular changes in lung cancers will provide new potential therapeutic targets for gene or antisense DNA therapy.

Recent clinical and laboratory evidence has emphasized the importance of programmed cell death in the response of cancer cells to treatment [67]. Programmed cell death is a cellular phenomenon involved in normal development, characterized by specific biochemical and morphological criteria [68]. Aberrations in this pathway are important in carcinogenesis [69]. Multiple endogenous and exogenous inducers of programmed cell death have been identified, including cytokines, DNA damaging chemotherapeutic agents and opioids; nicotine suppresses apoptosis *in vitro* in lung cancer cells [70]. These agents transmit signals through at least two poorly understood biochemical pathways, one of which depends on wild type p53 protein [71, 72].

The p53-dependent programmed cell death pathway (Figure 1) can be initiated by DNA damage, especially single strand breaks. Putative mechanisms include transcriptional control of specific genes and protein-protein interactions with multicomponent protein machines that are involved with DNA replication and repair [73]. In cells with wildtype p53, DNA damage-induced p53 expression leads to cell cycle arrest in the G1 phase, during which DNA repair might occur prior to DNA synthesis in S-phase. If repair is inadequate, wildtype p53 may then trigger programmed cell death as a protective mechanism. In cells with loss of p53 function due to mutation, this growth arrest and cell death would not occur. These cells therefore have a growth advantage, and are more likely to survive and produce daughter cells with additional mutations.

The hypothesis that tumors containing wild type p53 protein are more responsive to ionizing radiation and DNA damaging drugs is supported by direct laboratory data and some inferences derived from clinicopathological findings in human cancers [67]. Ionizing radiation and cancer

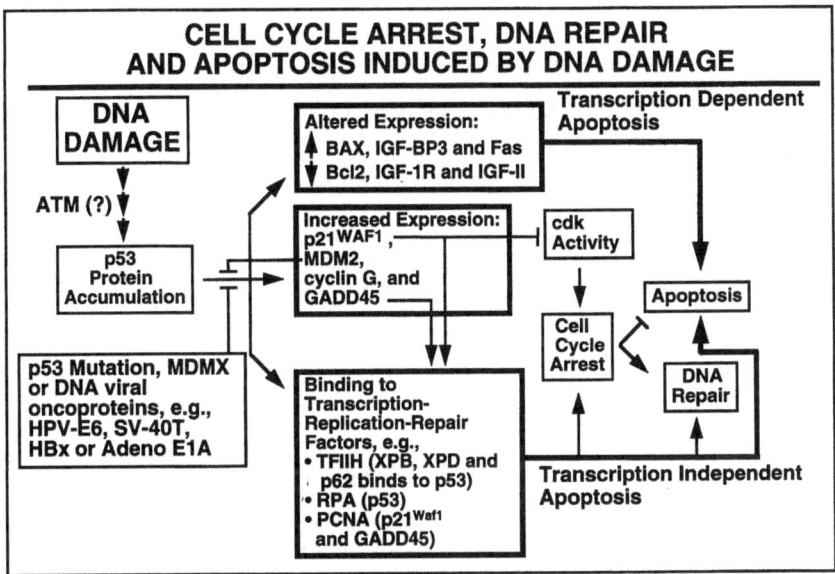

CELL CYCLE ARREST, DNA REPAIR AND APOPTOSIS INDUCED BY DNA DAMAGE

Figure 1. Events in the pathway of programmed cell death (apoptosis) include regulation by p53, bcl-2, bax, cdk, and other cell cycle pathways.

chemotherapeutic agents such as adriamycin, etoposide and cisplatin produce DNA damage and induce programmed cell death in sensitive cells [74]. Levels of normal p53 protein rise in cells thus damaged, and the presence of normal p53 protein is necessary for programmed cell death to occur in response to these agents [71, 72, 75]. After wildtype *p53* is transfected into *p53* null lung carcinoma cells, they acquire the ability to undergo programmed cell death in response to cisplatin *in vitro* and in nude mice [76]. The relationship between p53 function and response to chemo- or radiotherapy in human tumors *in vivo* has not yet been directly assessed, although one study in primary breast cancers suggests a negative correlation between elevated p53 levels (presumably representing mutant protein) and chemosensitivity *in vitro* [77].

Monoclonal antibodies against tumor-specific antigens have produced disappointing results in therapeutic trials for carcinomas. More detailed knowledge of the mechanisms of cell death and receptor signalling pathways suggests some new strategies. For example, anti-erbB-2 antibodies can inhibit and kill breast cancer lines overexpressing erbB-2 and could be used in erbB-2-overexpressing lung cancers. Proteins involved in programmed cell death (such as those in the bcl-2 pathway) are other potential targets for monoclonal antibodies [78].

References

1. Gazdar AF (1994) The molecular and cellular basis of human lung cancer. *Anticancer Res* 14: 261–267.
2. Greenblatt MS, Bennett WP, Hollstein M, Harris CC (1994) Mutations in the p53 tumor suppressor gene: clues to cancer etiology and molecular pathogenesis. *Cancer Res* 54: 4855–4878.
3. Carbone DP, Minna JD (1992) The molecular genetics of lung cancer. *Adv Intern Med* 37: 153–171.
4. Reddel RR, Ke Y, Kaighn ME, Malan-Shibley L, Lechner JF, Rhim JS, Harris CC (1988) Human bronchial epithelial cells neoplastically transformed by v-Ki-*ras*: Altered response to inducers of terminal squamous differentiation. *Oncogene Res* 3: 401–408.
5. Mabry M, Nakagawa T, Nelkin BD, McDowell E, Gesell M, Eggleston JC, Casero RA Jr, Baylin SB (1988) v-Ha-ras oncogene insertion: a model for tumor progression of human small cell lung cancer. *Proc Natl Acad Sci USA* 85: 6523–6527.
6. Mabry M, Nakagawa T, Baylin S, Pettengill O, Sorenson G, Nelkin B (1989) Insertion of the v-Ha-ras oncogene induces differentiation of calcitonin-producing human small cell lung cancer. *J Clin Invest* 84: 194–199.
7. Cuttitta F, Carney DN, Mulshine J, Moody TW, Fedorko J, Fischler A, Minna JD (1985) Bombesin-like peptides can function as autocrine growth factors in human small-cell lung cancer. *Nature* 316: 823–826.
8. Willey JC, Lechner JF, Harris CC (1984) Bombesin and the C-terminal tetradecapeptide of gastrin-releasing peptide are growth factors for normal human bronchial epithelial cells. *Exp Cell Res* 153: 245–248.
9. Montenarh M (1992) Functional implications of the growth-suppressor/oncoprotein p53 (Review). *Int J Oncol* 1: 37–45.
10. Levine AJ (1993) The tumor suppressor genes. *Annu Rev Biochem* 62: 623–651.
11. Lane DP (1994) On the expression of the p53 protein in human cancer. *Mol Biol Rep* 19: 23–29.
12. Lane DP, Benchimol S (1990) p53: oncogene or anti-oncogene. *Genes Dev* 4: 1–8.
13. Gerwin BI, Spillare E, Forrester K, Lehman TA, Kispert J, Welsh JA, Pfeifer AMA, Lechner JF, Baker SJ, Vogelstein B, et al. (1992) Mutant p53 can induce tumorigenic conversion of human bronchial epithelial cells and reduce their responsiveness to a negative growth factor, transforming growth factor type B1. *Proc Natl Acad Sci USA* 89: 2759–2763.
14. Reissmann PT, Koga H, Takahashi R, Figlin RA, Holmes EC, Piantadosi S, Cordon-Cardo C, Slamon DJ (1993) Inactivation of the retinoblastoma susceptibility gene in non-small cell lung cancer. The Lung Cancer Study Group. *Oncogene* 8: 1913–1919.
15. Gouyer V, Gazzeri S, Brambilla E, Bolon I, Moro D, Perron P, Benabid AL, Brambilla C (1994) Loss of heterozygosity at the RB locus correlates with loss of RB protein in primary malignant neuro-endocrine lung carcinomas. *Int J Cancer* 58: 818–824.
16. Okamoto A, Demetrick DJ, Spillare EA, Hagiwara K, Hussain SP, Bennett WP, Forrester K, Gerwin B, Serrano M, Beach DH, et al. (1994) Mutations and altered expression of genes regulating the cell cycle G1 checkpoint in human cancer. *Proc Natl Acad Sci USA* 91: 11045–11049.
17. Schauer IE, Siriwardana S, Langan TA, Sclafani RA (1994) Cyclin D1 overexpression vs. retinoblastoma inactivation: implications for growth control evasion in non-small cell and small cell lung cancer. *Proc Natl Acad Sci USA* 91: 7827–7831.
18. Whang-Peng J, Kao-Shan CS, Lee EC, Bunn PA, Carney DN, Gazdar AF, Minna JD (1982) Specific chromosome defect associated with human small-cell lung cancer; deletion 3p(14–23). *Science* 215: 181–182.
19. Rabbitts P, Douglas J, Daly M, Sundaresan V, Fox B, Haselton P, Wells F, Albertson D, Waters J, et al. (1989) Frequency and extent of allelic loss in the short arm of chromosome 3 in nonsmall-cell lung cancer. *Genes Chromosomes Cancer* 1: 95–105.
20. LaForgia S, Morse B, Levy J, Barnea G, Cannizzaro LA, Li F, Nowell PC, Boghosian-Sell L, Glick J, Weston A, et al. (1991) Receptor-linked protein-tyrosine-phosphatase, PTPy, is a candidate tumor suppressor at human chromosome region 3p21. *Proc Natl Acad Sci USA* 88: 5036–5040.
21. Houle B, Rochette-Egly C, Bradley WE (1993) Tumor-suppressive effect of the retinoic acid receptor beta in human epidermoid lung cancer cells. *Proc Natl Acad Sci USA* 90: 985–989.

22. D'Amico D, Carbone DP, Johnson BE, Meltzer SJ, Minna JD (1992) Polymorphic sites within the MCC and APC loci reveal very frequent loss of heterozygosity in human small cell lung cancer. *Cancer Res* 52: 1996–1999.

23. Lukeis R, Irving L, Garson M, Hasthorpe S (1990) Cytogenetics of non-small cell lung cancer: analysis of consistent non-random abnormalities. *Genes Chromosom Cancer* 2: 116–124.

24. Whang-Peng J, Knutsen T, Gazdar A, Steinberg SM, Oie H, Linnoila I, Mulshine J, Nau M, Minna JD (1991) Nonrandom structural and numerical chromosome changes in non-small-cell lung cancer. *Genes Chromosom Cancer* 3: 168–188.

25. Olopade OI, Buchhagen DL, Malik K, Sherman J, Nobori T, Bader S, Nau MM, Gazdar AF, Minna JD, Diaz MO (1993) Homozygous loss of the interferon genes defines the critical region on 9p that is deleted in lung cancers. *Cancer Res* 53: 2410–2415.

26. Kamb A, Gruis NA, Weaver-Feldhaus J, Liu Q, Harshman K, Tavtigian SV, Stockert E, Day RS, Johnson BE, Skolnick MH (1994) A cell cycle regulator potentially involved in genesis of many tumor types. *Science* 264: 436–440.

27. Weston A, Willey JC, Modali R, Sugimura H, McDowell EM, Resau J, Light B, Haugen A, Mann DL, Trump BF, et al. (1989) Differential DNA sequence deletions from chromosomes 3, 11, 13 and 17 in squamous cell carcinoma, large cell carcinoma and adenocarcinoma of the human lung. *Proc Natl Acad Sci USA* 86: 5099–5103.

28. Buchhagen DL (1991) Molecular mechanisms in lung pathogenesis. *Biochim Biophys Acta* 1072: 159–176.

29. Willey JC, Hei TK, Piao CQ, Madrid L, Willey JJ, Apostolakos MJ, Hukku B (1993) Radiation-induced deletion of chromosomal regions containing tumor suppressor genes in human bronchial epithelial cells. *Carcinogenesis* 14: 1181–1188.

30. Wyllie AH (1994) Apoptosis. Death gets a brake [news; comment]. *Nature* 369: 272–273.

31. Pezzella F, Turley H, Kuzu I, Tungekar MF, Dunnill MS, Pierce CB, Harris A, Gatter KC, Mason DY (1993) bcl-2 protein in non-small-cell lung carcinoma [see comments]. *N Engl J Med* 329: 690–694.

32. Bergh JC (1990) Gene amplification in human lung cancer. The myc family genes and other proto-oncogenes and growth factor genes. *Am Rev Respir Dis* 142: S20–S26.

33. Wodrich W, Volm M (1993) Overexpression of oncoproteins in non-small cell lung carcinomas of smokers. *Carcinogenesis* 14: 1121–1124.

34. Volm M, van Kaick G, Mattern J (1994) Analysis of c-fos, c-jun, c-erbB1, c-erbB2 and c-myc in primary lung carcinomas and their lymph node metastases. *Clin Exp Metastasis* 12: 329–334.

35. Shay JW, Wright WE, Werbin H (1993) Toward a molecular understanding of human breast cancer: a hypothesis. *Breast Cancer Res Treat* 25: 83–94.

36. Shirotani Y, Hiyama K, Ishioka S, Inyaku K, Awaya Y, Yonehara S, Yoshida Y, Inai K, Hiyama E, Hasegawa K, et al. (1994) Alteration in length of telomeric repeats in lung cancer. *Lung Cancer* 11: 29–41.

37. Singer MS, Gottschling DE (1994) TLC1: Template RNA compenent of saccharomyces cerevisiae telomerase. *Science* 266: 404–409.

38. Mendelsohn J, Lippman ME (1993) Principles of molecular cell biology of cancer: growth factors. *In:* DeVita VT, Hellman S, Rosenberg SA (eds) *Cancer: principles and practice of oncology.* Philadelphia: J.B. Lippincott, pp 114–133.

39. Jetten AM (1991) Growth and differentiation factors in tracheobronchial epithelium. *Am J Physiol* 260: L361–L373.

40. Noguchi M, Murakami M, Bennett W, Lupu R, Hui F Jr, Harris CC, Gerwin BI (1993) Biological consequences of overexpression of a transfected c-erbB-2 gene in immortalized human bronchial epithelial cells. *Cancer Res* 53: 2035–2043.

41. Kern JA, Schwartz D, Nordberg JA, Weiner DB, Greene MI, Torney L, Robinson RA (1990) p185neu expression in human lung adenocarcinomas predicts shortened survival. *Cancer Res* 50: 5184–5191.

42. Pfeifer A, Lechner JF, Masui T, Reddel RR, Mark GE, Harris CC (1989) Control of growth and squamous differentiation in normal human bronchial epithelial cells by chemical and biological modifiers and transferred genes. *Environ Health Perspect* 80: 209–220.

43. Saunders NA, Smith RJ, Jetten AM (1993) Regulation of proliferation-specific and differentiation-specific genes during senescence of human epidermal keratinocyte and mammary epithelial cells. *Biochem Biophys Res Commun* 197: 46–54.

44. Massague J, Cheifetz S, Laiho M, Ralph DA, Weis FM, Zentella A (1992) Transforming growth factor-beta. *Cancer Surv* 12: 81–103.
45. Uchida K, Nagatake M, Osada H, Yatabe Y, Kondo M, Mitsudomi T, Masuda A, Takahashi T (1996) Somatic in vivo alterations of the JV18-1 gene at 18q21 in human lung cancers. *Cancer Res* 56: 5583–5585.
46. Hahn SA, Schutte M, Hoque AT, Moskaluk CA, da Costa LT, Rozenblum E, Weinstein CL, Fischer A, Yeo CJ, Hruban RH, et al. (1996) DPC4, a candidate tumor suppressor gene at human chromosome 18q21.1. [see comments]. *Science* 271: 350–353.
47. Vignaud JM, Marie B, Klein N, et al. (1994) The role of platelet-derived growth factor production by tumor-associated macrophages in tumor stroma formation in lung cancer. *Cancer Res* 54: 5455–5463.
48. Ishibashi M, Fujisawa M, Furue H, Maeda Y, Fukayama M, Yamaji T (1994) Inhibition of growth of human small cell lung cancer by bromocriptine. *Cancer Res* 54: 3442–3446.
49. Vahakangas KH, Samet JM, Metcalf RA, Welsh JA, Bennett WP, Lane DP, Harris CC (1992) Mutations of p53 and ras genes in radon-associated lung cancer from uranium miners. *Lancet* 339: 576–580.
50. Sozzi G, Miozzo M, Donghi R, Pilotti S, Cariani CT, Pastorino U, Della Porta G, Pierotti MA (1992) Deletions of 17p and p53 mutations in preneoplastic lesions of the lung. *Cancer Res* 52: 6079–6082.
51. Sundaresan V, Ganly P, Hasleton P, Rudd R, Sinha G, Bleehen NM, Rabbitts P (1992) p53 and chromosome 3 abnormalities, characteristic of malignant lung tumours, are detectable in preinvasive lesions of the bronchus. *Oncogene* 7: 1989–1997.
52. Li ZH, Zheng J, Weiss LM, Shibata D (1994) c-k-ras and p53 mutations occur very early in adenocarcinoma of the lung. *Am J Pathol* 144: 303–309.
53. Gazdar AF (1994) Molecular changes preceding the onset of invasive lung cancers. *Lung Cancer* 11: 16–17 (Abstract).
54. Nuorva K, Soini Y, Kamel D, Autio-Harmainen H, Risteli L, Risteli J, Vahakangas K, Paakko P (1993) Concurrent p53 expression in bronchial dysplasias and squamous cell lung carcinomas. *Am J Pathol* 142: 725–732.
55. Bennett WP, Colby TV, Vahakangas KH, Soini Y, Takeshima Y, Metcalf RA, Welsh JA, Borkowski A, Jones R, Trump BE, et al. (1993) p53 protein accumulates frequently in early bronchial neoplasia. *Cancer Res* 53: 4817–4822.
56. Walker C, Robertson LJ, Myskow MW, Pendleton N, Dixon GR (1994) p53 expression in normal and dysplastic bronchial epithelium and in lung carcinomas. *Br J Cancer* 70: 297–303.
57. Hirano T, Franzen B, Kato H, Ebihara Y, Auer G (1994) Genesis of squamous cell lung carcinoma. Sequential changes of proliferation, DNA ploidy, and p53 expression. *Am J Pathol* 144: 296–302.
58. Folkman J (1994) Angiogenesis and breast cancer [editorial; comment]. *J Clin Oncol* 12: 441–443.
59. Dameron KM, Volpert OV, Tainsky MA, Bouck N (1994) Control of angiogenesis in fibroblasts by p53 regulation of thrombospondin-1. *Science* 265: 1582–1584.
60. Zabrenetzky V, Harris CC, Steeg PS, Roberts DD (1994) Expression of the extracellular matrix molecule thrombospondin inversely correlates with malignant progression in melanoma, lung and breast carcinoma cell lines. *Int J Cancer* 58: 1–5.
61. Mukhopadhyay T, Tainsky M, Cavender AC, Roth JA (1991) Specific inhibition of K-ras expression and tumorigenicity of lung cancer cells by antisense RNA. *Cancer Res* 51: 1744–1748.
62. Takahashi T, Carbone D, Nau MM, Hida T, Linnoila I, Ueda R, Minna JD (1992) Wild-type but not mutant p53 suppresses the growth of human lung cancer cells bearing multiple genetic lesions. *Cancer Res* 52: 2340–2343.
63. Goyette MC, Cho K, Fasching CL, Levy DB, Kinzler KW, Paraskeva C, Vogelstein B, Stanbridge EJ (1992) Progression of colorectal cancer is associated with multiple tumor suppressor gene defects but inhibition of tumorigenicity is accomplished by correction of any single defect via chromosome transfer. *Molec Cell Biol* 12: 1387–1395.
64. Fujiwara T, Cai DW, Georges RN, Mukhopadhyay T, Grimm EA, Roth JA (1994) Therapeutic effect of a retroviral wild-type p53 expression vector in an orthotopic lung cancer model [see comments]. *J Natl Cancer Inst* 86: 1458–1462.

65. Osaki T, Tanio Y, Tachibana I, Hosoe S, Kumagai T, Kawase I, Oikawa S, Kishimoto T (1994) Gene therapy for carcinoembryonic antigen-producing human lung cancer cells by cell type-spcific expression of herpes simplex virus thymidine kinase gene. *Cancer Res* 54: 5258–5261.

66. Freeman SM, Abboud CN, Whartenby KA, Packman CH, Koeplin DS, Moolten FL, Abraham GN (1993) The bystander effect: tumor regression when a fraction of the tumor mass is genetically modified. *Cancer Res* 53: 5274–5283.

67. Fisher DE (1994) Apoptosis in cancer therapy: crossing the threshold. *Cell* 78: 539–542.

68. Wyllie AH (1993) Apoptosis (the 1992 Frank Rose Memorial Lecture). *Br J Cancer* 67: 205–208.

69. Symonds H, Krall L, Remington L, Saenz-Robles M, Lowe S, Jacks T, Van Dyke T (1994) p53-Dependent apoptosis suppresses tumor growth and progression in vivo. *Cell* 78: 703–711.

70. Maneckjee R, Minna JD (1994) Opioids induce while nicotine suppresses apoptosis in human lung cancer cells. *Cell Growth Differ* 5: 1033–1040.

71. Lowe SW, Schmitt EM, Smith SW, Osborne BA, Jacks T (1993) p53 is required for radiation-induced apoptosis in mouse thymocytes. *Nature* 362: 847–849.

72. Clarke AR, Purdie CA, Harrison DJ, Morris RG, Bird CC, Hooper ML, Wyllie AH (1993) Thymocyte apoptosis induced by p53-dependent and independent pathways. *Nature* 362: 849–852.

73. Wang XW, Yeh H, Schaeffer L, Roy R, Moncollin V, Egly JM, Wang Z, Friedberg EC, Evans MK, Taffe BG, et al. (1995) p53 Modulation of TFIIH-associated nucleotide excision repair activity. *Nature Genet* 10: 188–195.

74. Hickman JA (1992) Apoptosis induced by anticancer drugs. *Cancer Metastasis Rev* 11: 121–139.

75. Lowe SW, Ruley HE, Jacks T, Housman DE (1993) p53-dependent apoptosis modulates the cytotoxicity of anticancer agents. *Cell* 74: 957–967.

76. Fujiwara T, Grimm EA, Mukhopadhyay T, Zhang WW, Owen-Schaub LB, Roth JA (1994) Induction of chemosensitivity in human lung cancer cells in vivo by adenovirus-mediated transfer of the wild-type p53 gene. *Cancer Res* 54: 2287–2291.

77. Petty RD, Cree IA, Sutherland LA, Hunter EM, Lane DP, Preece PE, Andreotti PE (1994) Expression of the p53 tumour suppressor gene product is a determinant of chemosensitivity. *Biochem Biophys Res Commun* 199: 264–270.

78. Vitetta ES, Uhr JW (1994) Monoclonal antibodies as agonists: an expanded role for their use in cancer therapy. *Cancer Res* 54: 5301–5309.

Clinical and Biological Basis of Lung Cancer Prevention
ed. by Y. Martinet, F.R. Hirsch, N. Martinet, J.-M. Vignaud
and J.L. Mulshine
© 1998 Birkhäuser Verlag Basel/Switzerland

CHAPTER 11
Neuropeptides, Signal Transduction and Small Cell Lung Cancer

Michael J. Seckl [1,2] and Enrique Rozengurt [*,1]

[1] *Imperial Cancer Research Fund, London, UK*
[2] *Department of Medical Oncology, Charing Cross Hospital, London, UK*

Introduction

Small cell lung carcinoma (SCLC) constitutes 25% of all lung cancers and despite initial sensitivity to chemotherapy and radiotherapy has a 5 year survival of less than 5%. Consequently there is an urgent need to develop new therapies and this is most likely to arise from a better understanding of the biology of the disease. There is increasing evidence that multiple neuro-peptides including bombesin/GRP, vasopressin, galanin, gastrin, brady-kinin and neurotensin can act as autocrine/paracrine growth factors for SCLC cell lines. Therefore, elucidation of the signalling pathways that lead from neuropeptide receptors to the nucleus where mitogenesis is induced may provide important clues for developing new therapeutic strategies.

---

*   Author for correspondence.

Many studies to identify the molecular pathways by which neuropeptide mitogens elicit cellular growth have exploited cultured murine Swiss 3T3 cells as a model system [1, 2]. These cells cease to proliferate when they deplete the medium of its growth-promoting activity, and can be stimulated to reinitiate DNA synthesis and cell division by the addition of various growth factors in serum-free medium [12]. In particular, bombesin [14], vasopressin [15], bradykinin [16], vasoactive intestinal peptide [17], endothelin [18] and vasoactive intestinal contractor [19] can act as growth factors for cultured 3T3 cells. An important feature of mitogenic signalling which has emerged from these and other studies is that cell proliferation can be stimulated through multiple, independent signal transduction pathways which act in a synergistic and combinatorial fashion. In what follows, some fundamental features of the mechanism of action of bombesin and other neuropeptides as growth factors in 3T3 cells will be discussed and subsequently the evidence for multiple neuropeptide growth factor action in SCLC will be considered. The review will then focus on the development of substance SP analogue broad spectrum neuropeptide antagonists as a novel SCLC therapy.

2. Early Signaling Events Induced by Bombesin

The early cellular and molecular responses elicited by bombesin and structurally related peptides have been elucidated in detail in Swiss 3T3 cells (Figure 1). Bombesin is a 14 amino acid peptide first isolated from the skin of the frog *Bombina bombina* [3]. Many bombesin-related peptides have subsequently been isolated from various species and classified into the three subfamilies bombesin, ranatensin and litorin according to their C terminal hexapeptide sequence homology. The principal mammalian counterparts are GRP and neuromedin B, members of the bombesin and ranatensin subfamilies, respectively.

2.1 Inositol Phosphatidyl Turnover, Ca^{2+} Mobilization and Activation of Protein Kinase C

Binding of neuropeptides such as bombesin/GRP to their receptors initiates a cascade of intracellular signals culminating in DNA synthesis 10 to 15 hours later. The bombesin/GRP receptor like many other neuropeptide receptors [4, 5] belongs to the superfamily of heterotrimeric G protein-coupled receptors. These are characterized by seven transmembrane domains which are thought to cluster to form a ligand binding pocket [4–7]. One of the earliest events to occur after the binding of bombesin to its specific receptor is the activation of the heterotrimeric G protein $G\alpha q$, which in turn stimulates the phospholipase $C\beta$ (PLCβ) isoform of PLC. This catalyses the hydrolysis of phosphatidyl inositol 4,5-bisphosphate

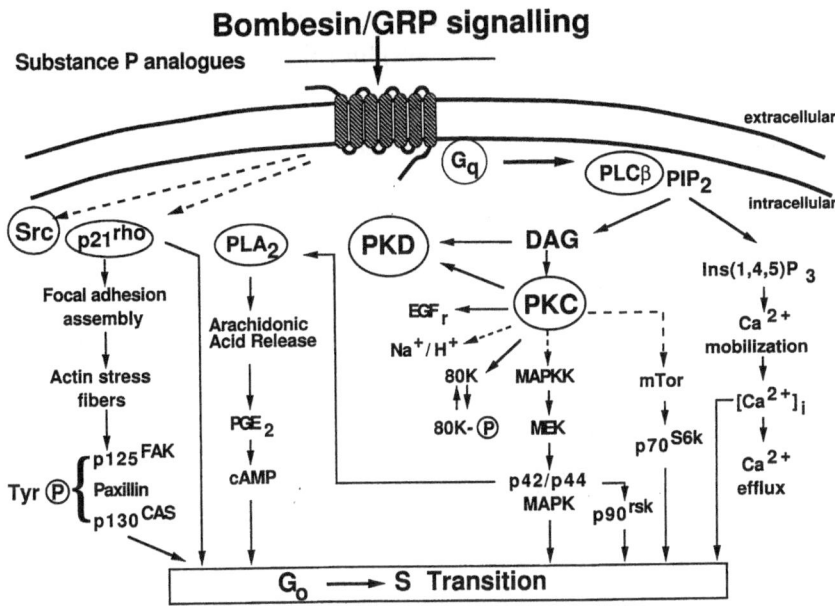

Figure 1. Bombesin-mediated signal transduction. Initiation of cell proliferation in Swiss 3T3 cells is stimulated by multiple signal transduction pathways that act in a synergistic and combinatorial fashion. The interactions have been well defined in these cells and provide experimental evidence for a model that involves multiple pathways. The mechanisms of action of neuropeptide growth factors are explained within the framework of this model. PLA$_2$, phospholipase A2; PLCβ, phospholipase Cβ; PIP$_2$, phosphatidylinositol 4,5-bisphosphate; DAG, diacylglycerol; p125^{FAK}, p125 focal adhesion kinase; MAPK, mitogen activated protein kinase, PGE$_2$, prostaglandin E$_2$; PKC, protein kinase C; PKD, protein kinase D; EGFr, epidermal growth factor receptor.

(PIP$_2$) in the plasma membrane to produce inositol 1,4,5-trisphosphate (IP$_3$) and 1,2-diacylglycerol (DG). IP$_3$ binds to a specific intracellular receptor which releases Ca^{2+} from internal stores [8]. Depletion of Ca^{2+} from internal stores (as induced by bombesin, other mitogenic neuropeptides and growth factors), could play a role as one of the synergistic signals that contribute to stimulating the transition from G$_0$ to DNA synthesis [9].

DAG, the other product of bombesin-induced PLC-mediated hydrolysis of PIP$_2$, directly activates protein kinase C (PKC) [10, 11]. In accordance with this, bombesin increases the phosphorylation of a major PKC substrate which is identical to myristolated alanine rich C kinase substrate and is termed 80K/MARCKS [12–15]. PKC activation induced by bombesin causes a translocation of 80K/MARCKS from the membrane to the cytosolic fraction [16] and a dramatic downregulation of the expression of mRNA and protein of the 80K/MARCKS substrate in Swiss 3T3 cells [14, 17, 18]. This result suggests that 80K/MARCKS, which appears to be a calmodulin- and actin-binding protein [19], may play a suppressor role in the control of cell proliferation. As shown in Figure 1, bombesin/GRP induces a variety of responses via PKC including the transmodulation of the epidermal growth factor (EGF) receptor [6].

2.2 Stimulation of Protein Kinase D by PKC

Protein kinase D (PKD) is a new cytosolic serine/threonine kinase that has been recently cloned [20]. It is distantly related to Ca^{2+}-regulated kinases but does not belong to any of the protein kinase subfamilies including PKC [21]. The sequence of PKD reveals several interesting structural motifs including a cysteine rich domain which binds DAG and phorbol esters [20, 22]. Indeed, DAG and phorbol esters directly stimulate PKD activity [20, 22]. The addition of serum or other growth factors including bombesin to living cells also stimulates PKD activation ([23] and unpublished observations). Interestingly, the pathway leading to the activation of PKD in living cells involves PKCs [23]. Thus PKD may function downsteam of PKCs in a novel signal transduction pathway.

2.3 Stimulation of Monovalent Ion Fluxes

The stimulation of the monovalent K^+, H^+ and Na^+ ion fluxes is a general early response seen in most types of quiescent cells stimulated to proliferate by multiple combinations of growth promoting factors (reviewed in [24]). Addition of bombesin and other neuropeptides to quiescent 3T3 cells also causes a rapid increase in the activity of the ouabain-sensitive Na^+/K^+ pump via PKC-dependent and independent pathways.

2.4 Stimulation of Mitogen-Activated Protein Kinase and Early Response Genes

Mitogen-activated protein (MAP) kinases are activated in response to a wide range of extracellular signals and are thought to play an important role in transducing growth signals. The two best characterized isoforms, p42^{MAPK} (ERK2) and p44^{MAPK} (ERK1) can be stimulated both by heterotrimeric G protein-linked receptors and receptors that possess intrinsic tyrosine kinase activity [25–27]. The pathway coupling receptor tyrosine kinases to the activation of MAP kinase is well understood and involves the stimulation of p21^{ras}, which activates an enzyme cascade consisting of Raf, MEK and finally MAP kinase [27]. In contrast, it is less clear how seven transmembrane domain receptors achieve activation of MP kinases. Bombesin stimulates MAP kinase and its upstream activating enzyme MEK via a PKC-dependent pathway without involving p21^{ras} or Raf in Swiss 3T3 cells [28–30]. However, in Rat-1 fibroblasts, 1-oleoyl-lyso-phosphatidic acid (LPA; like bombesin, signals via heterotrimeric G proteins), has been shown to activate MAP kinase via a Ras-dependent pathway which presumably involves Raf [31]. Similarly, both bombesin and neuromedin B induce MAPK activation via a Ras-dependent pathway in Rat-1 cells stably transfected with the respective receptors [32]. These data indicate that G protein-linked receptors may activate MAP kinase via separate pathways in different cells.

Bombesin and other neuropeptides rapidly and transiently induces the expression of the cellular oncogenes c-*fos* and c-*myc* in quiescent fibroblasts [33]. There is evidence implicating PKC activation in the sequence of events linking receptor occupancy and proto-oncogene induction [33]. Accordingly, bombesin-induced oncogene expression is markedly reduced by downregulation of PKC. As mentioned above, PKC activation leads to the activation of MAP kinase, which directly phosphorylates transcription factor regulators resulting in the increased expression of c-*fos* [26, 34].

2.5 Arachidonic Acid Release and Prostaglandin Synthesis: Differential Effects of Bombesin and Vasopressin

While bombesin and GRP stimulate DNA synthesis in the absence of other factors, vasopressin is mitogenic for Swiss 3T3 cells only in synergistic combination with other factors [35, 36]. Comparison of the early signal transduction events elicited by vasopressin with those of bombesin has shown that although most events appear identical there is at least one fundamental difference. Bombesin, but not vasopressin, induces a marked biphasic release of arachidonic acid into the extracellular medium [37, 38]. The arachidonic acid release by bombesin is likely to contribute to bombesin-induced mitogenesis because: (1) externally applied arachidonic acid potentiates mitogenesis induced by agents that stimulate polyphosphoinositide breakdown but not arachidonic acid release (e. g. vasopressin) [37]; (2) arachidonic acid released by bombesin is converted into E type prostaglandins which elevate intracellular levels of cyclic adenosine monophosphate (cAMP), which is a mitogenic signal for Swiss 3T3 cells (see Figure 1 and [39, 40]).

2.6 Bombesin Stimulation of Tyrosine Phosphorylation: Focal Adhesion Kinase (p125 FAK), Paxillin and p130 cas; Cytoskeletal Link

Although neuropeptide receptors do not possess intrinsic tyrosine kinase activity, they rapidly increase tyrosine phosphorylation of multiple substrates in quiescent Swiss 3T3 cells [41, 42]. These substrates include the focal adhesion-associated proteins p125 focal adhesion kinase (FAK), paxillin, p130cas and pp60src [43–46]. FAK is a cytosolic tyrosine kinase that is also tyrosine phosphorylated in response to other agents that regulate cell growth and differentiation, including bioactive lipids, growth factors and ligands of the integrin family [43, 47–51]. Thus, FAK appears to be a point of convergence in the action of multiple extracellular signals and could be involved in the regulation of cell shape, adhesion, growth and motility [47, 51, 52]. Furthermore, FAK may play a role in tumour metastasis formation and proliferation.

At present, it is unclear how neuropeptide receptors couple to tyrosine phosphorylation. Stimulation of FAK, paxillin and p130^{cas} tyrosine phosphorylation by bombesin and other neuropeptides is independent of PKC activation, Ca^{2+}-mobilization [43–45] and PI3 kinase activity [53]. Disruption of the actin cytoskeleton with cytochalasin D or high concentrations of platelet-derived growth factor (PDGF) blocks tyrosine phosphorylation. Furthermore, *Clostridium botulinum* toxin which specifically inactivates the small GTP binding Ras-related protein, p21^{rho}, blocks neuropeptide-induced actin cytoskeletal rearrangements and the induction of tyrosine phosphorylation [44, 54–56]. Thus, p21^{rho} is likely to mediate neuropeptide-induced tyrosine phosphorylation. This pathway appears to be distinct from that leading to MAPK activation in response to bombesin [57].

Neuropeptides also induce a rapid and transient activation of another cytosolic tyrosine kinase, pp60^{src} that is not dependent on either PLCβ-mediated pathways or the integrity of the actin cytoskeleton [46]. Hence, there appear to be two distinct pathways leading from the bombesin receptor to tyrosine kinase activation which are either dependent (FAK) or independent of the actin cytoskeleton (pp60^{src}).

The importance of tyrosine phosphorylation in neuropeptide mitogenic signalling has been investigated. The tyrphostins selectively inhibit tyrosine kinases and provide potential antiproliferative agents that block cell division through a novel mechanism [58]. In Swiss 3T3 cells, tyrphostin inhibits both bombesin stimulation of tyrosine phosphorylation, including FAK, and bombesin-induced DNA synthesis over a similar concentration range, suggesting that tyrosine phosphorylation may play a role in bombesin-mediated mitogenesis [59].

2.7 The Bombesin/GRP Receptor Transfected into Rat-1 Cells Couples to Multiple Pathways

It has been suggested that each of the signalling pathways elicited by bombesin (Figure 1) emanate form different bombesin receptor isoforms; in this way one bombesin receptor subtype may couple to tyrosine phosphorylation while another may couple to the PLCβ pathway [60]. However, a single bombesin receptor subtype transfected into Rat-1 cells can couple to multiple signaling pathways including Ca^{2+} mobilization,

80K/ MARCKS phosphorylation and tyrosine phosphorylation of FAK and paxillin [61]. The conclusion that a single receptor of the bombesin-like receptor family is linked to multiple intracellular pathways is further substantiated by similar results obtained with the transfected neuromedin B receptor in Rat-1 cells [62].

3. Neuropeptides and Small Cell Lung Carcinoma

The growth promoting effects of neuropeptides, and the elucidation of the signalling pathways that mediate their effects, assume an added importance since multiple neuropeptides may play a role in sustaining the proliferation of cancer cells. Indeed, bombesin/GRP has been implicated in carcinomas form lung, colon, prostate and breast. Interestingly, the neurosecretory granules of SCLC cells are now know to contain many different peptide growth factors [63–71]. In what follows, recent evidence implicating neuropeptide mediated proliferation in SCLC and the use of SP analogue broad spectrum neuropeptide antagonists as potential anticancer agents will be discussed.

3.1 Ca^{2+}-Mobilization in SCLC Cell Lines

Studies with SCLC have demonstrated that GRP stimulates mobilization of intracellular Ca^{2+} and inositol phosphate turnover in SCLC cells. These early events are similar to those previously elucidated in murine 3T3 cells (Figure 1). Subsequent work has shown that multiple neuropeptides including vasopressin, bradykinin, neurotensin, galanin, cholecystokinin and gastrin stimulate IP_3 production and/or Ca^{2+} mobilization in different SCLC cell lines [72–77]. The Ca^{2+}-mobilizing effects are mediated by distinct receptors, as shown by the use of specific antagonists and by the induction of homologous desensitization [72–75]. Collectively, these studies indicate that SCLC cells express many different neuropeptide receptors which are coupled to the mobilization of Ca^{2+}. Furthermore, the expression of these receptors is heterogeneous among SCLC cell lines.

3.2 Neuropeptides Stimulate MAPK Activation, Arachidonic Acid Mobilization and Tyrosine Phosphorylation in SCLC Cells

Several recent studies have revealed that human SCLC cells exhibit other early signalling pathways that are very similar to those induced by neuropeptides in Swiss 3T3 cells (Figure 1). SCLC cells express multiple diacylglycerol and phorbol ester-sensitive PKCs, including α, β, δ, and ε [78].

Activation of PKCs by phorbol esters has been demonstrated to stimulate MAP kinase and p90[rsk] activation [79], growth and transcription of GRP mRNA in SCLC cells [78]. Just as in Swiss 3T3 cells, PKC mediates both MAP kinase and p90[rsk] activation by neuropeptides in SCLC cells [79]. Furthermore, neuropeptides have been shown to cause rapid mobilization of arachidonic acid [80] and induction of tyrosine phosphorylation of multiple substrates migrating with an apparent Mr very similar to that seen in Swiss 3T3 cells [81].

3.3 Multiple Neuropeptides Stimulate Clonal Growth in SCLC Cells

In view of these findings, it has been hypothesized that SCLC growth is regulated by multiple autocrine and/or paracrine circuits involving Ca^{2+}-mobilizing neuropeptides [72–75, 82]. In accord with this hypothesis, multiple Ca^{2+}-mobilizing neuropeptides interact with specific receptors to promote the growth of different SCLC cell lines in semisolid medium in a dose-dependent fashion [73, 75, 82]. Furthermore, many of the peptides are produced by the SCLC cells or in adjacent tissues [63–71]. Thus, multiple Ca^{2+}-mobilizing neuropeptides, via distinct receptors, can act directly as growth factors for SCLC. Approaches designed to block SCLC growth must take into account this mitogenic complexity.

3.4 Blocking the Action of Multiple Neuropeptides: Broad Spectrum Antagonists

It follows from this discussion that antagonists capable of blocking the biological effects of multiple neuropeptides (i.e. broad spectrum neuropeptide antagonists) could provide an effective approach in the treatment of SCLC.

The substance P (SP) analogue [DArg[1], DPro[2], DTrp[7, 9], Leu[11]] SP (Table 1) provided the first clue that broad spectrum neuropeptide inhibition was possible. This analogue not only blocked the actions of SP but also inhibited the secretory effects of bombesin on a pancreatic cell preparation [83]. It was subsequently found to block ^{125}I-GRP binding, some bombesin-stimulated early signalling events, and mitogenesis in Swiss 3T3 cells [11, 33, 84–86]. It did not affect mitogenesis stimulated by polypeptide

Table 1. Comparative structures of bombesin, SP and some SP analogues

Bombesin	pGlu-Gln-Arg-Leu-Gly-Asn-Gln-Trp-Ala-Val-Gly-His-Leu-Met-NH$_2$
Substance P	Arg-Pro-Lys-Pro-Gln-Gln-Phe-Phe-Gly-Leu-Met-NH$_2$
Substance P	DArg-DPro-Lys-Pro-Gln-Gln-DTrp-Phe-DTrp-Leu-Leu-NH$_2$
Analogues	DArg-Pro-Lys-Pro-DPhe-Gln-DTrp-Phe-DTrp-Leu-Leu-NH$_2$
	DArg-Pro-Lys-Pro-DTrp-Gln-DTrp-Phe-DTrp-Leu-Leu-NH$_2$
	Arg-DTrg-MePhe-DTrp-Leu-Met-NH$_2$

growth factors, such as EGF and PDGF [84], but it was found to block vasopressin-stimulated mitogenesis [87]. Further SP analogues were therefore synthesized in order to clarify their mechanism of action and identify more potent antagonists that could be tested in SCLC [87–91].

Several interesting compounds were found and some are shown in Table 1. [Arg^6, DTrp$^{7, 9}$, MePhe^8]SP(6–11), [DArg^1, DPhe^5, DTrp$^{7, 9}$, Leu^{11}]SP and [DArg^1, DTrp$^{5, 7, 9}$, Leu^{11}]SP have been extensively investigated. All three inhibit signal transduction and DNA synthesis stimulated by bombesin, GRP, vasopressin and bradykinin by preventing agonist receptor binding in a reversible fashion [88–92]. However, the antagonists neither block DNA synthesis by PDGF, which stimulates Ca^{2+} mobilization through a different mechanism from neuropeptides (i.e. mediated by tyrosine phosphorylation rather than by a G protein), nor inhibit mitogenesis stimulated by vasoactive intestinal peptide, which induces cyclic AMP accumulation without Ca^{2+} mobilization [88–90]. Thus, the SP antagonist showed broad spectrum specificity against the neuropeptide mitogenes bombesin/GRP, vasopressin, bradykinin and endothelin, which act through distinct receptors in Swiss 3T3 cells but activate common signal transduction pathways (e.g. Figure 1). The facts that neuropeptide ligand binding is competitively inhibited, all downstream signalling events are reversibly blocked and that G protein activation is not independently affected by these SP analogues strongly indicates that they act at the receptor level [88–90, 92]. This hypothesis is supported by the fact that a deletion mutant of [DArg^1, DPhe^5, DTrp$^{7, 9}$, Leu^{11}]SP analogue lacking the terminal Leu loses its inhibitory effect against bombesin but not vasopressin-induced signal transduction and mitogenesis [90]. Nevertheless, the precise mechanism by which SP analogues inhibit the action of Ca^{2+}-mobilizing neuropeptides remains to be defined.

The compounds characterized as broad spectrum antagonists in Swiss 3T3 cells were tested as inhibitors of neuropeptide-mediated signals and growth in SCLC cell lines. The broad spectrum antagonists inhibited Ca^{2+} mobilization stimulated by GRP, vasopressin, bradykinin, CCK and galanin in diverse cell lines [73, 89, 91] and inhibited the growth of SCLC cell lines in liquid and semisolid media [73, 89, 91, 93, 94]. Moreover, the antagonists inhibited the growth SCLC tumours *in vivo* and the inhibitory effect was clearly maintained beyond the duration of administration [91, 94]. These results demonstrate that SP analogue broad spectrum neuropeptide antagonists may be of interest as a novel SCLC therapy. Indeed, on the basis of these and other studies, one of the SP analogues is now in a Phase I clinical study.

4. Conclusions

Neuropeptides are increasingly implicated in the control of cell proliferation and their mechanisms of action are attracting intense interest.

The peptides of the bombesin family, including GRP, bind to specific surface receptors and initiate a complex cascade of signalling events (Figure 1) that culminates in the stimulation of DNA synthesis and cell division in Swiss 3T3 cells in the absence of other growth promoting factors. These peptides also act as autocrine growth factors for certain SCLC cells. The results discussed here strongly suggest that multiple Ca^{2+}-mobilizing neuropeptides drive SCLC growth in an autocrine/paracrine fashion. Consequently, broad spectrum neuropeptide inhibitors that prevent the function of multiple Ca^{2+}-mobilizing receptors are of special interest. Indeed, certain SP analogues block neuropeptide-mediated signals in the 3T3 and SCLC cells and inhibit SCLC growth *in vitro* and *in vivo*. Thus, broad spectrum neuropeptide antagonists constitute potential anticancer agents.

References

1. Rozengurt E (1985) The mitogenic response of cultured 3T3 cells: integration of early signals and synergistic effects in a unified framework. *In:* Cohen P, Houslay M (ed.). *Molecular mechanisms of transmembrane signalling,* Elsevier, Amsterdam, pp 429–452.
2. Rozengurt E (1986) Early signals in the mitogenic response. *Science* 234: 161–166.
3. Anastasi A, Erspamer V, Bucci M (1971) Isolation and structure of bombesin and alytesin, two analogous active peptides form the skin of the European amphibians Bombina and Alytes. *Experientia* 27: 166–167.
4. Spindel ER, Giladi E, Brehm P, Goodman RJ, Segerson TP (1990) Cloning and functional characterization of complementary DNA encoding the murine fibroblast bombesin/gastrin-releasing peptide receptor. *Molec Endocrinol* 4: 1956–1963.
5. Battey JF, Way JM, Corjay MH, Shapira H, Kusario K, Harkins R, Wu JM, Slattery T, Mann E, Feldman RI(1991) Molecular cloning of the bombesin/GRP receptor from Swiss 3T3 cells. *Proc Natl Acad Sci USA* 88: 395–399.
6. Rozengurt E, Sinnett-Smith J (1990) Bombesin stimulation of fibroblast mitogenesis: specific receptors, signal transduction and early events. *Philos Trans R Soc Lond B Biol Sci* 327: 209–221.
7. Strosberg AD (1991) Structure/function relationship of proteins belonging to the family of receptors coupled to GTP-binding proteins. *Eur J Biochem* 196: 1–10.
8. Berridge MJ (1995) Inositol phosphate and calcium signalling. *Ann NY Acad Sci* 766: 31–43.
9. Charlesworth A, Rozengurt E (1994) Thapsigargin and di-*tert*-butylhydroquinone induce synergistic stimulation of DNA synthesis with phorbol ester and bombesin in Swiss 3T3 cells. *J Biol Chem* 269: 32528–32535.
10. Nishizuka Y (1988) The molecular heterogeneity of protein kinase C and its implications for cellular regulation. *Nature* 334: 661–665.
11. Erusalimsky J, Friedberg I, Rozengurt E (1988) Bombesin, diacylglycerol, and phorbol esters rapidly stimulate the phosphorylation of an Mr = 80,000 protein kinase C substrate in permiablized 3T3 cells. *J Biol Chem* 263: 19188–19194.
12. Rozengurt E, Rodriguez-Pena A, Smit KA (1983) Phorbol esters, phospholipase C, and growth factors rapidly stimulate the phosphorylation of a Mr 80,000 protein in intact quiescent 3T3 cells. *Proc Natl Acad Sci USA* 80: 7224–7248.
13. Erusalimsky JD, Brooks SF, Herget T, Morris C, Rozengurt E (1991) Molecular cloning and characterization of the acidic 80-kda protein kinase c substrate from rat brain identification as a glycoprotein. *J Biol Chem* 266: 7072–7080.
14. Brooks SF, Herget T, Erusalimsky JD, Rozengurt E (1991) Protein kinase C activation potentially down-regulates the expression of its major substrate 80K, in Swiss 3T3 cells. *EMBO J* 10: 2497–2505.

15. Herget T, Brooks SF, Broad S, Rozengurt E (1992) Relationship between the major protein kinase C substrates acidic 80-kDa protein-kinase-C substrate (80K) and myristoylated alanine-rich C-kinase substrate (MARCKS). *Eur J Biochem* 209: 7–14.
16. Herget T, Broad S, Rozengurt E (1994) Overexpression of the myristoylated alanine-rich C-kinase substrate in Rat1 cells increases sensitivity to calmodulin antagonists. *Eur J Biochem* 225: 549–556.
17. Brooks S, Herget T, Broad S, Rozengurt E (1992) The expression of 80K/MARCKS, a major substrate of KPC, is down-regulated through both PKC-dependent and -independent pathways. *J Biol Chem* 267: 14212–14218.
18. Herget T, Brooks SF, Borad S, Rozengurt E (1993) Expression of the major protein kinase C substrate, the acidic 80-kilodalton myristoylated alanine-rich C kinase substrate, increases sharply when Swiss 3T3 cells move out of cycle and enter G_0. *Proc Natl Acad Sci USA* 909: 2945–2949.
19. Blackshear PJ (1993) The MARCKS family of cellular protein kinase C substrates. *J Biol Chem* 268: 1501–1504.
20. Valverde AM, Sinnett-Smith J, Van Lint J, Rozengurt E (1994) Molecular cloning and characterization of proteinkinase D: a target for diacylglycerol and phorbol esters with a distinctive catalytic domain. *Proc Natl Acad Sci USA* 91: 8572–8576.
21. Rozengurt E, Sinnett-Smith J, Van Lint J, Valverde AM (1995) Protein kinase D (PKD): a novel target for diacylglycerol and phorbol esters. *Mutat Res* 333: 153–160.
22. Van Lint J, Sinnett-Smith J, Rozengurt E (1995) Expression and characterization of PKD, a phorbol-ester and diacylglycerol-stimulated serine protein kinase. *J Biol Chem* 270: 1455–1461.
23. Zugaza JL, Sinnett-Smith J, Van Lint J, Rozengurt E (1996) Protein kinase D (PKD) activation in intact cells through a proteinkinase C-dependent signal transduction pathway. *EMBO J* 15: 6220–6230.
24. Rozengurt E, Mendoza SA (1986) Early stimulation of Na^+/H^+ antiport, Na^+/K^+ pump activity and Ca^{2+} fluxes in fibroblast mitogenesis. *In:* Mandel I, Benos D (eds): *Current topics in membranes and transport,* vol 27, Academic Press, San Diego, pp 163–191.
25. Crews CM, Erikson RL (1993) Extracellular signals and reversible protein phosphorylation: what to Mek of it all. *Cell* 74: 215–217.
26. Davis R (1993) The mitogen-activated protein kinase signal transduction pathway. *J Biol Chem* 268: 14553–14556.
27. Marshall CJ (1995) Specificity of receptor tyrosine kinase signaling: transient versus sustained extracellular signal-regulated kinase action. *Cell* 80: 179–185.
28. Pang L, Decker SJ, Saltiel AR (1993) Bombesin and epidermal growth factor stimulate the mitogen-activated protein kinase through different pathways in Swiss 3T3 cells. *Biochem J* 289: 283–287.
29. Mitchell FM, Heasley LE, Quian N-X, Zamarripa J, Johnson GL (1995) Differential modulation of Bombesin-stimulated phospholipase Cβ and mitogen-activated protein kinase activity by [D-Arg¹, D-Phe⁵, D-Trp⁷,⁹, Leu¹¹] substance P. *J Biol Chem* 270: 8623–8628.
30. Seufferlein T, Withers DJ, Rozengurt E (1996) Reduced requirement of MAPK activity for entry into the S phase of the cell cycle in Swiss 3T3 fibroblasts stimulated by bombesin and insulin. *J Biol Chem* 271: 21471–21477.
31. Cook S, Rubinfeld B, Albert I, McCormick F (1993) RapV12 antagonizes Ras-dependent activation of ERK1 and ERK2 by LPA and EGF in Rat-12 fibroblasts. *EMBO J* 12: 3475–3485.
32. Charlesworth A, Rozengurt E (1997) Bombesin and neuromedin B stimulate the activation of p42ᵐᵃᵏ and p74ʳᵃᶠ⁻¹ via a protein kinase C-independent pathway. *Oncogene* (in press).
33. Rozengurt E, Sinnett-Smith J (1988) Early signals underlying the induction of the proto-oncogenes c-fos and c-myc in quiescent fibroblasts: studies with peptides of the bombesin family and other growth factors. *Prog Nucleic Acid Res Mol Biol* 35: 261–295.
34. Treisman R (1992) The serum response element. *TIBS* 17: 423–426.
35. Rozengurt E, Legg A, Pettican P (1979) Vasopressin stimulation of mouse 3T3 cell growth. *Proc Natl Acad Sci USA* 76: 1284–1287.
36. Rozengurt E, Sinnett-Smith J (1983) Bombesin stimulation of DNA synthesis and cell division in cultures of Swiss 3T3 cells. *Proc Natl Acad Sci USA* 80: 2936–2940.
37. Millar JB, Rozengurt E (1990) Chronic desensitization to bombesin by progressive down-regulation of bombesin receptors in Swiss 3T3 cells: distinction from acute desensitization. *J Biol Chem* 265: 12052–12058.

38. Domin J, Rozengurt E (1993) Platelet-derived growth factor stimulates a biphasic mobilization of arachidonic acid in Swiss 3T3 cells. The role of phospholipase A_2. *J Biol Chem*

39. Rozengurt E (1995) Polypeptide and neuropeptide growth factors: signalling pathways and role in cancer. *In:* Peckham M, Pinedo H, Veronesi U (eds): *The Oxford Textbook of Oncology,* Oxford University Press, pp 12–20.

40. Withers DJ, Bloom SR, Rozengurt E (1995) Dissociation of cAMP-stimulated mitogenesis from activation of the mitogen-activated protein kinase cascade in Swiss 3T3 cells. *J Biol Chem* 270: 21411–21419.

41. Zachary I, Gil J, Lehmann W, Sinnett-Smith J, Rozengurt E (1991) Bombesin, vasopressin and endothelin rapidly stimulate phosphorylation in intact Swiss 3T3 cells. *Proc Natl Acad Sci USA* 88: 4577–4581.

42. Zachary I, Sinnett-Smith J, Rozengurt E (1991) Stimulation of tyrosine kinase activity in anti-phosphotyrosine immune complexes of Swiss 3T3 cell lysates occurs rapidly after addition of bombesin, vasopressin, and endothelin to intact cells. *J Biol Chem* 266: 24126–24133.

43. Zachary I, Sinnett-Smith J, Turner CE, Rozengurt E (1993) Bombesin, vasopressin, and endothelin rapidly stimulate tyrosine phosphorylation of the focal adhesion-associated protein paxillin in Swiss 3T3 cells. *J Biol Chem* 268: 22060–22065.

44. Sinnett-Smith J, Zachary I, Valverde AM, Rozengurt E (1993) Bombesin stimulation of p125 focal adhesion kinase tyrosine phosphorylation: Role of protein kinase C, Ca^{2+} mobilization and the actin cytoskeleton. *J Biol Chem* 268: 14261–14268.

45. Casamassima A, Rozengurt E (1997) Tyrosine phosphorylation of p130[cas] by bombesin, lysophosphatidic acid, phorbol esters and PDGF: signalling pathways and formation of p130[cas]-Crk complex. *J Biol Chem* 272: 9363–9370.

46. Rodriquez-Fernandez JL, Rozengurt E (1996) Bombesin, bradykinin, vasopressin and phorbol esters rapidly and transiently activate src family tyrosine kinases in Swiss 3T3 cells. *J Biol Chem* 271: 27895–27901.

47. Zachary I, Rozengurt E (1992) Focal Adhesion Kinase (p125[FAK]): A point of convergence in the action of neuropeptides, integrins and oncogenes. *Cell* 71: 891–894.

48. Rankin S, Rozengurt E (1994) Platelet-derived growth factor modulation of focal adhesion kinase (p125[FAK]) and paxillin tyrosine phosphorylation in Swiss 3T3 cells. *J Biol Chem* 269: 704–710.

49. Seufferlein T, Rozengurt E (1994) Lysophosphatidic acid stimulates tyrosine phosphorylation of focal adhesion kinase, paxillin and p130: signalling pathways and crosstalk with platelet-derived growth factor. *J Biol Chem* 269: 9345–9351.

50. Seufferlein T, Rozengurt E (1994) Sphingosine induces p125[FAK] and paxillin tyrosine phosphorylation, actin stress fiber formation, and focal contact assembly in Swiss 3T3 cells. *J Biol Chem* 269: 27610–27617.

51. Rozengurt E (1995) Convergent signaling in the action of integrins, neuropeptides, growth factors and oncogenes. *Cancer Surveys* 24: 81–96.

52. Llic D, Furuta Y, Kanazawa S, Takeda N, Sobue K, Nakatsuji N, Nomura S, Fujimoto J, Okada M, Yamamoto T (1995) Enhanced focal adhesion contact formation in cells from FAK-deficient mice. *Nature* 377: 539–544.

53. Rankin S, Hosshmand-Rad R, Claesson-Welsh L, Rozengurt E (1996) Requirement for phosphatidylinositol 3'-kinase activity in platelet-derived growth factor-stimulated tyrosine phosphorylation of p125 focal adhesion kinase and paxillin. *J Biol Chem* 271: 7829–7834.

54. Ridley AJ, Hall A (1992) The small GTP-binding protein rho regulates the assembly of focal adhesions and actin stress fibers in response to growth factors. *Cell* 70: 389–399.

55. Rankin S, Morii N, Narumiya S, Rozengurt E (1994) Botulinum C3 exoenzyme blocks the tyrosine phosphorylation of p125[FAK] and paxillin induced by bombesin and endothelin. *FEBS Letters* 354: 315–319.

56. Seckl MJ, Morii N, Narumiya S, Rozengurt E (1995) GTPγS stimulates tyrosine phosphorylation of p125[FAK] and paxillin in permeabilized Swiss 3T3 cells: role of *rho* p[21]. *J Biol Chem* 270: 6984–6990.

57. Seufferlein T, Withers DJ, Mann D, Rozengurt E (1996) Dissociation of mitogen-activated protein kinase activation from p125 focal adhesion kinase tyrosine phosphorylation in Swiss 3T3 cells stimulated by bombesin, lysophosphatidic acid, and platelet-derived growth factor. *Molec Biol Cell* 1865–1875.

58. Levitzki A (1992) Tyrphostins: tyrosine kinase blockers as novel antiproliferative agents and dissectors of signal transduction. *FASEB J* 6: 3275–3282.
59. Seckl MJ, Rozengurt E (1993) Tyrphostin inhibits bombesin stimulation of tyrosine phosphorylation, c-fos expression and DNA synthesis in Swiss 3T3 cells. *J Biol Chem* 268: 9548–9554.
60. Bold RJ, Lowry PS, Ishizuka J, Battey JF, Townsend CM Jr., Thompson JC (1994) Bombesin stimulates the in vitro growth of a human gastric cancer cell line. *J Cell Physiol* 161: 519–525.
61. Charlesworth A, Broad S, Rozengurt E (1996) The bombesin/GRP receptor transfected into Rat-1 fibroblasts couples to phospholipase C activation, tyrosine phosphorylation of p125^{FAK} and paxillin and cell proliferation. *Oncogene* 12: 1337–1345.
62. Lach EB, Borad S, Rozengurt E (1995) Mitogenic signaling by transfected Neuromedin B receptors in Rat-1 cells. *Cell Growth Diff* 6: 1427–1435.
63. Sorenson GD, Pettengill OS, Brimk-Johnsen T, Cate CC, Maurer LH (1981) Hormone production by cultures of small-cell carcinoma of the lung. *Cancer* 47: 1289–1296.
64. Maurer LH (1985) Ectopic hormone syndrome in small cell carcinoma of the lung. *Oncology* 4: 1289–1296.
65. Wood SM, Wood JR, Ghatei MA, Lee YC, O'Shaughnessy D, Bloom SR (1981) Bombesin, somatostatin and neurotensin-like immunoreactivity in bronchial carcinoma. *J Clin Endocrinol Metab* 53: 1310–1312.
66. North WG, Maurer LH, Valtin H, O'Donnell JF (1980) Human neurophysins as potential tumour markers for small cell lung carcinoma of the lung: application of specific radioimununoassays. *J Clin Endocrinol Metab* 51: 892–896.
67. Gazdar AF, Carney DN (1984) Endocrine properties of small cell lung carcinoma of the lung. *In:* WB Saunders (ed.) *The endocrine lung in health and disease,* Becker KI, Philadelphia, pp 501–508.
68. Goedert M, Reeve JG, Emson PC, Bleehen NM (1984) Neurotensin in human small cell lung cancer. *Br J Cancer* 50: 179–183.
69. Sausville E, Carney D, Battey J (1985) The human vasopressin gene is linked to the oxytoxin gene and is selectively expressed in a cultured lung cancer cell line. *J Biol Chem* 260: 10236–10241.
70. Cuttitta F, Carney DN, Mulshine J, Moody TW, Fedorko J, Fischler A, Minna JD (1985) Bombesin like peptides can function as autocrine growth factors in human small cell lung cancer. *Nature* 316: 823–826.
71. Mahmoud S, Staley J, Taylor J, Bogden A, Moreau J-P, Coy D, Avis I, Cuttitta F, Mulshine JL, Moody TW (1991) [Psi13, 14] bombesin analogues inhibit growth of small cell lung cancer *in vitro* and *in vivo*. *Cancer Res* 51: 1798–1802.
72. Woll PJ, Rozengurt E (1989) Multiple neuropeptides mobilize calcium in small cell lung cancer: effects of vasopressin, bradykinin, cholecystokinin, galanin and neurotensin. *Biophys Biochem Res Commun* 164: 66–73.
73. Sethi T, Rozengurt E (1991) Galanin stimulates Ca^{2+} mobilization, inositol phosphate accumulation, and clonal growth in small cell lung cancer cells. *Cancer Res* 51: 1674–1679.
74. Sethi T, Rozengurt E (1992) Gastrin stimulates Ca^{2+} mobilization and clonal growth in small cell lung cancer cells. *Cancer Res* 52: 6031–6035.
75. Sethi T, Herget T, Wu SV, Walsh JH, Rozengurt E (1993) CCKA and CCKB receptors are expressed in small cell lung cancer lines and mediate Ca^{2+} mobilization and clonal growth. *Cancer Res* 53: 5208–5213.
76. Bunn PA, Dienhart DG, Chan D, Puck TT, Tagawa M, Jewett PB, Braunschweiger E (1990) Neuropeptide stimulation of calcium flux in human lung cancer cells: delineation of alternative pathways. *Proc Natl Acad Sci USA* 87: 2162–2166.
77. Bunn PA, Chan D, Dienhart DG, Tolley R, Tagawa M, Jewett PB (1992) Neuropeptide signal transduction in lung cancer: clinical implications of bradykinin sensitivity and overall heterogeneity. *Cancer Res* 52: 24–31.
78. Jones CLA, Beck LK, Brozna JP, Holley M, Dempsey EJ, Kane MA (1995) Properties of classic protein kinase C in human small cell lung carcinoma NCl-H 345 cells. *Cell Growth and Diff* 6: 1627–1634.
79. Seufferlein T, Rozengurt E (1996) Galanin, neurotensin and phorbol esters rapidly stimulate activation of mitogen activated protein kinase in small cell lung cancer cells. *Cancer Res* 56: 5758–5764.

80. Avis IM, Jett M, Boyle T, Vos MD, Moody T, Treston AM, Martinez A, Mulshine JL (1996) Growth control of lung cancer by interruption of 5-lipoxygenase-mediated growth factor signaling. *J Clin Invest* 97: 806–813.
81. Tallett A, Chilvers ER, Hannah S, Dransfield I, Lawson MF, Haslett C, Sethi T (1996) Inhibition of neuropeptide-stimulated tyrosine phosphorylation and tyrosine kinase activity stimulates apoptosis in small cell lung cancer cells. *Cancer Res* 56: 4255– 4263.
82. Sethi T, Rozengurt E (1991) Multiple neuropeptides stimulate clonal growth of small cell lung cancer: effects of bradykinin, vasopressin, cholecystokinin, galanin, and neurotensin. *Cancer Res* 51: 3621–3623.
83. Jenson RT, Jones SW, Folkers K, Gardner JD (1984) A synthetic peptide that is a bombesin receptor antagonist. *Nature* 309: 61–63.
84. Zachary I, Rozengurt E (1985) High affinity receptors for the bombesin family in Swiss 3T3 cells. *Proc Natl Acad Sci* 82: 7616–7620.
85. Sinnett-Smith J, Lehmann W, Rozengurt E (1990) Bombesin receptor in membranes from Swiss 3T3 cells. *Biochem J* 265: 80–84.
86. Mendoza SA, Schneider JA, Lopez-Rivas A, Sinnett-Smith JW, Rozengurt E (1986) Early events elicited by bombesin and structurally related peptides in quiescent Swiss 3T3 cells. II. Changes in Na^+ and Ca^{2+} fluxes, Na^+/K^+ pump activity and intracellular pH. *J Cell Biol* 102: 2223–2233.
87. Zachary I, Rozengurt E (1986) A substance P antagonist also inhibits the specific binding of vasopressin and bombesin-related peptides in Swiss 3T3 cells. *Biochem Biophys Res Commun* 137: 135–141.
88. Woll PJ, Rozengurt E (1988) [D-Arg^1, D-Phe^5, D-Trp^{7,9}, Leu^{11}] Substance P, a potent bombesin antagonist in murine Swiss 3T3 cells, inhibits the growth of small cell lung cancer cells *in vitro*. *Proc Natl Acad Sci USA* 85: 1859–1863.
89. Woll PJ, Rozengurt E (1990) A neuropeptide antagonist that inhibits the growth of small cell lung cancer *in vitro*. *Cancer Res* 50: 3968–3973.
90. Seckl MJ, Higgins TE, Rozengurt E (1996) [DArg^1, DTrp^{5,7,9}, Leu^{11}] Substance P coordinately and reversibly inhibits bombesin and vasopressin induced signal transduction pathways in Swiss 3T3 cells. *J Biol Chem* 271: 29453–29460.
91. Seckl MJ, Higgins T, Widmer F, Rozengurt E (1997) [DArg^1, DTrp^{5,7,9}, Leu^{11}] Substance P: a novel and potent inhibitor of signal transduction and growth *in vitro* and *in vivo* in small cell lung cancer cells. *Cancer Res* 57: 51–54.
92. Seckl MJ, Newman RH, Freemont PS, Rozengurt E (1995) Substance P related antagonists inhibit vasopressin and bombesin but not GTPγS stimulated inositol phosphate production in Swiss 3T3 cells. *J Cell Physiol* 163: 87–95.
93. Sethi T, Langdon SP, Smyth JF, Rozengurt E (1992) Growth of small cell lung cancer cells: stimulation by multiple neuropeptides and inhibition by broad spectrum antagonists *in vitro* and *in vivo*. *Cancer Res* 52 (Suppl): 2737–2742.
94. Langdon SP, Sethi T, Ritchie A, Muir M, Smyth J, Rozengurt E (1992) Broad spectrum neuropeptide antagonists inhibit the growth of small cell lung cancer *in vivo*. *Cancer Res* 52: 4554–4557.

Clinical and Biological Basis of Lung Cancer Prevention
ed. by Y. Martinet, F.R. Hirsch, N. Martinet, J.-M. Vignaud
and J. L. Mulshine
© 1998 Birkhäuser Verlag Basel/Switzerland

CHAPTER 12
In Vitro Analysis of Bombesin/Gastrin-Releasing Peptide Receptor (bb2) Ligand Binding and G-Protein Coupling

Glenn S. Kroog[1], Mark R. Hellmich[1], Mark A. Akeson[1], Robert T. Jensen[2], John K. Northup[3] and James F. Battey[1,*]

[1] *Laboratory of Molecular Biology, National Institute on Deafness and Other Communication Disorders, National Instituts of Health, Rockville, Maryland, USA*
[2] *Digestive Diseases Branch, National Institute of Diabetes and Digestive and Kidney Diseases, National Instituts of Health, Bethesda, Maryland, USA*
[3] *Laboratory of Cell Biology, National Institute of Mental Health, National Instituts of Health, Bethesda, Maryland, USA*

1. Summary

Bombesin/gastrin releasing peptide receptors (GRP-R, or bb2) mediate a broad spectrum of biological responses including secretion of other peptide hormones, gastric acid secretion, smooth muscle contraction, modulation of neuron firing rate, and growth regulation of both normal and neoplastic cells. Of particular interest, bombesin and its receptor have been shown to promote the growth of some human lung carcinoma cells by an autocrine mechanism, a phenomenon that is thought to play a pivotal role in the pathogenesis and progression of these tumors. These observations make the bb2 receptor a potentially important target for early intervention and prevention strategies. To develop these strategies, it is essential to under-

---

* Author for correspondence.

stand the initial events in receptor mediated signal transduction: ligand binding and activation of G_q, a cognate heterotrimeric G protein for this receptor. We have developed *in vitro* assays for both ligand binding and G protein activation, which allow a quantitative analysis of the molecular pharmacology of both processes. In addition to providing important insights into the pharmacology of bb2, these *in vitro* assays provide a means to evaluate the utility and efficacy of compounds or drugs which may interfere with ligand binding and/or receptor/G-protein coupling.

2. Introduction

Bombesin is an amidated tetradecapeptide, originally identified in extracts from frog skin as an agent promoting smooth muscle contractility [1]. In mammals, there are two bombesin-like peptides known at present: gastrin-releasing peptide (GRP)[2] and neuromedin B (NMB)[3]. These peptides elicit a broad range of responses, including secretion of gastrointestinal, adrenal and pituitary hormones, gastric acid secretion, regulation of smooth muscle contraction, and modulation of neuron firing rate. In the central nervous system, bombesin-like peptides are thought to regulate homeostasis, body temperature, metabolism and behavior [4, 5]. The mammalian bombesin-like peptide, GRP, can stimulate the airway growth and development of rhesus monkey lung [6], which shows that lung tissue can be stimulated to grow by bombesin under some circumstances. Bombesin-like peptides can also serve as mitogens in Swiss 3T3 fibroblasts [7], Rat-1 fibroblasts expressing a transfected bombesin receptor gene [8, 9], and human bronchial epithelial cells expressing a transfected bombesin receptor gene [10]. Some small cell lung cancer cells also secrete biologically active bombesin-like peptides, resulting in autocrine growth stimulation [11]. Since nonmalignant pulmonary endocrine cells synthesize bombesin peptides, it is thought that bombesin-mediated growth stimulation may be a relatively early step in neoplastic transformation and tumor progression. These observations suggest that the bombesin growth signaling pathway may be a useful target for early intervention strategies aimed at early detection and prevention of lung tumors.

Bombesin-like peptides exert their effects by binding to a family of heptahelical G protein-coupled receptors. Three human bombesin receptors have so far been isolated and characterized: a GRP-preferring receptor (GRP-R, or bb2) [12], a NMB-preferring receptor (NMB-R, or bb1) [12] and bombesin receptor subtype 3 (BRS-3, or bb3) [13] which has several orders of magnitude lower affinity for GRP, NMB and bombesin. All three receptors have a similar signal transduction cascade after binding an agonist ligand, including heterotrimeric G protein activation leading to activation of phospholipase C, elaboration of inositol 1,4,5-trisphosphate, calcium mobilization from intracellular stores, and consequent activation of protein kinase C [14–16]. In addition, rapid tyrosine phosphorylation of p125 focal adhesion kinase and other proteins that modulate the cytoskeleton follows bombesin receptor activation [17, 18], although the relationship between these two signal transduction pathways remains to be elucidated. After binding an agonist, the bombesin receptor is rapidly phosphorylated [19] and internalized [15, 20, 21], events which probably lead to termination of the receptor-catalyzed exchange of GDP for GTP on heterotrimeric G proteins and a reduction of receptor responses to subsequent challenges by agonists.

To understand in detail the initial events in the bombesin receptor signal transduction pathway, we have developed *in vitro* assays which define (in quantitative terms) the molecular pharmacology of ligand binding and subsequent receptor-catalyzed activation of heterotrimeric G proteins. These assays provide important insights into the biochemistry of these processes; in addition, they can be used to identify and evaluate the mechanism of action, efficacy and potency of agents that may interfere with the first two biochemical events in GRP-R signalling.

3. Materials and Methods

3.1. Materials

Dulbecco's modified Eagle's medium (DMEM), fetal bovine serum and aminoglycoside G418 were obtained from BRL Life Technologies, Inc. (Gaithersburg, MD). The GRP-R agonists GRP and bombesin were purchased from Peninsula Laboratories (Belmont, CA). Purified squid $G\alpha_q$ was prepared as described by Hartman and Northup [22]. Purified bovine brain $\beta\gamma$ was prepared as described previously [23]. AEBSF(4-(2-Aminoethyl)-benzenesulfonyl fluoride) was purchased from ICN Biomedical, Inc. (Aurora, OH). Nitrocellulose filters were obtained from Millipore Corporation (Bedford, MA). All other chemicals used in these experiments were reagent grade. $[^{125}I]$-$[D\text{-}Tyr^6]Bn(6-13)$ methyl ester ($[^{125}I]$-Tyr-ME), the radiolabelled GRP-R antagonist used in whole cell binding studies, was prepared as described previously [24, 25]. ^{35}S-GTPγS was purchased from NEN/DuPont (Boston, MA).

3.2 Cell Culture

The cells used for these assays were Balb/c 3T3 cells transfected with an epitope-tagged mouse GRP-R cDNA (5ET-4), or Balb/c 3T3 cells transfected with the wildtype mouse GRP-R (BN7.9). The epitope-tagged GRP-R behaves identically to the wildtype GRP-R when assayed for ligand binding, coupling, internalization and desensitization [19]. The cells were maintained in DMEM containing 300 µg/ml G418 and 10% (v/v) fetal bovine serum, and grown at 37 °C in 5% CO_2.

3.3 Whole Cell Binding Assay

On the day before binding is performed, transfected cells are plated at 10^4 cells/well in 24-well microtiter dishes (Costar), and binding buffer (BB) is prepared. BB consists of 140 mM NaCl, 5 mM KCl, 0.1% (w/v) bovine serum albumin, 1 mM $CaCl_2$, 0.03% (w/v) bacitracin, 50 mM HEPES pH 7.4. On the day the assay is performed, the protease inhibitors AEBSF and leupeptin are added to the BB at final concentrations of 100 µM and 1 µg/ml respectively. Immediately before beginning the binding assay, growth medium is removed from each well, and the cells are washed with 1 ml BB, followed by a 5 minute incubation with 0.5 ml BB supplemented with protease inhibitors. Following this incubation, 0.5 ml BB supplemented with protease inhibitors, and 25000 cpm [^{125}I]-Tyr-ME (about 13 pM concentration) is added. In some cases unlabelled peptide ligands as indicated are added to each well. Binding proceeds at room temperature (23 °C) for the indicated times, and is terminated by removal of the buffer containing radioligand. The cells are washed with 1 ml BB without inhibitors three times. After the three washes, the cells are detached by incubation in 0.2 ml 0.2 M NaOH, 1% (w/v) sodium dodecyl sulfate for 5 minutes. The cells and debris are removed by serial pipetting of the 0.2 ml detachment solution until all cells are in solution. The detachment solution is transferred to a tube appropriate for gamma counting, and the well washed one final time with 0.25 ml BB without protease inhibitors. The wash is transferred to the tube containing detachment solution, and the 0.45 ml volume is counted in a gamma counter (Cobra II, Packard Instrument Company, Downers Grove, IL 60515). Curve fitting and data analysis for the ligand binding experiments were performed using the LIGAND program [26] and a Macintosh LCII computer.

3.4 Membrane Preparation for Coupling Assay

To measure GRP-R coupling to heterotrimeric G proteins, it was necessary to prepare a GRP-R containing membrane fraction with minimal residual background GTP binding activity. 5-ET4 cells adhering to growth dishes were washed twice with 10 ml phosphate buffered saline at room temperature, and incubated at 4 °C for 15 minutes in hypotonic solution A (10 mM HEPES pH 7.4, 1 mM EGTA) fortified with 100 µM AEBSF. Swollen cells were harvested by scraping, homogenized in a Dounce homogenizer (15 strokes with a tight pestle), and nuclei and cell debris removed by centrifugation at $750 \times$ g for 10 minutes at $4\,°C$. A post-nuclear membrane fraction (P2) was pelleted by centrifugation at $75\,000 \times$ g for 30 minutes at $4\,°C$. The P2 pellet was suspended in solution A supplemented with the chaotropic agent urea at 6 M concentration, and membranes were incubated on ice for 30 minutes. The membranes were collected by centrifugation at $75\,000 \times$ g for 30 minutes at $4\,°C$, extracted a second time with solution A fortified with 6 M urea on ice, collected by centrifugation at $75\,000 \times$ g for 30 minutes at $4\,°C$, washed once with solution A alone, and resuspended in solution A supplemented with 12% (w/v) sucrose. Aliquots of chaotrope-extracted membranes were frozen on dry ice and stored at $-80\,°C$ until used for coupling assays.

3.5 Assay for GRP-R Coupling to Heterotrimeric G proteins

The first event in G protein-coupled receptor coupling to heterotrimeric G protein is the receptor-catalyzed exchange of GTP for GDP bound to the $G\alpha$ subunit. In our experiments, GRP-R mediated nucleotide exchange was determined *in vitro* using a procedure modified from the method of Fawzi et al. [27]. Membranes containing GRP-R (final concentration about 3 nM GRP-R) were incubated in a 50 µL binding reaction buffer containing 20 mM HEPES pH 7.5, 100 mM NaCl, 3 mM $MgSO_4$, 1 mM DTT, 1 mM EDTA, 1 µM GDP, 0.3% (w/v) BSA, 400000 cpm [^{35}S]GTPγS, with or without 280 nM $G\alpha_q$, 1 µM $\beta\gamma$, and/or 1 µM GRP as indicated. Binding proceeded at 30°C for 10 minutes, and was terminated by addition of 2 ml ice-cold solution B (20 mMTris-HCl, pH 8.0, 100 mM NaCl, 25 mM $MgCl_2$). After addition of ice-cold solution B, the bound [^{35}S]GTPγS was collected by filtration using a nitrocellulose filter and a vacuum manifold. Filters were washed four times, each time using a 2 ml aliquot of ice-cold solution B, dried, and counted by liquid scintillation using a beta counter (Wallac 1219). The counts bound reported in this manuscript are the mean of three independent experiments.

4. Results

4.1 Binding Properties of [^{125}I]-Tyr-ME Radioligand

Ligand binding to a receptor is the first event in a cascade of biochemical reactions of signal transduction. It is therefore important to establish a reliable assay to measure ligand binding that can give accurate, quantitative results. Figure 1A shows a time course for binding of the [^{125}I]-Tyr-ME radioligand to the GRP-R expressed in the transfected Balb/c 3T3 cell line 5-ET4. We elected to use a pure GRP-R antagonist as the radioligand in this

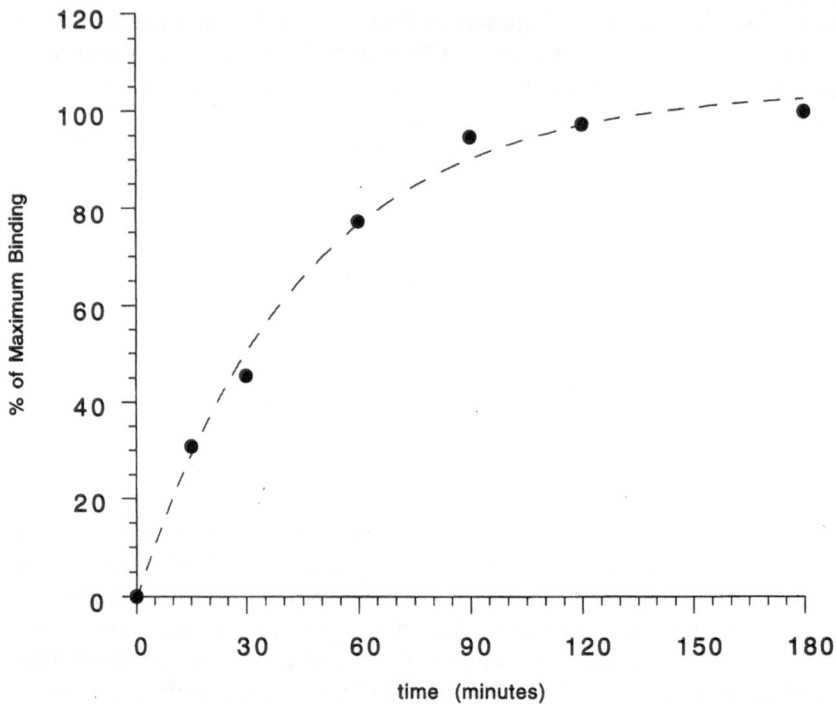

Figure 1A. Time course of [^{125}I]-Tyr-ME radioligand binding to (1A), and dissociation from (1B), the GRP-R. Figure 1A shows the rate and extent of binding of the radioligand over a 180 minute time period. Equilibrium binding is achieved by about 90–120 minutes, and there is no evidence for instability of the radioligand.

whole cell binding assay to avoid internalization of the radioligand, which occurs within minutes of agonist binding to the receptor in whole cells [15, 20, 21]. Internalization would confuse the quantitative analysis of radioligand binding to GRP-R by generating a pool of radioligand inside the cell that is associated with the cells but is not bound to GRP-R in the cell membrane. The binding reaches a plateau after about 90–120 minutes at room temperature, indicating the amount of binding where the GRP-R binding and dissociation rates are at dynamic equilibrium in the presence of 13 pM radioligand tracer. There is no change in this plateau if the binding assay progresses for as long as 4 hours, consistent with structural stability of the radioligand during the time required to come to equilibrium binding.

To confirm ligand stability, we compared the high performance liquid chromatographic properties of the radioligand after binding for eight hours with the radioligand before exposure to the binding assay. Over 95% of the radioligand incubated in a binding reaction for up to eight hours elutes in

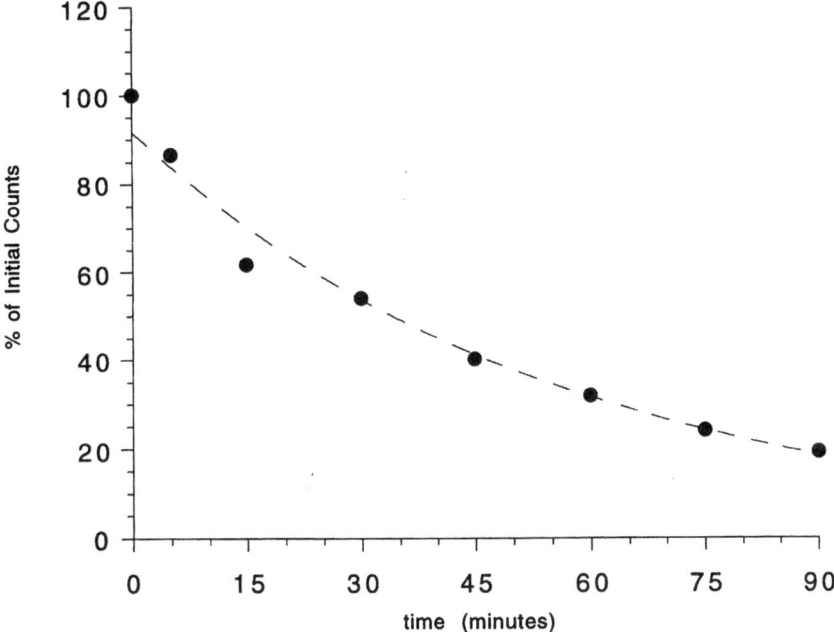

Figure 1 B. The time course of dissociation of radioligand bound to the GRP-R. About half of the radioligand has dissociated by 38 minutes. Data shown in this figure are representative of experiments repeated at least three times.

the same fractions as the radioligand before binding, confirming the structural integrity of the radioligand in this binding assay (data not shown).

In Figure 1B, the GRP-R is brought to dynamic equilibrium by binding to about a 13 pM radioligand for two hours, after which time 1 µM unlabelled ME or bombesin is added to the binding assay. By following the time dependent decrease in radioligand bound in the assay, we can determine quantitatively the off-rate of bound radioligand [28]. Radioligand dissociation from the GRP-R is relatively rapid, with a $t_{1/2}$ of 38 minutes. By taking into account the specific activity of the radioligand (2200 Ci/ mmole), these data allow a calculation of the off-rate constant k_2, which is about 3.0×10^{-4} sec^{-1}, and the on-rate constant k_1, which is about 5.1×10^6 M^{-1} sec^{-1} [28]. The dissociation constant K_d can be calculated as the ratio of $k_2/k_1 = 6.0 \times 10^{-11}$ M, or 60 pM, indicating that this radioligand antagonist has a very high (sub nM) affinity for GRP-R in this whole cell radioligand binding assay.

Figure 2A shows a typical ligand displacement analysis of binding to the GRP-R in the presence of varying concentrations of unlabelled ligand. Note that about half of the binding is inhibited by addition of 100 pM unlabelled ligand, consistent with a K_d value of about 100 pM. In Figure 2B, the same binding data are plotted to give a Scatchard curve, and the best

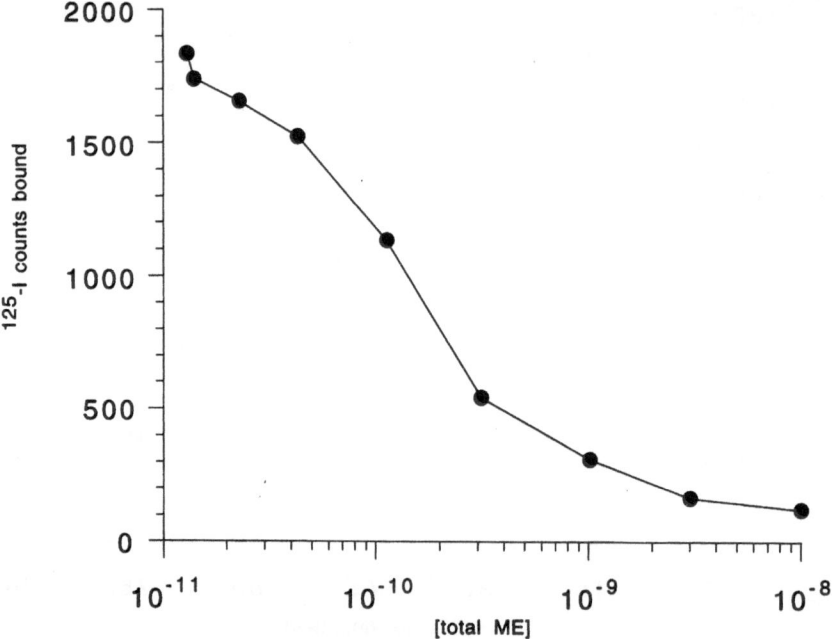

Figure 2A. Quantitative displacement analysis of [^{125}I]-Tyr-ME radioligand binding in the presence of varying concentrations of unlabelled ME. Figure 2A shows the displacement curve for radioligand binding, with about half of the binding inhibited by addition of approximately 10^{-10} M ME. Values on the abscissa are indicated as M/l.

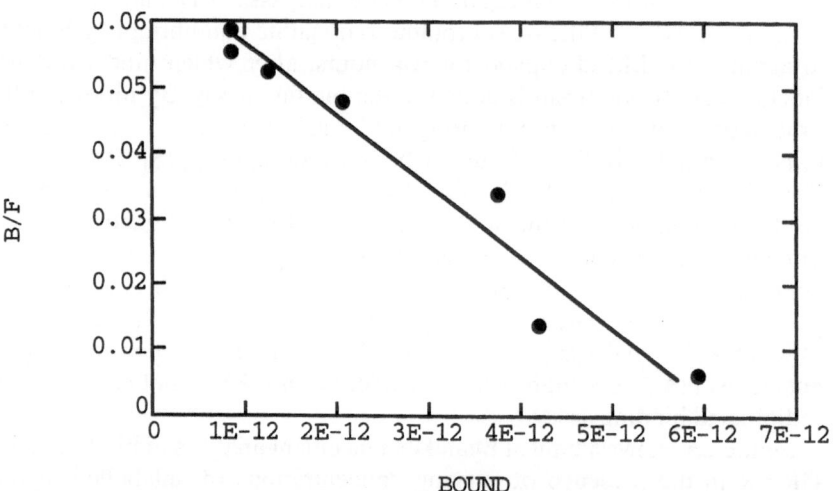

Figure 2B. Shows the same data from Figure 2A plotted in Scatchard format, indicating a single high affinity binding site with a K_d of 0.92×10^{-10} M. Data shown in this figure are representative of experiments repeated at least three times.

linear fit predicts K_d of 92 pM, and a B_{max} of about 2×10^5 receptors/cell. These measurements of K_d are in close agreement with that derived independently from the kinetic data in Figure 1 ($K_d = 60$ pM).

The [^{125}I]-Tyr-ME radioligand has been shown to function as a pure antagonist, with no evidence for partial agonism [24]. If this radioligand is in fact a pure antagonist, there should be no internalization of bound radioligand. This lack of internalization is supported by the kinetic data shown in Figure 1B, where the majority of radioligand bound to the receptor over a two hour time period at room temperature is competed off by unlabelled radioligand within two hours. These results are consistent with the majority of the bound radioligand remaining at the cell surface, and not internalized within the cell. To confirm that the bound [^{125}I]-Tyr-ME radioligand antagonist is not internalized, we determine that >99% of the bound [^{125}I]-Tyr-ME radioligand can be removed by treating the cells with 0.2 M acetic acid (pH 2.5)/0.5 M NaCl for 5 minutes at 22 °C. In contrast, when the radioligand is an agonist such as [^{125}I]-Tyr^4-bombesin, about 30% of the label remains associated with the cells after treatment with acid, which confirms that this agonist radioligand is internalized after binding (data not shown).

4.2 GRP-R Coupling to G_q in Vitro

Heterotrimeric G proteins that couple to G protein-coupled receptors are composed of the products of three distinct gene families, each of which encodes α, β or γ subunits. When activated by agonist binding, the receptor catalyzes the release of GDP from the $G\alpha$ subunit of the heterotrimer, which in turn leads to dissociation of the heterotrimer into distinct α and $\beta\gamma$ subunits, and GTP binding to the α subunit. Thus, receptor coupling can be measured by assaying the agonist stimulated binding of a nonhydrolysable GTP analog (such as [^{35}S]GTPγS) to the $G\alpha$ subunit.

At least 20 distinct mammalian $G\alpha$ subunits are known at present, and have been classified according to sequence homology and intracellular effector regulation [29, 30]. In mammals, the G_q subfamily of G proteins has been shown to be insensitive to pertussis toxin, and to activate phospholipase C and stimulate phosphoinositide hydrolysis [31, 32], the initial events known to be involved in GRP-R signal transduction [33]. Based on this information, we chose $G\alpha_q$ as a logical coupling partner for the GRP-R coupling assay. Squid transducin, a member of the G_q subfamily, is the major heterotrimeric G protein in the squid photoreceptor [34], which makes this a good source for purification of active $G\alpha_q$ with appropriate post-translational lipid modifications.

Table 1 shows the results of GRP-R-catalysed exchange binding of radiolabelled [^{35}S]GTPγS for GDP, a measure of receptor coupling. Note that the radioligand bound remained at background levels (<5000 cpm) in the absence of agonist. GRP-stimulated nucleotide exchange levels above

Table 1 GRP-R coupling to $G\alpha_q$. The binding of ^{35}S-GTPγS is measured after addition of different combinations of heterotrimeric G protein subunits, with or without addition of GRP (a GRP-R agonist). Note that any binding observed over background required addition of GRP, $G\beta\gamma$ and $G\alpha_q$. The numbers reported in this figure are CPM bound during the assay, and are representative of data from experiments repeated at least three times.

GRP-R Coupling to $G\alpha_q$

GRP(1 µM)	+	−
Membranes alone	4840	4346
Membranes + α_q	6321	4462
Membranes + $\beta\gamma$	3433	5466
Membranes + α_q + $\beta\gamma$	46321	5756

this background required the presence of $G\alpha_q$, $\beta\gamma$ and agonist, as predicted from the model of receptor-G protein interaction. When all G protein subunits and agonist are present, nucleotide exchange is catalysed, resulting in the binding of >40000 cpm of [^{35}S]GTPγS (Table 1). This reaction is saturable for addition of both $G\alpha_q$ and $\beta\gamma$ [35] and the EC$_{50}$ for GRP-stimulated exchange of [^{35}S]GTPγS is 3.5 nM [35], in close agreement with the reported K_d of 3.1 ± 1.4 nM for GRP-R expressed in Balb/c 3T3 cells [15]. Taken together, these data indicate that this assay reconstitutes GRP-R coupling to G_q *in vitro*, and that the coupling can be measured using the nucleotide exchange of [^{35}S]GTPγS for GDP bound to the $G\alpha_q$ subunit.

5. Discussion

We have developed *in vitro* assays to characterize the first two biochemical events involved in GRP-R signal transduction, ligand binding and G protein coupling. The ligand binding assay is a reliable tool to determine both steady state and kinetic parameters of GRP-R interaction with ligands. In addition, it establishes binding conditions where the [^{125}I]-Tyr-ME radioligand interacts with GRP-R with high affinity. This radioligand is stable in the binding assay for long periods, compared to the time required for binding to come to dynamic equilibrium in the presence of low concentrations of ligand (13 pM). The [^{125}I]-Tyr-ME radioligand is an antagonist which will not rapidly internalize after receptor binding, in contrast to radioligand agonists for GRP-R such as [^{125}I]-Tyr^{4}Bombesin or [^{125}I]GRP used in other GRP-R binding assays. For this reason, the [^{125}I]-Tyr-ME radioligand is better suited for studies designed to measure binding, or inhibition of binding, to GRP-R expressed in intact cells. Furthermore, this assay could be adapted to characterize molecules that interfere with binding, or for screening libraries of nonpeptide small molecules that function as pure antagonists for GRP-R binding. These specific GRP-R antagonists would prove very useful in determining the function of GRP-R in complex organ systems such as the brain or digestive tract, and might also prove useful in early intervention strategies where GRP-R mediated growth is an important step in establishing growth deregulation, neoplasia or tumor progression.

We have also developed an assay to measure GRP-R coupling *in vitro*, which is the step in GRP-R signal transduction immediately after agonist binding. Our studies indicate that GRP-R coupling, as measured by exchange of [^{35}S]GTPγS for GDP bound to the α subunit of G_q, requires GRP agonist, α_q and $\beta\gamma$ subunits as expected. In future studies, it will be interesting to see if there are any differences in coupling properties observed when the four mammalian $G\alpha_q$ family members (α_q, α_{11}, α_{14} and $\alpha_{15/16}$) are compared. This study awaits the expression and purification of adequate amounts of these four $G\alpha$ proteins, an effort currently underway in our laboratories. This assay system also provides an experimental test of the selectivity of GRP-R coupling to G_q, a selectivity brought into question by reports of pertussis toxin sensitive GRP-R signalling in guinea pig lung membranes [36] suggesting GRP-R signal transduction mediated through G_i and/or G_o. In addition, it can be adapted to compare the coupling properties of GRP-R (bb2) to the two other known mammalian bombesin receptor subtypes, NMB-R (bb1) and BRS-3 (bb3). A study using antisense oligonucleotides to deplete *Xenopus* oocytes of individual members of the $G\alpha_q$ family revealed differences in the coupling requirements for GRP-R and NMB-R expressed in these cells [37]. *In vitro* reconstitution of receptor coupling may well reveal qualitative and quantitative differences between G protein receptor interactions that would be difficult, if not impossible, to appreciate by analyzing coupling *in vivo*. As in the radioligand binding assay, the *in vitro* coupling assay provides a means to analyze quantitatively the properties of compounds postulated either to augment or interfere with receptor coupling, such as mastoparan [38, 39], or to screen for compounds that modulate GRP-R signal transduction at the level of coupling. Compounds that interact at the level of coupling may be of great interest in the future, since multiple neuropeptides have been observed to activate similar signal transduction pathways in small cell lung carcinoma cells [40].

There is growing documentation of associations between amino acid sequence changes in G protein coupled receptors and a variety of inherited human disorders [41, 42]. In fact, a recent case report of a patient with autism carrying a balanced reciprocal translocation disrupting the human GRP-R has raised the possibility that GRP-R mutations may be in part responsible for this disorder [43]. Well-characterized assays for receptor function will allow a rigorous analysis of any allelic variants in the GRP-R, or other G protein-coupled receptors, to distinguish between an allelic variant that alters receptor function and one which is functionally neutral.

Acknowledgments

The authors gratefully acknowledge Mr. Samuel Mantey for his expertise in preparation of the [^{125}I]-Tyr-ME radioligand used in these studies, and for technical assistance in the high pressure liquid chromatography analysis of radioligand before and after binding.

References

1. Anastasi A, Erspamer V, Bucci M (1971) Isolation and structure of bombesin and alytesin, two analogous active tetradecapeptides from the skin of the European amphibians *Bombina* and *Alytes. Experientia* 27: 166–167.
2. McDonald TJ, Jornvall H, Nilsson G, Vagne M, Ghatei M, Bloom SR, Mutt V (1979) Characterization of a gastrin releasing peptide from porcine non-antral gastric tissue. *Biochem Biophys Res Comm* 90: 227–233.
3. Minamino N, Kangawa K, Matsuo H (1983) Neuromedin B: a novel bombesin-like peptide identified in porcine spinal cord. *Biochem Biophys Res Comm* 114: 541–548.
4. Lebacq-Verheyden AM, Trepel J, Sausville EA, Battey JF (1990) Bombesin and gastrin-releasing peptide: neuropeptides, secretogogues, and growth factors. *In:* Sporn MB, Roberts AB (eds): *Handbook of Experimental Pharmacology, Vol. 95/II. Peptide Growth Factors and Their Receptors II,* Springer-Verlag, Berlin Heidelberg, pp 71–124.
5. Spindel ER (1986) Mammalian bombesin-like peptides. *Trends Neurosci* 9: 130–133.
6. Li K, Nagalla SR, Spindel ER (1994) A rhesus monkey model to characterize the role of gastrin-releasing peptide (GRP) in lung development: evidence for stimulation of airway growth. *J Clin Invest* 94: 1605–1615.
7. Rozengurt E, Sinnett-Smith J (1983) Bombesin stimulation of DNA synthesis and cell division in cultures of Swiss 3T3 cells. *Proc Natl Acad Sci USA* 80: 2936–2940.
8. Charlesworth A, Broad S, Rozengurt E (1996) The bombesin/GRP receptor transfected into Rat-1 fibroblasts couples to phospholipase C activation, tyrosine phosphorylation of p125 FAK and paxillin and cell proliferation. *Oncogene* 12(6): 1337–1345.
9. Lach EB, Broad S, Rozengurt E (1995) Mitogenic signalling by transfected neuromedin B receptors in Rat-1 cells. *Cell Growth Diff* 6(11): 1427–1435.
10. Cuttitta F, Carney DN, Mulshine J, Moody TW, Fedorko J, Fischler A, Minna J (1985) Bombesin-like peptides can function as autocrine growth factors in human small-cell lung cancer. *Nature* 316: 823–826.
11. Moustafa A, Tsao M-S, Battey JF, Viallet J (1995) Expression of the gastrin-releasing peptide receptor confers a growth response to bombesin in immortalized human bronchial epithelial cells. *Cancer Res* 55: 1853–1855.
12. Corjay MH, Dobrzanski D, Way J, Viallet J, Shapira H, Worland P, Sausville EA, Battey JF (1991) Two distinct bombesin receptor subtypes are expressed and functional in human lung carcinoma cells. *J Biol Chem* 266: 18771–18779.
13. Fathi Z, Corjay M, Shapira H, Wada E, Benya R, Mantey S, Jensen R, Viallet J, Sausville EA, Battey JF (1993) BRS-3: a novel bombesin receptor subtype selectively expressed in testis and lung carcinoma cells. *J Biol Chem* 268: 5979–5984.
14. Benya R, Wada E, Battey JF, Fathi Z, Wang L-H, Mantey S, Coy DH, Jensen RT (1992) Neuromedin B receptors retain functional expression when transfected into Balb 3T3 fibroblasts: analysis of binding kinetics, stoichiometry, modulation by guanine nucleotide binding proteins, signal transduction, and comparison with natively expressed receptors. *Molec Pharmacol* 42: 1058–1068.
15. Benya R, Fathi Z, Kusui T, Pradham T, Battey JF, Jensen RT (1994) Gastrin-releasing peptide receptor-induced internalization, down-regulation, desensitization, and growth: possible role for cyclic AMP. *Molec Pharmacol* 46: 235–245.
16. Benya R, Kusui T, Pradham T, Battey JF, Jensen RT (1995) Expression and characterization of cloned human bombesin receptors. *Molec Pharmacol* 47: 10–20.
17. Zachary I, Sinnett-Smith J, Turner CE, Rozengurt E (1993) Bombesin, vasopressin, and endothelin rapidly stimulate tyrosine phosphorylation of the focal adhesion-associated protein paxillin in Swiss 3T3 cells. *J Biol Chem* 268: 22060–22065.

18. Sinnett-Smith J, Zachary I, Valverde AM, Rozengurt E (1993) Bombesin stimulation of p125 focal adhesion kinase tyrosine phosphorylation: role of proteinkinase C, calcium mobilization, and the actin cytoskeleton. *J Biol Chem* 268: 14261–14268.

19. Kroog G, Sainz E, Worland P, Jensen RT, Battey JF (1995) The gastrin-releasing peptide receptor (GRP-R) is rapidly phosphorylated by a kinase other than protein kinase C (PKC) after exposure to agonist. *J Biol Chem* 270: 8217–8224.

20. Benya R, Fathi Z, Battey JF, Jensen RT (1993) Specific serines and threonines in the gastrin-releasing peptide receptor carboxy terminus mediate agonist-stimulated internalization. *J Biol Chem* 268: 20285–20290.

21. Benya R, Kusui T, Shikado F, Battey JF, Jensen RT (1994) Desensitization of neuromedin B receptors (NMB-R) on native and NMB-R transfected cells involves down-regulation and internalization. *J Biol Chem* 269: 11721–11728.

22. Hartman J, Northup JK (1996) Functional reconstitution of 5HT2c receptors in situ with αq and inverse agonism of 5HT2c receptor antagonists. *J Biol Chem* 271: 22591–22597.

23. Sternweis P, Robishaw JD (1984) Isolation of two proteins with high affinity for guanine nucleotides from membranes of bovine brain. *J Biol Chem* 259: 13806–13813.

24. Mantey S, Frucht H, Coy DH, Jensen RT (1993) Characterization of bombesin receptors using a novel, potent, radiolabelled antagonist that distinguishes bombesin receptor subtypes. *Molec Pharmacol* 43: 762–774.

25. Wang L-H, Mantey S, Lin JT, Frucht H, Jensen RT (1993) Ligand binding, internalization, degradation and regulation by guanine nucleotides of bombesin receptor subtypes: a comparative study. *Biochim Biophys Acta* 175: 232–242.

26. Munson PJ, Rodbard D (1980) LIGAND: A versatile computerized approach for characterization of ligand-binding systems. *Anal Biochem* 107: 220–239.

27. Fawzi AB, Northup JK (1990) Guanine nucleotide binding characteristics of transduction: essential role of rhodopsin for rapid exchange of guanine nulceotides. *Biochemistry* 29: 3804–3812.

28. Limbird LE (1986) *Cell surface receptors: a short course on theory and methods,* Martinus Nijhoff Publishing, Boston.

29. Helper JR, Gilman AG (1992) G proteins. *Trends Biochem Sci* 17: 383–387.

30. Wilkie TM, Gilbert DJ, Olsen AS, Chen X-N, Amatruda TT, Korenberg JR, Trask BJ, de Jong P, Reed RR, Simon MI, et al. (1992) Evolution of the mammalian G protein α subunit multigene family. *Nature Genet* 1: 85–91.

31. Smrcka AV, Helper JR, Brown KO, Sternweis PC (1991) Regulation of polyphosphoinositide-specific phospholipase C activity by purified G$_q$. *Science* 251: 804–807.

32. Taylor SJ, Chae HZ, Rhee SG, Exton JH (1991) Activation of the β1 isozyme of phospholipase C by α subunits of the G$_q$ class of G proteins. *Nature* 350: 516–518.

33. Brown KD, Blay J, Irvine RF, Heslop JP, Berridge MJ (1984) Reduction of epidermal growth factor receptor affinity by heterologous ligands: evidence for a mechanism involving the breakdown of phosphoinositide and the activation of protein kinase C. *Biochem Biophys Res Comm* 123: 377–384.

34. Pottinger JD, Ryba NJ, Keen JN, Findlay JB (1991) The identification and purification of the heterotrimeric GTP-binding protein from squid (Loligo forbesi) photoreceptors. *Biochem J* 279: 323–326.

35. Hellmich MR, Battey JF, Northup JK (1997) Selective reconstitution of gastrin-releasing peptide receptor with Gα$_q$. *Proc Natl Acad Sci USA* 94: 751–756.

36. Lach E, Trifilieff A, Scherrer D, Gies J-P (1994) Association of guinea pig lung bombesin receptors with pertussis toxin-sensitive guanine nucleotide binding proteins. *Eur J Pharmacol* 269: 87–93.

37. Shapira H, Way J, Lipinsky D, Oron Y, Battey JF (1994) Neuromedin B receptor, expressed in *Xenopus laevis* oocytes, selectively couples to Gα$_q$ and not Gα$_{11}$. *FEBS Lett* 348: 89–92.

38. Higashijima T, Uzu S, Nakajima T, Ross EM (1988) Mastoparan, a peptide toxin from wasp venom, mimics receptors by activating GTP-binding regulatory proteins (G proteins). *J Biol Chem* 263: 6491–6494.

39. Higashijima T, Burnier J, Ross EM (1990) Regulation of G$_i$ and G$_o$ by mastoparan, related amphiphilic peptides, and hydrophobic amines: mechanism and structural determinants of activity. *J Biol Chem* 265: 14176–14186.

40. Woll PJ, Rozengurt E (1989) Multiple neuropeptides mobilize calcium in small cell lung cancer: effects of vasopressin, bradykinin, cholecystokinin, galanin, and neurotensin. *Biochem Biophys Res Comm* 164: 66–73.
41. Clapham DE (1993) Mutations in G protein-linked receptors: novel insights on disease. *Cell* 75: 1237–1239.
42. Spiegel AM (1996) Defects in G protein-coupled signal transduction in human disease. *Ann Rev Physiol* (in press).
43. Ishikawa-Brush Y, Powell JF, Bolton P, Francis F, Lehrach H, Monaco AP (1995) Disruption of the GRPR gene and translocation breakpoint sequence associated with multiple exostoses and autism. *Am J Hum Genet* 57: A56, abstract #292.

Clinical and Biological Basis of Lung Cancer Prevention
ed. by Y. Martinet, F. R. Hirsch, N. Martinet, J.-M. Vignaud
and J. L. Mulshine
© 1998 Birkhäuser Verlag Basel/Switzerland

CHAPTER 13
DNA Methylation Changes in Lung Cancer

Samir M. Hanash[1,*], Bruce Richardson[2], Rork Kuick[1],
Katharina Wimmer[1], Didier H. Thoraval[1], Barbara Lamb[1],
Yoshihiro Nambu[3] and David G. Beer[3]

[1] *Department of Pediatrics, University of Michigan, Ann Arbor, Michigan, USA*
[2] *Department of Internal Medicine, University of Michigan, Ann Arbor, Michigan, USA*
[3] *Department of Surgery, University of Michigan, Ann Arbor, Michigan, USA*

1. Summary

Recent evidence has suggested a role for DNA methylation changes and for DNA (cytosine 5-) methyltransferase in some aspect of tumor development. Limited data are currently available related to changes in the methylation process in lung cancer. Using a novel two-dimensional genome scanning approach to detect gene dosage alterations in tumors, we have identified loci that exhibited hypermethylation and others that exhibited hypomethylation in lung adenocarcinoma. The data suggest that some of the methylation changes observed are unlikely to be due to methylation errors. Full implementation of the genome scanning approach will probably uncover a large number of loci affected by methylation change in lung carcinogenesis.

2. Introduction

In eukaryotic cells, DNA methylation refers primarily to the postsynthetic methylation of deoxycytosine (dC) at the 5 position to form 5-deoxy-

---

* Author for correspondence.

methylcytosine (d^{m}C) [1]. DNA methylation is implicated in a number of biological processes, including imprinting and X chromosome inactivation. Nearly all d^{m}C is found in the dinucleotide CpG, although only 70% to 80% of the CpG pairs are methylated. Most unmethylated CpG pairs are found in GC-rich sequences referred to as CpG islands, while the majority of the methylated pairs are found elsewhere in the genome. CpG islands are approximately 1 kb long, and are almost always located near coding sequences of genes [2]. CpG islands contain multiple binding sites for transcription factors, and function as promoters for the associated gene(s) [2]. Nearly all "housekeeping" genes, and some tissue specific genes, contain CpG islands [3]. Current estimates indicate that there are approximately 45 000 CpG islands per haploid genome in humans [4]. Approximately 56% of human genes are associated with CpG islands [4].

While the role of DNA methylation in different biological processes is increasingly appreciated, the significance of methylation changes observed in cancer mostly remains to be determined. In mature cells, DNA methylation patterns are maintained through mitosis by the enzyme DNA (cytosine-5-) methyltransferase (DNA MTase) [5]. During mitosis, DNA MTase recognizes hemimethylated CpG dinucleotides in the parent and daughter DNA strands, and catalyzes the transfer of the methyl group from S-adenosylmethionine to the cytosine residues in the unmethylated daughter DNA strand, producing symmetrically methylated sites and maintaining methylation patterns [6]. Since DNA methylation patterns may affect gene expression and are heritable through mitosis, yet do not involve sequence mutations, DNA methylation has been referred to as an "epigenetic" mechanism of gene regulation [7]. *De novo* methylation of unmethylated DNA sequences also occurs. Examples include cells recovering from treatment with DNA hypomethylating agents and changes occurring during gametogenesis [8]. However, the mechanisms regulating *de novo* methylation are poorly understood. A few CpG islands have been investigated in aging and found to be methylated [2, 9, 10]. However, the extent of CpG island methylation changes in aging is unknown.

DNA methylation has been implicated in carcinogenesis. Reduced d^{m}C levels have been described in a variety of malignancies [11]. Hypomethylation of proto-oncogenes has been reported in liver tumors, leukemias and colorectal cancer [12] and may contribute to malignant transformation by modifying proto-oncogene expression. The methylation of normally unmethylated CpG islands has also been associated with a variety of human tumors [12]. For example, hypermethylation of the *Rb* gene may contribute to neoplastic transformation in retinoblastoma by inactivating its tumor suppressor function. DNA methylation can also lead to point mutations as a result of deamination of d^{m}C to form thymine. Repair mechanisms may then repair the mismatched guanidine to adenosine, causing a point mutation. This process is further accelerated by DNA MTase overexpression, which may be an early event in the transformation of certain cells [13, 14]. The estimated mutation rate of CpG dinucleotides is 10 to 40 times that of other dinucleotides [12], and this mutation has been implicated in 25% to 33% of *p53* mutations in human tumors [12]. Finally, regional DNA hypomethylation has been related to sequence specific strand breaks and deletions, which can also contribute to malignant transformation [15, 16].

3. DNA Methylation and Lung Cancer

Knowledge of methylation changes in lung cancer is very limited. Unique methylation changes associated with lung cancer have yet to be identified and most current knowledge is of a general nature. However, a recent study suggests, that in lung cancer, methylation of some CpG islands may be related to the specific type of carcinogen exposure. The estrogen receptor (*ER*) gene contains a CpG island which is methylated in different cancers [17–19]. In a study of *ER* gene methylation in lung tumors, promoter methylation was detected in 4 of 11 tumors from nonsmokers and 7 of 35 tumors from smokers [20]. A significant difference in *ER* methylation was also observed in a rodent lung tumor model. Lung tumors induced by a tobacco carcinogen had a low incidence of *ER* methylation relative to spontaneous and plutonium-induced tumors, which had a very high incidence [20].

The role of MTase in tumor initiation or development has been of interest, particularly in view of the demonstration that disruption of MTase in knockout mice results in partial protection from colon tumor development when crossed with *min* mice that have susceptibility to colon tumors [21]. Additionally, overexpression of the murine MTase in NIH 3T3 cells was shown to cause transformation [22]. In a mouse model of lung carcinogenesis, Belinsky et al. [23] examined MTase levels in mice that exhibit high or low susceptibility for lung tumor formation. They reported increased levels of MTase in the target alveolar type II cells in the high susceptibility mice after carcinogen exposure. While it could be suggested that an increase in MTase activity is associated with tumor development and might represent an important step in carcinogenesis, it is likely that the increase in MTase activity observed is partly attributable to an increase in the proliferative activity of the target cells. For example, a recent study of colon tumors showed limited upregulation of MTase activity in colon cancer commensurate with increased cell proliferation [24]. We have also observed a marked increased in MTase activity, following mitotic stimulation of resting T cells with PHA (phyto-haemagglutinin) (Richardson et al., manuscript in preparation).

4. Analysis of Methylation Changes in Lung Tumors
by Two-Dimensional Separations of *Not*I Genomic Digests

The effects of methylation are most consistently observed in CpG islands, where methylation has a strong correlation with transcriptional suppression [25], and lack of methylation is usually required for expression of the associated gene [26]. These observations, together with the common localization of CpG islands in gene promoters, make CpG islands ideal landmarks for genome scanning approaches to detect changes in DNA methylation.

The identification of loci that undergo methylation changes in the genome of cancer cells, apart from the analysis of candidate genes, has been limited by the lack of suitable means to search for methylation alterations across the genome. We have implemented a computerized approach initially developed by our group for protein 2D analysis [27–29] for the analysis of 2D separations of enzyme digested genomic DNA [30–32]. By using different combinations of restriction enzymes and/or different electrophoretic conditions, the number of independent fragments in a human genomic DNA sample that can be analyzed in multiple 2D patterns can reach several thousand. The approach relies on radioisotope labelling of genomic fragments at cleavage sites specific for a rare cutting restriction enzyme. The labelled genomic digests are separated in a first dimension, followed by *in situ* digestion prior to second-dimension separation. The reliance on the rare cleaving restriction enzyme *Not*I to digest genomic DNA prior to labelling, allows visualization of DNA fragments that occur preferentially in CpG islands of the genome. Because of the localization of CpG islands in proximity to transcribed sequences, the 2D patterns obtained with this enzyme are highly targeted to a functional component of the genome [33, 34]. Thus, there is a strong likelihood that *Not*I fragments detected in 2D gels represent sequences in genes.

An important application of this approach is the study of genomic alterations in cancer, including chromosomal deletions, amplifications and methylation changes, by measuring fragment intensities. We have previously shown that loss of one of the two genomic copies encoding for a fragment could be detected without the need for reliance on heterozygosity [31, 32]. The 2D genome scanning approach is being implemented by our group for the study of genomic alterations in lung tumors. Our current findings pertaining to DNA methylation changes in lung adenocarcinomas are reviewed. For the studies described, whole genomic DNA of tumor tissue and normal control tissue is digested with the enzyme *Not*I and a second six base pair cutting enzyme such as *Eco*RV or *Bgl*II [32, 35]. The protruding ends produced by the methylation-sensitive CpG specific enzyme *Not*I are isotopically labelled. About 1 µg of the resulting DNA fragments are subjected to disc agarose gel electrophoresis to separate fragments in the 1.0 to 5.0 and 5.0 to 12.0 kb range. The separated DNA fragments are subsequently subjected to further *in situ* cleavage with a third frequently-cutting restriction enzyme (*Hin*fI or *Pst*I) and electrophoresed in a second dimension in polyacrylamide gels. The resulting fragments are visualized using phosphor storage technology. The digitized images are analyzed using software we have previously developed [27–29].

5. Hypomethylation of Repetitive DNA Sequences in Lung Adenocarcinoma

To date we have analysed 17 lung adenocarcinomas by 2D genome scanning. Representative patterns of a tumor and of normal lung tissue from the same patients are shown in Figure 1. Multicopy fragments observed in patterns of normal DNA are largely attributed to ribosomal DNA (rDNA) genes [32]. The transcribed portion of the rDNA results in some 20 labelled fragments visible on each gel as multicopy spots. We have mapped these spots to the sequences responsible for their occurrence on the gels, based partly on direct sequencing of fragments [32]. Some fragments display a shift in their position, to a larger size, attributable to methylation at specific *Not*I sites (Figure 2). 14 of the 17 tumors analysed displayed

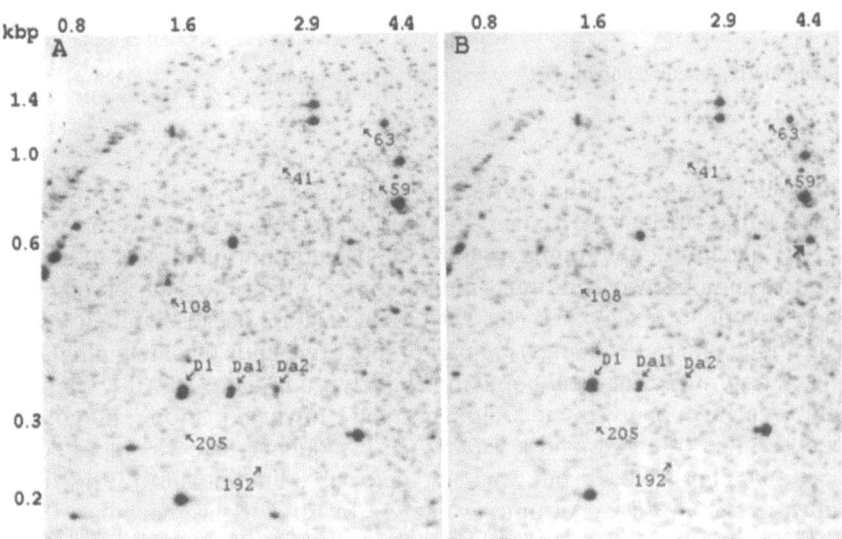

Figure 1. 2D separation of genomic digests of normal lung (A) and tumor (B) from the same patient. Hypomethylation of the D fragment of rDNA is evident by decreased intensity of Da1 and Da2 in the tumor. Numbered spots correspond to chromosome 1 fragments that exhibited reduced intensity in same tumor. The multicopy fragment indicated with a large arrow in the tumor is a part of the ErbB2 amplicon present in this tumor.

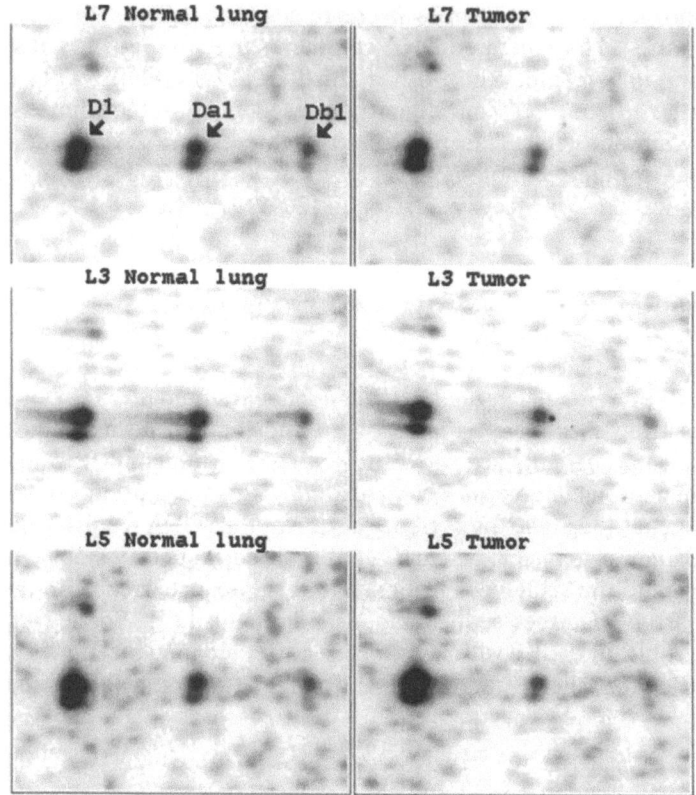

Figure 2. Hypomethylation of rDNA D fragment in three tumors.

diminished intensity of the shifted rDNA fragments, consistent with hypomethylation of their *Not*I sites. In addition, in two tumors, we have observed one multicopy fragment that was absent in normal tissue. In one of
the two tumors, two additional multicopy fragments were observed. The
three fragments (designated Nbl-1, Nbl-2, and Nbl-3 because of their initial
detection in neuroblastomas) are part of repetitive units that are methylated
in a variety of normal cell populations analyzed to date [36–38]. Cloning
and sequence analysis of fragment Nbl-1 revealed strong homology
between this fragment and a subtelomeric sequence that was reported to
occur in chimpanzees but was not detectable in humans [39]. Nbl-2
units occur in the centromeric region of many chromosomes [38].
A third fragment, Nbl-3, was also detected in multicopies in neuroblastoma by our group [38] and in melanoma, colon cancer and pancreatic
cancer by another group [37]. The appearance of all three fragments in 2D
gels was demonstrated to be due to demethylation of cytosine at the *Not*I
sites.

6. Hypermethylated CpG Islands in Lung Adenocarcinomas

We have undertaken a detailed analysis of fragments derived from chromosome 1 that are observed in our standard 2D patterns obtained with *Not*I, *Eco*RV and *Hin*fI. Flow cytometry has provided the means to purify single chromosomes [40]. In a previous study, we have shown that the availability of single chromosome preparations allows the 2D separation of restriction fragments of specific chromosomes and the identification of corresponding fragments in whole genomic patterns [41]. A total of 346 fragments in whole genomic 2D patterns were assigned with high confidence to chromosome 1 based on their comigration with chromosome 1 fragments. The intensities of 183 fragments assigned to chromosome 1 in the range 1.0–5.0 kb were investigated in lung adenocarcinoma 2D patterns. Reduction in fragment intensity or complete absence of a fragment could be due to deletion or cytosine methylation at its *Not*I site. Analysis of fragments in 12 lung adenocarcinomas and corresponding normal lung tissue was undertaken. Six chromosome 1 fragments were found to exhibit reduced intensity in two or more tumor samples, compared to their intensity in the control samples (Table 1, Figure 3). Fragment 41 was previously cloned and shown to map to 1p13–21 [41]. It comprises a novel sequence. The availability of the cloned fragment 41 allowed us to undertake Southern analysis to determine if the fragment is deleted or if its absence in tumor 2D patterns was due to hypermethylation. Southern analysis confirmed *Not*I site methylation in tumors that exhibited diminished intensity of fragments 41 by 2D analysis (unpublished data). The availability of a large number of genomic 2D patterns of esophageal tumors allowed us to determine whether the six fragments also exhibited changes in esophageal adenocarcinomas. Among the six fragments that exhibited reduced intensity in lung adenocarcinomas, two also exhibited reduced intensity in esophageal adenocarcinoma. It is also noteworthy that two of

Table 1. Chromosome 1 fragments with reduced intensity in lung adenocarcinomas *

	L2	L4	L5	L6	L7	L8	L10	L11
041	2/1	2/1	2/1	2/1	2/1	–	–	2/1
059p	2/1	–	1/1	1/1	2/1	–	–	2/1
063	2/1	2/1	–	2/1	–	–	–	??
108	2/1	–	2/1	–	–	–	–	2/1
193	–	–	–	–	–	2/1	–	2/1
205p	h/1	h/h	–	–	–	h/h	h/1	–

* Tumors are identified with the letter L. Absence of a change is designated as –. A designation of 2/1 indicates that the intensity in a tumor is half that in normal tissue. Two fragments (59 and 205) exhibit polymorphism. One allele is detectable in 2D gels for 59, whereas two alleles are detectable for 205. A designation of h/1 indicates that one allele is detectable in the tumor, whereas the normal tissue shows heterozygosity.

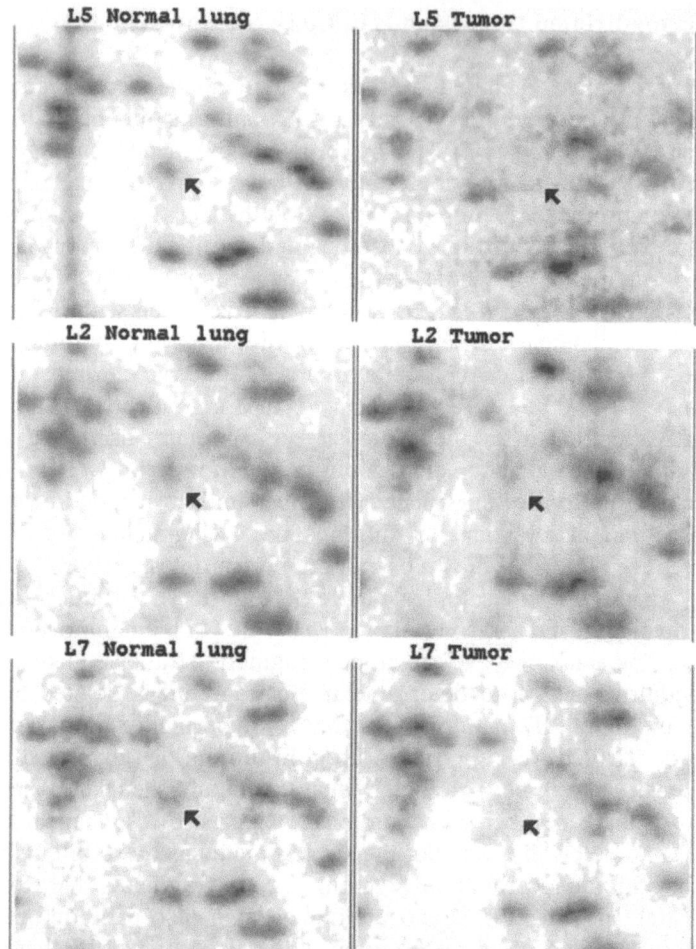

Figure 3. Closeup section of 2D patterns of three tumors that exhibited reduced intensity of fragment 41 (arrow) relative to corresponding normal controls.

these fragments were missing from the A549 lung adenocarcinoma cell line 2D patterns [42].

7. Conclusion

While the results of the 2D genome scanning to date are descriptive in nature, they are quite informative with respect to the methylation process. They do establish that in lung adenocarcinomas, as in a number of other tumor types we have analysed, some CpG islands become hypermethylated while others are hypomethylated. It is unlikely that the methylation changes are simply the result of stochastic errors in methylation as previously suggested. One example is the demethylation of repetitive units. Our findings indicate that only a fraction of the Nbl-1 repetitive units exhibits demethylation at the *Not*I sites. If the change in cytosine methylation were a random process, it would follow that the multiple copies of the repetitive sequence would be randomly demethylated. However, the data indicate that a tandem subset is demethylated. Thus it would appear that factors other than the sequence motif or random errors are responsible for the change in methylation status. The identification of a CpG island containing a *Not*I fragment that was reduced in intensity in lung tumors, and the demonstration of hypermethylation of its *Not*I site by Southern analysis, indicate that the 2D approach will be informative for studies of methylation changes in lung tumors. The fragment was among 6 of 183 fragments analysed that exhibited reduced intensity in tumors. As the study is expanded to include all *Not*I fragments detectable in 2D patterns, the full extent of methylation changes observed in 2D patterns of tumors will be appreciated. The identity of affected loci will be determined by current sequencing experiments.

References

1. Adams RLP, Burdon RH (1985) DNA methylation in the cell. *In:* Rich A (ed): *Molecular Biology of DNA Methylation*, Springer-Verlag, New York, pp 9–18.
2. Antequera F, Bird A (1993) CpG islands. *In:* Jost JP, Saluz HP (eds): *DNA Methylation: Molecular Biology and Biological Significance,* Birkhäuser Verlag, Basel, pp 169–185.
3. Yeivin A, Razin A (1993) Gene methylation patterns and expression. *In:* Jost JP, Haluz HP (eds): *DNA Methylation: Molecular Biology and Biological Significance.* Birkhäuser Verlag, Basel, pp 523–568.
4. Antequera F, Bird A (1993) Number of CpG islands and genes in the human and mouse. *Proc Natl Acad Sci USA* 90: 11995–11999.
5. Bestor T, Laudano A, Mattaliano R, Ingram V (1988) Cloning and sequencing of a cDNA encoding DNA methyltransferase of mouse cells. *J Molec Biol* 203: 971–983.
6. Adams RLP, Burdon RH (1985) S-Adenosyl-L-methionine – donor of methyl groups. *In:* Razin A, Cedar H, Riggs AD (eds): *Molecular Biology of DNA Methylation.* Springer-Verlag, New York, pp 31–41.
7. Stein WD (1980) The epigenetic address: A model for embryological development. *Journal of Theoretical Biology* 82: 663–677.
8. Adams RLP, Lindsay H, Reale A, Seivwright C, Kass S, Cummings M et al. (1993) Regulation of *de novo* methylation. *In:* Jost JP, Saluz HP (eds): *DNA Methylation: Molecular Biology and Biological Significance.* Birkhäuser Verlag, Basel, pp 487–509.
9. Issa J-PJ, Ottaviano YL, Celano P, Hamilton SR, Davidson NE, Baylin SB (1994) Methylation of the oestrogen receptor CpG island links ageing and neoplasia in human colon. *Nature Genetics* 7: 536–540.
10. Watanabe S, Kawai J, Hirotsune S, Suzuki H, Hirose K, Taga C, Ozawa N, Fushiki S, Hayashizaki Y (1995) Accessibility to tissue-specific genes from methylation profiles of mouse brain genomic DNA. *Electrophoresis* 16: 218–226.
11. Spruck CH, Rideout WM, Jones PA (1993) DNA methylation and cancer. *In:* Jost JP, Saluz HP (eds): *DNA Methylation: Molecular Biology and Biological Significance.* Birkhäuser Verlag, Basel, pp 487–509.
12. Laird PW, Jaenisch R (1994) DNA methylation and cancer. *Hum Molec Genet* 3: 1487–1495.
13. Counts JL, Goodman JI (1995) Alterations in DNA methylation may play a variety of roles in carcinogenesis. *Cell* 83: 13–15.

14. Yebra MJ, Bhagwat AS (1995) Role of cytosine methyltransferases in causing C to T mutations. *Biochem* 34: 14752–14757.
15. Breit TM, Wolvers-Tettero ILM, van Dongen JJM (1994) Lineage specific demethylation of *tal*-1 gene breakpoint region determines the frequency of *tal*-1 deletion in $\alpha\beta$ lineage T cells. *Oncogene* 9: 1847–1853.
16. Pogribny IP, Basnakian AG, Miller BJ, Lopatina NG, Poirier LA, James SJ (1995) Breaks in genomic DNA and within the *p53* gene are associated with hypomethylation in livers of folate/methyl-deficient rats. *Cancer Res* 55: 1894–1901.
17. Ottaviano YL, Issa J-PJ, Parl FF, Smith HS, Baylin SB, Davidson NE (1994) Methylation of the estrogen receptor gene CpG island marks loss of estrogen receptor expression in human breast cancer cells. *Cancer Res* 54: 2552–2555.
18. Millikin D, Meese E, Vogelstein B, Witkowski C, Trent J (1991) Loss of heterozygosity for loci on the long arm of chromosome 6 in human malignant melanoma. *Cancer Res* 51: 5449–5453.
19. Issa J-PJ, Zehnbauer BA, Civin CI, Collector MI, Sharkis SJ, Davidson NE, Kaufmann SH, Baylin SB (1996) The estrogen receptor CpG island is methylated in most hematopoietic neoplasms. *Cancer Res* 56: 973–977.
20. Issa J-PJ, Baylin SB, Belinsky SA (1996) Methylation of the estrogen receptor CpG island in lung tumors is related to the specific type of carcinogen exposure. *Cancer Res* 56: 3655–3658.
21. Laird PW, Jackson-Grusby L, Fazeli A, Dickinson SL, Jung WE, Li E, Weinberg RA, Jaenisch R (1995) Suppression of intestinal neoplasia by DNA hypomethylation. *Cell* 81: 197–205.
22. Wu J, Issa J-PJ, Herman J, Basset Jr. DE, Nelin BD, Baylin SB (1993) Expression of an exogenous eukaryotic DNA methyltransferase gene induces transformation of NIH 3T3 cells. *Proc Natl Acad Sci USA* 90: 8891–8895.
23. Belinsky SA, Nikula KJ, Baylin SB, Issa J-PJ (1996) Increased cytosine DNA-methyltransferase activity is target-cell-specific and an early event in lung cancer. *Proc Natl Acad Sci USA* 93: 4045–4050.
24. Lee PJ, Washer LL, Law DJ, Boland CR, Horon IL, Feinberg AP (1996) Limited up-regulation of DNA methyltransferase in human colon cancer reflecting increased cell proliferation. *Proc Nat Acad Sci USA* 93: 10366–10370.
25. Triboli C, Tamanini F, Patrosso C, Milanesi L, Villa A, Pergolizzi R, Maestrini E, Rivella S, Blone S, Mancini M, et al. (1992) Methylation and sequence analysis around Eagi sites: Identification of 28 new CpG islands in XQ24-XQ28. *Nucl Acids Res* 20: 727–733.
26. Stein R, Razin A, Cedar H (1982) *In vitro* methylation of the hamster adenine phosphoribosyltransferase gene inhibits its expression in mouse L cells. *Proc Natl Acad Sci USA* 79: 3418–3422.
27. Skolnick MM, Sternberg SR, Neel JV (1982) Computer programs for adapting two-dimensional gels to the study of mutation. *Clin Chem* 28: 969–978.
28. Skolnick MM, Neel JV (1986) An algorithm for comparing two-dimensional electrophoretic gels, with particular reference to the study of mutation. *In:* Harris H, Hirschhorn K (eds): *Advances in Human Genetics.* Plenum Press, New York, pp 55–160.
29. Kuick R, Skolnick MM, Neel JV, Hanash SM (1991) An automatic spot matching algorithm for two-dimensional electrophoresis. *Electrophoresis* 12: 736–746.
30. Hatada I, Hayashizaki Y, Hirotsune S, Komatsubara H (1991) A genomic scanning method for higher organisms using restriction sites as landmarks. *Proc Natl Acad Sci USA* 88: 9523–9527.
31. Asakawa J, Kuick R, Neel JV, Kodaira M, Satoh C, Hanash SM (1994) Genetic variation detected by quantitative analysis of end-labeled genomic DNA fragments. *Proc Natl Acad Sci USA* 91: 9052–9056.
32. Kuick R, Asakawa J, Neel JV, Satoh C, Hanash SM (1995) High yield of restriction fragment length polymorphisms in two-dimensional separations of human genomic DNA. *Genomics* 25: 345–353.
33. Larsen F, Gundersen G, Lopez R, Prydz H (1992) CpG islands as gene markers in the human genome. *Genomics* 13: 1095–1107.
34. Lindsay S, Bird AP (1987) Use of restriction enzymes to detect potential gene sequences in mammalian DNA. *Nature* 327: 336–338.

35. Asakawa J, Kuick R, Neel JV, Kodaira M, Satoh C, Hanash SM (1995) Quantitative and qualitative genetic variation in two-dimensional DNA gels of human lymphocytoid cell lines. *Electrophoresis* 16: 241–252.
36. Thoraval D, Asakawa J, Kodaira M, Chang C, Radany E, Kuick R, Lamb B, Richardson B, Neel JV, Glover T et al. (1996) A methylated human 9 Kb repetitive sequence on acrocentric chromosomes is homologous to a subtelomeric repeat in chimpanzee. *Proc Natl Acad Sci USA* 93: 4442–447.
37. Miwa W, Yashima K, Sekine T, Sekiya T (1995) Demethylation of a repetitive DNA sequence in human cancers. *Electrophoresis* 16: 227–232.
38. Thoraval DH, Asakawa J-I, Wimmer K, Kuick R, Lamb B, Richardson B, Ambros P, Glover T, Hanash S, et al. (1996) Demethylation of repetitive DNA sequences in neuroblastoma. *Genes Chromosom Cancer* 17: 234–244.
39. Royle N, Hill M, Jeffreys A (1992) Isolation of telomere junction fragments by anchored polymerase chain reaction. *Proc Royal Soc London: Series B* 247: 57–61.
40. Fawcett JJ, Longmire JL, Martin JC, Deaven LL, Cram LS (1994) Large-scale chromosome sorting. *Methods Cell Biol* 42: 319–330.
41. Wimmer K, Thoraval D, Asakawa J, Kuick R, Kodaira M, Lamb B, Fawcett J, Glover T, Cran S, Hanash S (1996) Two-dimensional separation and cloning of chromosome 1 *Notv-Eco-*RI-derived genomic fragments. *Genomics* 38: 124–134.
42. Giard DJ, Aaronson SA, Todaro GJ, Arnstein P, Kersey JH, Dosik H, Parks WP (1973) *In vitro* cultivation of human tumors: Establishment of cell lines derived from a series of solid tumors. *J Natl Cancer Inst* 51: 1417–1423.

Clinical and Biological Basis of Lung Cancer Prevention
ed. by Y. Martinet, F. R. Hirsch, N. Martinet, J.-M. Vignaud
and J. L. Mulshine

CHAPTER 14
K-*ras* Mutations as Molecular Markers of Lung Cancer

Daniel R. Jacobson

Department of Medicine and Kaplan Cancer Center, New York University Medical Center, and Medical and Research Services, New York Department of Veterans Affairs Medical Center, New York, NY, USA

1. Genetic Abnormalities in Lung Cancer and Potential Use as Tumor Markers

In recent years, molecular tumor markers have found increasing clinical application in a variety of tumors. In lung cancer, however, they are still primarily research tools, and are only beginning to move towards clinical application. In general, molecular genetic tumor markers may be of potential use in at least four distinct clinical settings: 1) for diagnostic purposes, when a malignancy is suspected, and molecular studies are performed on biopsy specimens or biological fluids such as bronchoalveolar lavage (BAL) fluid or sputum [1–4]; 2) for the early diagnosis of disease relapse following therapy for malignancy [5, 6]; 3) for improved pathological staging of malignancy, where the application of sensitive tumor markers may improve the ability to detect micrometastases [7–10]; 4) for cancer screening, in asymptomatic populations [11]. DNA-based tumor markers may eventually come to play a role in all four areas in lung cancer.

According to current concepts of carcinogenesis, malignancies develop because of an accumulation of abnormalities in genes that affect cell growth and differentiation (oncogenes and tumor suppressor genes); single genetic abnormalities are insufficient to cause cancer, but may alter cellular growth, leading to an increased propensity for the acquisition of additional genetic abnormalities, any of which can potentially be used diagnostically. Among the various genes which often contain abnormalities in lung cancer, the K-*ras* oncogene and the *p53* tumor suppressor gene appear at present to be most suitable as potential clinical tumor markers, because of their prevalence in none-small cell lung cancer (NSCLC) and the relative ease of detecting them [12–14]. Other genes often containing abnormalities in a large percentage of lung cancer cases include the retinoblastoma (*rb*) gene, which often exhibits deletions, mutations, or translocations, and the *myc* and HER2/*neu* genes, which are often overexpressed. In addition, various chromosomal regions contain deletions in many cases of lung cancer; these genomic segments, including segments of chromosomes 3p, 5q, and 9p, appear to contain tumor suppressor genes (or, in the case of 3p, multiple tumor suppressor genes [15, 16]), which play a role in lung carcinogenesis. The genetic changes associated with lung cancer have been reviewed in detail elsewhere [17–21].

Ras mutations, and other somatic genetic abnormalities found in large percentages of lung cancer cells, clearly offer potentially powerful tools for detection of cancer in many clinical settings. For example, one group, using a highly sensitive mutation detection assay, detected K-*ras* mutations in sputum prior to the diagnosis of lung adenocarcinoma [11]. Similarly, we have demonstrated that K-*ras* mutations can be detected in BAL fluid obtained from patients under evaluation for suspected lung cancer, and that molecular genetic studies can be more sensitive than routine histological and cytological examination for detecting carcinoma [1]. These types of studies have raised hopes that molecular assays may soon be routinely applied to clinical material [22]. However, there are still technical obstacles and unanswered biological questions which must be addressed before *ras* mutations will ready for routine clinical application.

2. *Ras* Mutations in Lung Cancer: Biology and Technology

The *ras* oncogene family includes three highly conserved functional genes, N-*ras*, K-*ras*, and H-*ras*, which encode related proteins of 189 amino acids, termed p21. The ras proteins possess GTPase activity and function in signal transduction. Point mutations confer transforming properties on the *ras* genes; nearly all oncogenic *ras* mutations have occurred in codons 12, 13, and 61 [23, 24]. Oncogenic mutations yield p21 proteins with altered GTP binding, leading to constitutive activation. Many cases of lung adenocarcinoma contain mutations within K-*ras* codon 12; thus, an assay for mutations in this codon should be of use as a tumor marker. In the largest published series of *ras* mutations in human lung cancer, from the Netherlands Cancer Institute, K-*ras* codon 12 mutations were found in 43/181 (24%) of lung adenocarcinomas, and mutations in other *ras* codons were much less common; several other studies have reported similar results (reviewed in [12]). A crucial technical issue, however, is that the reported prevalence of *ras* mutations in lung cancer depends not only upon their true prevalence, but also upon the relationship in each specimen between the percentage of cells carrying a mutation and the sensitivity of the mutation-detection assay used; thus, in evaluating these studies and studies attempting to apply K-*ras* mutations as clinical tumor markers, we must consider the sensitivity of the assays used. If a *ras* mutation is present in only a fraction of the malignant cells, or if the DNA studied is isolated from a clinical sample containing both normal and malignant cells, the total number of copies of mutant *ras* alleles in the sample may be much less than the number of normal-sequence alleles, and if an insensitive assay for *ras* mutations is used in this setting, then false negative results may occur (reviewed in [12] and [25]).

In recent years, most investigators studying *ras* mutations have used assays based on the polymerase chain reaction (PCR) of *ras* exon 1 (containing codons 12 and 13) and exon 2 (containing codon 61) followed by allele-specific oligonucleotide hybridization (ASO-h), for which a mutation must be present in at least 10% of the corresponding *ras* alleles to be detected [25–27]. Other groups detected K-*ras* mutations using assays based on restriction analysis [28], PCR/single strand conformation polymorphism analysis [29] or PCR/denaturing gradient gel electrophoresis [30], which are no more sensitive than PCR/ASO-h [31, 32].

Since cancer is a clonal disease, one might expect that in *ras* mutation-positive cases, the mutation would be contained in all cells of the tumor, but this issue has not been examined in lung cancer. Indeed, in one malignancy in which this question has been rigorously studied, acute myelogenous leukemia (AML), N-*ras* mutations are often contained in only a fraction of the leukemic cells [33–35]. In general, after several genetic changes occur, cells may acquire a growth advantage over their normal counterparts and may appear histologically premalignant, but may not yet have acquired all the features of malignant cells, such as the ability to metastasize. As additional genetic changes accumulate, cells undergo further biological changes. If, as suggested by some lung cancer data [36], *ras* mutations are not among the first genetic changes acquired by pulmonary cells during their evolution into cancer cells, but rather are only acquired after clonal growth is established, then as in AML, these mutations might appear in only a fraction of the tumor cells.

Another important technical issue complicating attempts to detect oncogene mutations in clinical samples is that resected lung cancer specimens generally contain both tumor cells and normal pulmonary cells; DNA isolated from such specimens is derived from both populations. For example, the Netherlands Cancer Institute series included specimens containing as few as 25% malignant cells [37], while another study included samples containing as few as 20% cancer cells, which the investigators acknowledged may have led to some false negative results [26]. Thus, both the presence of *ras* mutations in only a fraction of the malignant cells, and the mixture of normal with malignant cells in clinical samples could lead to the preparation of DNA containing a mutation in only a small fraction of the total number of *ras* alleles. As long as the minimum percentage of mutant alleles which is detectable by an assay is larger than the percentage of mutant alleles present in some DNA samples, false negative results must arise.

With these concerns in mind, we ascertained the prevalence of K-*ras* codon 12 mutations in lung adenocarcinoma, using a more sensitive assay (Figure 1). We reexamined some of the DNA samples from the Netherlands Cancer Institute series and, in several cases, detected mutations which had

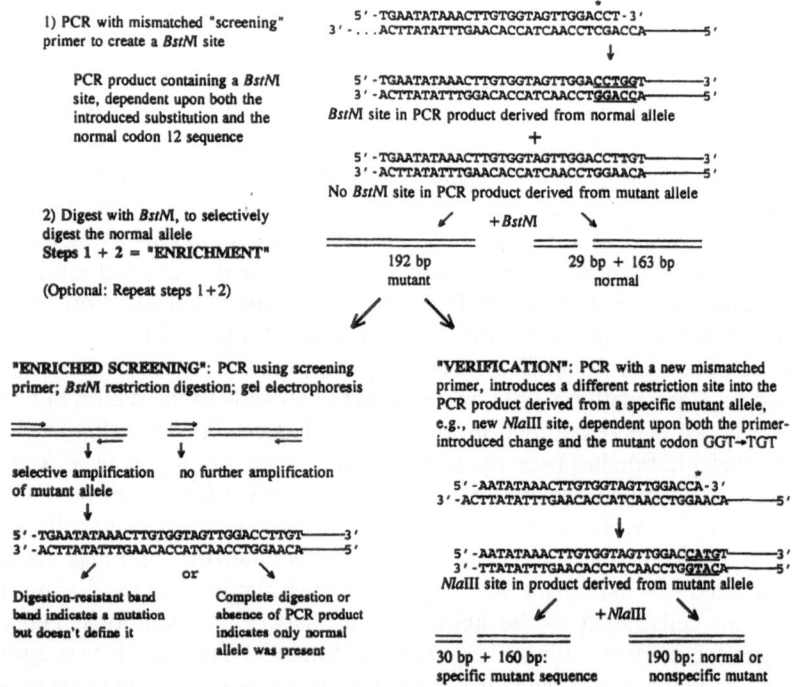

Figure 1. The PCR-PIREMA strategy, as applied to K-*ras* codon 12, and verification of one mutation, in this case TGT. Prior to the first round of enrichment, we typically perform PCR using fully matched primers flanking the exon [1, 12]; this leads to increased yield, but may not always be necessary. PCR is performed using a 5' ("screening") primer containing a mismatch from the DNA being amplified, which introduces a *Bst*NI restriction site into PCR products derived from a normal-sequence allele, while an allele containing a mutation at position 1 or 2 of codon 12 forms a digestion-resistant product. PCR products are *Bst*NI-digested, leaving the products derived from mutant alleles. These two steps may be repeated, with potential gain in sensitivity, but loss of specificity (see text). Further amplification followed by *Bst*NI digestion is performed, and analyzed by agarose gel electrophoresis ("enriched screening"); a digestion-resistant band indicates that a mutant allele was present originally, but does not identify the mutation. To identify the mutation, PCR is performed on the enriched product using different mismatched "verification" primers which introduce new restriction sites into the PCR products derived from specific mutant alleles. A PCR product which cuts with a verification enzyme confirms that a specific mutation is present. The verification primers and enzymes used to identify K-*ras* codon 12 mutations are listed in Table 1. Verification strategies have been designed for all K- and N-*ras* codon 12, 13, and 61 mutations [25]. PCR conditions are as described [12].

been missed by PCR/ASO-h; we estimated that mutations were actually present in 48% of the cases, or twice as many as had been detectable using PCR/ASO-h [12]. Consistent with these results, we also found K-*ras* codon 12 mutations in 56% of previously unstudied lung adenocarcinoma specimens at our institution [12]. Two other small studies which used highly sensitive mutation assays also reported *ras* mutations in over 50% of lung adenocarcinoma cases [11, 38]. Our data and those of others therefore indicate that at least 50% of lung adenocarcinomas contain a point mutation in K-*ras* codon 12, suggesting that these mutations may prove to be more widely applicable as clinical tumor markers than would be expected from studies which used less sensitive assays. Furthermore, the suggestion that significant numbers of cases of lung adenocarcinoma have *ras* mutations in only a small percentage of the cancer cells (as implied by the detection of these mutations by a highly sensitive assay but not by PCR/ASO-h) suggests that *ras* mutations are not an early event, but are more likely to be a secondary event in a subclone of the tumor, as has been argued for AML [39]. This concept is consistent with the association of *ras* mutations with increased tumor growth and invasiveness, as suggested by the poorer prognosis of mutation-positive than mutation-negative cases treated by surgical resection [26, 30, 40–42]. These studies also emphasize the importance of considering the technical aspects of mutation detection assays when drawing biological conclusions.

3. *Ras* Mutations as Tumor Markers: Application to Early Diagnosis and Screening

Several groups of investigators have recognized that for many purposes, and certainly for clinical studies aiming to diagnose cancer by detecting mutations in biological specimens, "standard" assays such as PCR/ASO-h are not sensitive enough, and that a mutation, even if present, will remain hidden in a much larger number of normal alleles. One approach to this problem, taken by several research groups including our own, has been to use a technique often called "enriched PCR" (in our lab, termed PCR-primer-introduced restriction with enrichment of mutant alleles, PCR-PIREMA) [12, 25, 43 – 50]. Our assay, as used to detect mutations in K-*ras* codon 12, is depicted schematically in Figure 1. The concept underlying this method is that PCR is performed using a primer which introduces a restriction site (for the enzyme *Bst*NI) into PCR products derived from the mutant, but not normal allele. This product is digested with *Bst*NI, after which only PCR products containing a mutation should remain uncleaved, and thus available for further amplification. Additional PCR is then performed, selectively amplifying the mutant allele, and the product is analysed for mutations, either by further PCR and restriction analysis (as in Figure 1, "enriched screening" and "verification"), or by other methods such as ASO-h or sequencing.

We have used this assay to study whether detection of K-*ras* codon 12 mutations in BAL fluid obtained from patients undergoing evaluation for suspected lung cancer is of potential clinical value [1]. The enrichment for mutant alleles provided by PCR-PIREMA was essential, because cancer cells, when present in BAL fluid, are mixed with many genetically normal nucleated cells (alveolar macrophages, white blood cells, and bronchial epithelial cells) [51]. In the patients we have studied, detection of a K-*ras* mutation in BAL fluid has been both highly sensitive and specific for diagnosing mutation-positive cases of adenocarcinoma. In all cases where we have detected a mutation in BAL fluid, the patient was eventually diagnosed with lung cancer, or, in a few cases, has been lost to followup without a definitive diagnosis being established. In addition, in several cases, mutations have been detected in BAL fluid obtained during otherwise nondiagnostic procedures, i.e. when the BAL fluid and all biopsies obtained were read as cytologically and histologically negative for malignancy, and cancer was not diagnosed histologically until later in the patient's course [1]. In all cases, mutation analysis was at least as sensitive as cytological examination of BAL fluid. These results suggest that molecular analysis of BAL fluid offers potential for widespread clinical application, and may lead to earlier diagnoses of lung cancer. An obvious next step is to investigate whether this assay also will enable detection of K-*ras* mutations in sputum specimens; if so, it may offer a tool not only for earlier diagnosis in patients clinically suspected of having lung cancer, but also for lung cancer screening programs of asymptomatic populations.

The potential of identifying cancer-associated mutations in sputum prior to the diagnosis of lung cancer is illustrated by a study in which 15 patients who provided sputum specimens as part of a randomized trial of lung cancer screening later developed lung cancer. The primary tumors of ten of the patients contained a mutation in K-*ras* codon 12 or in *p53*. In eight patients, the identical mutation was detected in at least one sputum sample a month or more prior to the clinical diagnosis, which clearly demonstrates the potential of screening sputum samples for mutations. A drawback to this study was that it used a mutation detection method which may be too labor-intensive and expensive for routine application to large numbers of clinical samples: after DNA was isolated from sputum, PCR was performed, the PCR products were cloned into a bacteriophage vector, transferred to nylon filters, and the filters were assayed for mutant clones by ASO-h [11].

4. Technical Limitations

The development of enriched PCR assays has not yet led to their widespread use, and several groups, after publishing one or two studies using the method, have apparently abandoned it. The individual steps outlined in

Figure 1 appear to be straightforward, and on paper, the technique would appear to offer a method for achieving unlimited sensitivity for mutation detection. What, then, is the difficulty?

We and others have found that the biggest technical obstacle arises from the fact that after amplification with a mismatched primer, *Bst*NI digestion and reamplification, the PCR products become resistant to *Bst*NI digestion even if no mutation was present in the original starting material. This means, on "enriched screening" (Figure 1), all samples, including normal controls, may contain a digestion-resistant band, regardless of the amount of *Bst*NI in the reaction. While true mutants may be distinguishable from normals by the fact that the digestion-resistant band is more intense in the true mutants, any degree of incomplete digestion in the normal controls changes the assay from a qualitative to quantitative assay, and leads to some questionable results. The appearance of visibly digestion-resistant bands may be inconsistent from sample to sample and experiment to experiment, which complicates the interpretation of data. If, in an effort to visualize low-level mutations, two rounds of enrichment are performed (repeating steps 1 and 2 prior to analysis), the problem of digestion-resistant bands appearing in all lanes becomes even more noticeable.

This difficulty arises from the high misincorporation rate of *Taq* polymerase (on the order of 1 error per $10^4 - 10^5$ bases, under "standard" PCR conditions) [52]. During PCR, occasional errors made by the polymerase when copying the first and second bases of codon 12 can change a normal codon into a mutant. This error rate is not be high enough to lead to a visible digestion-resistant band on agarose gel electrophoresis if no enrichment for mutant alleles is performed, so after a single round of PCR and *Bst*NI digestion (without enrichment), normal PCR products appear to cut completely. The enrichment process, however, enriches not only for PCR products derived from authentic mutant alleles present originally, but also for PCR products containing mutations in codon 12 introduced as errors during PCR, which change the PCR product from *Bst*NI-sensitive to *Bst*NI-resistant. These digestion-resistant products are then further amplified in subsequent PCR reactions.

When it became apparent that *Taq* polymerase infidelity might be the explanation for the digestion-resistance of normal controls on enriched screening, it seemed that a possible solution lay in attempting to improve the polymerase fidelity. *Taq* polymerase does not have a proofreading activity, while other heat-stable polymerases with proofreading activity have a higher fidelity; however, a proofreading enzyme would be expected to remove the mismatched base in the primer which is necessary for creation of the *Bst*NI site, so this approach is not an option. "Standard" PCR conditions (200 µM each nucleotide and 1.5–2.0 mM MgCl$_2$ concentrations) maximize the speed of polymerization and lead to maximal PCR product yield and fastest permissible cycling times. These advantages (the overriding considerations for many experiments) are obtained at the expense, however, of optimal polymerase fidelity [52]. Decreased concentrations of nucleotides and $MgCl_2$ in the PCR reaction lead to increased *Taq* polymerase fidelity [52], so we investigated these variables (and others, such as cycling times and temperatures) in an effort to improve assay sensitivity and specificity. We have empirically established conditions with lowered nucleotide and $MgCl_2$ concentrations which improve *Taq* polymerase fidelity and still provide sufficient yield [12], leading to an assay with improved reliability.

Although we have improved *Taq* polymerase fidelity (leading to improved assay results), we have not been able to eliminate polymerase errors completely (probably an impossibility), so false positive digestion-resistant bands always remain a possibility for individual samples. This is particularly the case if two rounds of enrichment, which may help visualize a mutation on the verification step, are performed (Figure 1). Our approach to this problem is twofold: first, if a sample appears to contain a mutation on "enriched screening", we always determine the specific mutation present. Our method for determining the specific mutation is to perform further PCR and restriction analysis, termed "verification" (usually using a primer which introduces another mismatch, Table 1). Other methods of determining the specific mutation present, including ASO-h and sequencing, have been used by other groups. As another important precaution, we confirm all test results at least twice (or, in cases where a result is questionable, more times) from the beginning. As *Taq* polymerase errors

Table 1. K-*ras* codon 12 screening and verification primers and enzymes

Primer	Primer sequence	Site
s-GGT	5′ TGAATATAAACTTGTGGTAGTTGGA**CC**Tggtgg...	*BstNI*
v-AGT[a]	5′ TGAATATAAACTTGTGGTAGTTGGAC**C**Tagtgg...	*BfaI*
v-CGT	5′ TGAATATAAACTTGTGGTAGTTGGAC**CA**cgtgg...	*BbrPI*
v-TGT[b]	5′ TGAATATAAACTTGTGGTAGTTGGAC**CA**tgtgg...	*NlaIII*
v-GTT[b]	5′ TGAATATAAACTTGTGGTAGTTGGA**CCA**gttgg...	*BsrI*
v-GCT[b]	5′ TGAATATAAACTTGTGGTAGTTGGAC**CA**gctgg...	*PvuII*
v-GAT	5′ TGAATATAAACTTGTGGTAGTTGG**TCA**Tgatgg...	*BspHI*

Primer names indicate whether a screening "s-" or verification "v-" primer is used, and the specific mutation detected. Primer sequences are capitalized; lowercase letters indicate bases incorporated during PCR. Mismatched bases are in boldface. Bases comprising newly-created restriction sites are underlined. The screening primer can be used both in screening/enrichment and as a verification primer for the mutated codon AGT; the CGT verification primer can also be used, with different restriction enzymes, to verify mutant codons TGT, GTT, and GCT. Thus, the total number of verification primers (and verification PCR reactions) required is fewer than the number of mutations which can be verified: [a]identical sequence to the primer above; [b]identical sequence to the screening primer. All position 3 mutations are silent, and need not be screened for.

should be somewhat random (although certain misincorporations are more common than others) [52, 53], any sample which repeatedly demonstrates the same mutation can be considered to be definitively positive. Mutation detection based solely upon the results of enriched PCR and *BstN*I digestion, without further analysis to determine the specific mutation present in each sample, is, in our experience, less reliable.

Other methods have also been used to detect a small proportion of mutant *ras* alleles in a background of many more normal alleles. One approach has used allele-specific PCR (also termed "mutant-allele-specific amplification", "PCR amplification of specific alleles", and other names) [9, 54–56]. In this method, a particular mutant allele is PCR-amplified using a primer with a 3′ nucleotide which matches the mutant base and thus contains a 3′ mismatch from the normal allele. The difficulty with this method is that many studies have determined that while "allele-specific" PCR can be made to amplify *preferentially* one allele over another, it is difficult or impossible to make allele-specific PCR *completely* allele-specific [54, 57, 58]; if even a single molecule of the normal allele is successfully amplified despite a 3′ primer mismatch in an early round of PCR, this PCR product would serve as a perfectly matched template for subsequent rounds of PCR, and could lead to a false positive signal.

The multitude of methods used to detect low level *ras* mutations indicates the imperfection of all currently used methods, and further development will undoubtedly continue in many directions. Furthermore, all of the assays described above remain somewhat labor-intensive and costly for routine clinical application. As a practical matter, while additional technical improvements are needed, our experience is that with the precautions and caveats discussed above, enriched PCR-based methods provide a powerful tool for analysis of clinical samples.

5. Biological Limitations

In addition to the technical considerations discussed above, important biological questions about the specificity of *ras* mutations for lung cancer remain unanswered. No person has ever been reported with a germline activating *ras* mutation, and somatic *ras* mutations have been considered oncogenic, implying a close association with malignancy, or at least abnormal growth properties. A key question, however, is whether the presence of a K-*ras* codon 12 point mutation in DNA isolated from pulmonary-derived tissue *always* indicates that lung cancer must be present in the tissue from which the DNA was isolated. If so, such mutations should have strong potential for clinical use as tumor markers. On the other hand, if *ras* mutations can occur in normal pulmonary tissue, or at least in tissue which is not irrevocably destined to develop cancer, then the clinical interpretation of finding a mutation in BAL fluid or sputum becomes problematic.

Recent data have begun to address this issue. One group studied DNA samples isolated from paired malignant lung tumors and non malignant lung tissue specimens obtained from the same patient at bronchoscopy or thoracotomy [59, 60]. The non malignant lung samples were taken from a site as distant as possible from the primary tumor. As expected, many of the primary adenocarcinomas contained K-*ras* codon 12 mutations, but in several cases, a K-*ras* codon 12 mutation was found also in the histologically normal tissue not adjacent to the tumor. The specific mutation in the tumor did not always correspond to the mutation in the normal tissue, and a mutation was also found in normal tissue from one patient whose primary tumor (a squamous cell carcinoma) was mutation-negative. Furthermore, two specimens from patients with pulmonary infection or inflammation, but no evidence of malignancy anywhere in the pulmonary tree, had mutations in histologically normal tissue. These results, if confirmed in larger numbers of patients, would bring into question the specificity of *ras* mutations in lung tissue for cancer. Similarly, another group also reported finding K-*ras* mutations in several normal appearing lung tissues (again, mostly from patients with lung cancer), although they did not determine the specific mutations present, which would have solidified the genetic relationship between the tumors and normal tissues, and made their data more convincing [61].

Another group looked for K-*ras* mutations in paired regions of lung adenocarcinoma and atypical alveolar hyperplasia (AAH), as well as in histologically normal lung tissue adjacent to the regions of AAH, obtained from 28 patients [62]. Samples of AAH, which may be a preneoplastic precursor to lung adenocarcinoma [63], were identified as microscopic growths of cytologically atypical cuboidal to columnar cells along the alveolar septa in the absence of significant inflammation and fibrosis of the surrounding lung parenchyma, and were not studied if they were directly adjacent to a primary tumor. Eight of 19 primary adenocarcinoma specimens contained a K-*ras* codon 12 mutation, as did 16 of 41 AAH specimens removed from the same patients. The mutation status of the carcinoma and AAH specimens from the same patient usually did not correlate, suggesting that many AAH were independent mutation-containing lesions, and raising the question of whether mutation-containing AAH can occur in patients without evidence of adenocarcinoma. On the other hand, three AAH specimens from patients without malignancy were also studied (one with a hyalinized granuloma, one with interstitial lung disease, and one resected because of trauma), and no mutation was found in these samples. Thus, although K-*ras* mutations were found in regions of the lung not appearing to harbor cancer, no mutation was found in tissue from a patient without lung cancer somewhere in the pulmonary tree.

Analogous questions have been addressed in other malignancies, particularly colon cancer. Thus, K-*ras* codon 12 mutations have been found in about 50% of colon adenocarcinoma cases, and have also been reported in small hyperplastic or dysplastic lesions [64–70]. In analogy with the situation in lung cancer, many, but not all such samples studied had been removed from patients with adenocarcinoma elsewhere in the colon. Studies on colon cancer may or may not be directly applicable to lung cancer, but they support the concept that *ras* mutations need not be specific for fully developed cancer. Further investigation in these areas is needed before clinicians will be able to use *ras* mutation status in making patient care decisions.

6. Clinical Significance and the Application of "Early" versus "Late" Genetic Changes as Lung Cancer Tumor Markers

Regardless of the ultimate specificity of *ras* mutations for cancer, it does appear that, in many cases, *ras* mutations occur relatively "late" in lung carcinogenesis, usually after the development of other, "early" clonal genetic abnormalities which have been associated with dysplasia or hyperplasia [36, 71–73]. The question of whether a genetic marker occurring early or late during lung carcinogenesis is "better" as a clinical tumor marker depends upon the proposed use of the marker.

One potential setting is in lung cancer screening. To date, most lung cancer screening programs (using X-rays and/or sputum cytology) have demonstrated no impact on lung cancer mortality; therefore, such screening is generally not recommended for patients outside a research setting [74–76]. In contrast, screening programs for other common malignancies, such as colon, breast, and cervical cancer, appear to decrease cancer-related mortality, and are generally recommended [77, 78]. Thus, it appears that the ineffectiveness to date of lung cancer screening appears to result from the insensitivity of the screening tests used, rather than a flaw in the concept of screening. In previous screening studies using sputum samples, the only test performed on the samples obtained was microscopic examination for visible, intact tumor cells. One approach to improving lung cancer detection will be the application of molecular genetic tumor markers, perhaps including *ras* mutations, to sputum and/or BAL fluid samples.

Ultimately, genetic changes in occurring at the earliest stages of lung carcinogenesis may be of the greatest use for identifying patients at high risk of developing lung cancer, and people with evidence of these changes in sputum or BAL fluid may be candidates for cancer chemoprevention trials and intensified cancer surveillance. Patients found to harbor genetic changes associated with later stages of carcinogenesis may be candidates for aggressive attempts to identify an underlying malignancy, or even possibly definitive therapy based on the presence of the tumor marker alone. For example, a patient found to have a *ras* mutation in BAL fluid obtained from one pulmonary lobe, and mutation-negative fluid obtained from the other lobes, could be deemed a candidate for surgical resection even if histological and radiographic evidence of malignancy cannot be obtained. The optimal clinical use of each marker awaits further data on their biological specificity for cancer, as well as improvements in the sensitivity, specificity, reproducibility, and cost of the assays used to identify cancer-associated genetic changes.

Acknowledgements

I thank Charles Fishman, Nancy Mills, Tibor Moskovits, Peter Leonardi, Sibyl Anderson and Julia Xu for their invaluable contributions to the mutation assay development and its application to lung cancer studies. The assistance of John Scholes, Michael Ittman, Jaishree Jagirdar, Jane Denuto, William Rom, Sjoerd Rodenhuis and Bert Top in procuring clinical samples is gratefully acknowledged. I thank Joel Buxbaum and Harold Ballard for helpful conversations and useful critiques of the manuscript. This work was supported in part by American Cancer Society Institutional Grant #IRG-14-35, National Cancer Institute core grant P30 CA16087, and American Cancer Society Research Grant #CN-155.

References

1. Mills NE, Fishman CL, Scholes J, Anderson SE, Rom WN, Jacobson DR (1995) Detection of K-*ras* oncogene mutations in bronchoalveolar lavage fluid for lung cancer diagnosis. *J Natl Cancer Inst* 87: 1056–1060.
2. Mao L, Schoenberg MP, Scicchitano M, Erozan YS, Merlo A, Schwab D, Sidransky D (1996) Molecular detection of primary bladder cancer by microsatellite analysis. *Science* 271: 659–662.
3. Kawasaki ES (1992) The polymerase chain reaction: its use in the molecular characterization and diagnosis of cancers. *Cancer Invest* 10: 417–429.
4. Ronai Z, Yakubovskaya M (1995) PCR in clinical diagnosis. *J Clin Lab Anal* 9: 269–283.
5. Miller WH Jr, Kakizuka A, Frankel SR, Warrell RP Jr, DeBlasio A, Levine K, Evans RM, Dimitrovsky E (1992) Reverse transcription polymerase chain reaction for the rearranged retinoic acid receptor α clarifies diagnosis and detects minimal residual disease in acute promyelocytic leukemia. *Proc Natl Acad Sci USA* 89: 2694–2698.
6. Schilder RJ (1995) Molecular markers and stem-cell transplants: are they made for each other? *J Clin Oncol* 13: 1052–1054.
7. Brennan JA, Mao L, Hruban RH, Boyle JO, Eby YJ, Koch WM, Goodman SN, Sidransky D (1995) Molecular assessment of histopathological staging in squamous-cell carcinoma of the head and neck. *N Engl J Med* 332: 429–435.
8. Katz AE, Olsson CA, Raffo AJ, Cama C, Perlman H, Seaman E, O'Toole KM, McMahon D, Benson MC, Buttyan R (1994) Molecular staging of prostate cancer with the use of an enhanced reverse transcriptase-PCR assay. *Urology* 43: 765–775.
9. Hayashi N, Ito I, Yanagisawa A, Kato Y, Nakamori S, Imakoka S, Watanabe H (1995) Genetic diagnosis of lymph-node metastasis in colorectal cancer. *Lancet* 345: 1257–1259.
10. Schoenfeld A, Luqmani Y, Smith D, O'Reilly S, Shousha S, Sinnett HD, Coombes RC (1994) Detection of breast cancer micrometastases in axillary lymph nodes by using polymerase chain reaction. *Cancer Res* 54: 2986–2990.
11. Mao L, Hruban RH, Boyle JO, Tockman M, Sidransky D (1994) Detection of oncogene mutations in sputum precedes diagnosis of lung cancer. *Cancer Res* 54: 1634–1637.
12. Mills NE, Fishman CL, Rom WN, Dubin N, Jacobson DR (1995) Increased prevalence of K-*ras* oncogene mutations in lung adenocarcinoma. *Cancer Res* 55: 1444–1447.
13. Greenblatt MS, Bennett WP, Hollstein M, Harris CC (1994) Mutations in the *p53* tumor suppressor gene: clues to cancer etiology and molecular pathogenesis. *Cancer Res* 54: 4855–4878.
14. Krawczak M, Smith-Sorensen B, Schmidtke J, Kakkar VV, Cooper DN, Hovig E (1995) Somatic spectrum of cancer-associated single basepair substitutions in the TP53 gene is determined mainly by endogenous mechanisms of mutation and by selection. *Hum Mutation* 5: 48–57.

15. Wei MH, Latif F, Bader S, Kashuba V, Chen JY, Duh FM, Sekido Y, Lee CC, Geil L, Kuzmin I, et al. (1996) Construction of a 600-kilobase cosmid clone contig and generation of a transcriptional map surrounding the lung cancer tumor suppressor gene (TSG) locus on human chromosome 3p21.3: progress toward the isolation of a lung cancer TSG. *Cancer Res* 56: 1487–1492.
16. Sozzi G, Veronese ML, Negrini M, Baffa R, Coticelli MG, Inoue H, Tornielli S, Pilotti S, De Gregorio L, Pastorino U, et al. (1996) The *FHIT* gene at 3p14.2 is abnormal in lung cancer. *Cell* 85: 17–26.
17. Jacobson DR, Fishman CL, Mills NE (1995) Molecular genetic tumor markers in the early diagnosis and screening of non-small-cell lung cancer. *Ann Oncol* 6 (Suppl. 3): S3–S8.
18. Gazdar AF (1994) The molecular and cellular basis of human lung cancer. *Anticancer Res* 13: 261–268.
19. Minna JD (1993) The molecular biology of lung cancer pathogenesis. *Chest* 103; Suppl: 449S–456S.
20. Sabichi AL, Birrer MJ (1993) The molecular biology of lung cancer: application to early detection and prevention. *Oncol (USA)* 7: 19–26.
21. Giaccone G (1996) Oncogenes and antioncogenes in lung tumorigenesis. *Chest* 109: 130S–134S.
22. Birrer MJ (1995) Translational research and epithelial carcinogenesis: molecular diagnostic assays now-molecular screening assays soon? *J Natl Cancer Inst* 87: 1041–1043.
23. Kiaris H, Spandidos DA (1995) Mutations of *ras* genes in human tumours (review). *Internat J Oncol* 7: 413–421.
24. Lowy DR (1993) Function and regulation of ras. *Ann Rev Biochem* 62: 851–891.
25. Jacobson DR, Mills NE (1994) A highly sensitive assay for mutant *ras* genes and its application to the study of presentation and relapse genotypes in acute leukemia. *Oncogene* 9: 553–563.
26. Sugio K, Ishida T, Yokoyama H, Inoue T, Sugimachi K, Sasazuki T (1992) *ras* gene mutations as a prognostic marker in adenocarcinoma of the human lung without lymph node metastasis. *Cancer Res* 52: 2903–2906.
27. Farr CJ, Saiki RK, Erlich HA, McCormick F, Marshall CJ (1988) Analysis of *RAS* gene mutations in acute myeloid leukemia by polymerase chain reaction and oligonucleotide probes. *Proc Natl Acad Sci USA* 85: 1629–1633.
28. Mitsudomi T, Viallet J, Mulshine JL, Linnoila RI, Minna JD, Gazdar AF (1991) Mutations of *ras* genes distinguish a subset of non-small-cell lung cancer cell lines from small-cell lung cancer cell lines. *Oncogene* 6: 1353–1362.
29. Suzuki Y, Orita M, Shiraishi M, Hayashi K, Sekiya T (1990) Detection of *ras* gene mutations in human lung cancers by single-strand conformation polymorphism analysis of polymerase chain reaction products. *Oncogene* 5: 1037–1043.
30. Silini EM, Bosi F, Pellegata NS, Volpato G, Romano A, Nazari S, Tinelli C, Ranzani GN, Solcia E, Fiocca R (1994) K-ras gene mutations: an unfavorable prognostic marker in stage I lung adenocarcinoma. *Virchows Archiv* 424: 367–373.
31. Mitsudomi T, Steinberg SM, Nau MM, Carbone D, D'Amico D, Bodner S, Oie HK, Linnoila RI, Mulshine JL, Minna JD, et al. (1992) *p53* gene mutations in non-small-cell lung cancer cell lines and their correlation with the presence of *ras* mutations and clinical features. *Oncogene* 7: 171–180.
32. Ridanpää M, Husgafvel-Pursiainen K (1993) Denaturing gradient gel electrophoresis (DGGE) assay for K-*ras* and N-*ras* genes: detection of K-*ras* point mutations in human lung tumour DNA. *Hum Molec Genet* 2: 639–644.
33. Toksoz D, Farr CJ, Marshall CJ (1987) Ras gene activation in a minor proportion of the blast population in acute myeloid leukemia. *Oncogene* 1: 409–413.
34. Syvänen AC, Söderlund H, Laaksonen E, Bengtström M, Turunen M, Palotie A (1992) N-*ras* gene mutations in acute myeloid leukemia: accurate detection by solid-phase mini-sequencing. *Int J Cancer* 50: 713–718.
35. Bashey A, Gill R, Levi S, Farr CJ, Clutterbuck JL, Millar JL, Pragnell IB, Marshall CJ (1992) Mutational activation of the N-*ras* oncogene assessed in primary clonogenic culture of acute myeloid leukemia (AML): implications for the role of N-*ras* mutation in AML pathogenesis. *Blood* 79: 981–989.
36. Sugio K, Kishimoto Y, Virmani AK, Hung JY, Gazdar AF (1994) K-*ras* mutations are a relatively late event in the pathogenesis of lung carcinomas. *Cancer Res* 54: 5811–5815.

37. Rodenhuis S, Slebos RJC, Boot AJM, Evers SG, Mooi WJ, Wagenaar SS, van Bodegom PC, Bos JL (1988) Incidence and possible clinical significance of K-*ras* oncogene activation in adenocarcinoma of the human lung. *Cancer Res* 48: 5738–5741.
38. Reynolds SH, Anderson MW (1991) Activation of proto-oncogenes in human and mouse lung tumors. *Env Health Persect* 93: 145–148.
39. Toksoz D, Farr CJ, Marshall CJ (1989) *Ras* genes and acute myeloid leukemia. *Br J Haematol* 71: 1–6.
40. Slebos RJC, Kibbelaar RE, Dalesio O, Kooistra A, Stam J, Meijer CJLM, Wagenaar SS, Vanderschueren RGJRA, van Zandwijk N, Mooi Wj, et al. (1990) K-*ras* oncogene activation as a prognostic marker in adenocarcinoma of the lung. *N Engl J Med* 323: 561–565.
41. Mitsudomi T, Steinberg SM, Oie HK, Mulshine JL, Phelps R, Viallet J, Pass H, Minna JD, Gazdar AF (1991) *ras* gene mutations in non-small cell lung cancers are associated with shortened survival irrespective of treatment intent. *Cancer Res* 51: 4999–5002.
42. Rosell R, Li S, Anton A, Moreno I, Martinez E, Vadell C, Mate JL, Ariza A, Monzo M, Font A, et al. (1994) Prognostic value of K-*ras* genotypes in patients with advanced non-small cell lung cancer receiving carboplatin with either intravenous or chronic oral dose etoposide. *Internat J Oncol* 5: 169–176.
43. Chen J, Viola MV (1991) A method to detect *ras* point mutations in small subpopulations of cells. *Anal Biochem* 195: 51–56.
44. Kahn SM, Jiang W, Culberston TA, Weinstein IB, Williams GM, Tomita N, Ronai Z (1991) Rapid and sensitive nonradioactive detection of mutant K-*ras* genes via 'enriched' PCR amplification. *Oncogene* 6: 1079–1083.
45. Levi S, Urbano-Ispizua A, Gill R, Thomas DM, Gilbertson J, Foster C, Marshall CJ (1991) Multiple K-*ras* codon 12 mutations in cholangiocarcinomas demonstrated with a sensitive polymerase chain reaction technique. *Cancer Res* 51: 3497–3502.
46. Todd AV, Ireland CM, Iland HJ (1991) Allele-specific enrichment: a method for the detection of low level N-*ras* gene mutations in acute myeloid leukemia. *Leukemia* 5: 160–161.
47. Kondo H, Sugano K, Fukayama N, Kyogoku A, Nose H, Shimada K, Ohkkura H, Ohtsu A, Yoshida S, Shimosato Y (1994) Detection of point mutations in the K-*ras* oncogene at codon 12 in pure pancreatic juice for diagnosis of pancreatic carcinoma. *Cancer* 73: 1589–1594.
48. Minamoto T, Ronai Z, Yamashita N, Ochiai A, Sugimura T, Mai M, Esumi H (1994) Detection of Ki-*ras* mutation in non-neoplastic mucosa of Japanese patients with colorectal cancers. *Internat J Oncol* 4: 397–401.
49. Fleischhacker M, Lee S, Spira S, Takeuchi S, Koeffler HP. (1995) DNA aneuoploidy in morphologically normal colons from patients with colon cancer. *Mod Path* 8: 360–365.
50. Loktionov A, O'Neill IK (1995) Early detection of cancer-associated gene alterations in DNA isolated from rat feces during intestinal tumor induction with 1,2-dimethylhydrazine. *Internat J Oncol* 6: 437–445.
51. Merchant RK, Schwartz DA, Helmers RA, Dayton CS, Hunninghake GW (1992) Bronchoalveolar lavage cellularity: the distribution in normal volunteers. *Am Rev Respir Dis* 146: 448–453.
52. Eckert KA, Kunkel TA (1991) DNA polymerase fidelity and the polymerase chain reaction. *PCR Meth Appl* 1: 17–24.
53. Keohavong P, Ling L, Dias C, Thilly WG (1993) Predominant mutations induced by the *Thermococcus litoralis*, Vent DNA polymerase during DNA amplification in vitro. *PCR Meth Appl* 2: 288–292.
54. Cha RS, Zarbl H, Keohavong P, Thilly WG (1992) Mismatch amplification mutation assay (MAMA): application to the c-H-*ras* gene. *PCR Meth Appl* 2: 14–20.
55. Takeda S, Ichii S, Nakamura Y (1993) Detection of K-*ras* mutation in sputum by mutant-allele-specific amplification (MASA). *Hum Mutation* 2: 112–117.
56. Hasegawa Y, Takeda S, Ichii S, Koizumi K, Maruyama M, Fujii A, Ohta H, Nakajima T, Okuda M, Baba S, et al. (1995) Detection of K-*ras* mutations in DNAs isolated from feces of patients with colorectal tumors by mutant-allele-specific amplification (MASA). *Oncogene* 10: 1441–1445.
57. Newton CR, Graham A, Heptinstall LE, Powell SJ, Summers C, Kalsheker N, Smith JC, Markham AF (1989) Analysis of any point mutation in DNA. The amplification refractory mutation system (ARMS). *Nucl Acids Res* 17: 2503–2516.

58. Sarker G, Cassady J, Bottema C, Sommer S (1990) Characterization of polymerase chain reaction amplification of specific alleles. *Anal Biochem* 186: 64–68.
59. Nelson MA, Wymer J, Clements N Jr (1996) Detection of K-ras gene mutations in non-neoplastic lung tissue and lung cancers. *Cancer Lett* 103: 115–121.
60. Clements NC Jr, Nelson MA, Wymer JA, Savage C, Aguirre M, Garewal H (1995) Analysis of K-*ras* gene mutations in malignant and nonmalignant endobronchial tissue obtained by fiberoptic bronchoscopy. *Am J Respir Crit Care Med* 152: 1374–1378.
61. Yakubovskaya MS, Spiegelman V, Luo FC, Malaev S, Salnev A, Zbvorovskaya I, Gasparyan A, Polotsky B, Machaladze Z, Trachtenberg AC, et al. (1995) High frequency of K-*ras* mutation in normal appearing lung tissues and sputum of patients with lung cancer. *Int J Cancer* 63: 810–814.
62. Westra WH, Baas IO, Hruban RH, Askin FB, Wilson K, Offerhaus JA, Slebos RJ (1996) K-*ras* oncogene activation in atypical alveolar hyperplasias of the human lung. *Cancer Res* 56: 2224–2228.
63. Kerr KM, Carey FZ, King G, Lamb D (1994) Atypical alveolar hyperplasia: relationship with pulmonary adenocarcinoma, p53, and c-*erb*B-2 expression. *J Pathol* 174: 249–256.
64. Vogelstein B, Fearon ER, Hamilton SR, Kern SE, Preisinger AC, Leppert M, Nakamura Y, White R, Smits AMM, Bos JL (1988) Genetic alterations during colorectal-tumor development. *N Engl J Med* 319: 525–532.
65. Pretlow TP, Brasitus TA, Fulton NC, Cheyer C, Kaplan EL (1993) K-ras mutations in putative preneoplastic lesions in human colon. *J Natl Cancer Inst* 85: 2004–2007.
66. Yamashita N, Minamoto T, Ochiai A, Onda M, Esumi H (1995) Frequent and characteristic K-*ras* activation and absence of p53 protein accumulation in aberrant crypt foci of the colon. *Gastroenterol* 108: 434–440.
67. Yamashita N, Minamoto T, Ochiai A, Onda M, Esumi H (1995) Frequent and characteristic K-ras activation in aberrant crypt foci of colon. Is there preference among K-ras mutants for malignant progression? *Cancer* 75(6 suppl): 1527–1533.
68. Jackson PE, Hall CN, Badawi AF, O'Connor PJ, Cooper DP, Povey AC (1996) Frequency of Ki-*ras* mutation and DNA alkylation in colorectal tissue from individuals living in Manchester. *Molec Carcinogen* 16: 12–19.
69. Pretlow TP (1995) Aberrant crypt foci and K-*ras* mutations: earliest recognized players or innocent bystanders in colon carcinogenesis? *Gastroenterol* 108: 600–603.
70. Ajiki T, Fujimori T, Ikehara H, Saitoh Y, Maeda S (1995) K-*ras* gene mutation related to histological atypias in human colorectal adenomas. *Biotechnic & Histochem* 70: 90–94.
71. Smith AL, Hung J, Walker L, Rogers TE, Vuitch F, Lee E, Gazdar AF (1996) Extensive areas of aneuploidy are present in the respiratory epithelium of lung cancer patients. *Br J Cancer* 73: 203–209.
72. Kishimoto Y, Sugio K, Hung JY, Virmani AK, McIntire DD, Minna JD, et al. (1995) Allele-specific loss in chromosome 9p loci in preneoplastic lesions accompanying non-small cell lung cancers. *J Natl Cancer Inst* 87: 1224–1229.
73. Miozzo M, Sozzi G, Musso K, Pilotti S, Incarbone M, Pastorino U, Pierotti MA (1996) Microsatellite alterations in bronchial and sputum specimens of lung cancer patients. *Cancer Res* 56: 2285–2288.
74. Richert-Boe KE, Humphrey LL (1992) Screening for cancers of the lung and colon. *Arch Intern Med* 152: 2398–2404.
75. McDougall JC (1994) Lung cancer: to screen or not to screen? *Arch Intern Med* 154: 945.
76. Wolpaw DR (1996) Early detection in lung cancer. Case finding and screening. *Med Clin N Am* 80: 63–82.
77. Toribara NW, Sleisenger MH (1995) Screening for colorectal cancer. *N Engl J Med* 332: 861–867.
78. Miller AB (1995) An epidemiological perspective on cancer screening. *Clin Biochem* 28: 41–48.

Clinical and Biological Basis of Lung Cancer Prevention
ed. by Y. Martinet, F. R. Hirsch, N. Martinet, J.-M. Vignaud
and J. L. Mulshine
© 1998 Birkhäuser Verlag Basel/Switzerland

CHAPTER 15
Sheep Lung Adenomatosis: A Model of Virally Induced Lung Cancer

Caroline Leroux, Monique Lyon, Bénédicte Etienne, Robert Loire and Jean-François Mornex*

Laboratoire d'Immunologie et de biologie pulmonaire, INSERM CJF 93-08, Hôpital Louis Pradel et Université Claude Bernard, Lyon, France
Laboratoire associé de recherches sur les lentivirus chez les petits ruminants, INRA et Ecole nationale vétérinaire, Lyon, France

1. Introduction

Sheep lung adenomatosis is a contagious tumor of the lung. It is present in all continents [1, 2], it can be reproduced by intratracheal inoculation of tumor tissue or fluid and it is caused by a retrovirus (Jaagsiekte sheep retrovirus) that is endogenously present in sheep.

2. Epidemiology and Clinical Presentation

Adenomatosis is generally introduced into flocks by the acquisition of infected sheep or rams. It was initially described in South Africa in the late 1890s [3, 4] and is present worldwide. Initial descriptions are somewhat confusing with regard to maedi (lentiviral induced lung disease) [3]. The incidence of adenomatosis is close to 5% of the animals [5]. The incubation period in naturally infected animals is 2 to 4 years. Surprisingly, the disease is observed shortly after experimental induction. It can be detected 5 to 12 months after intratracheal inoculation in lambs.

---

* Author for correspondence.

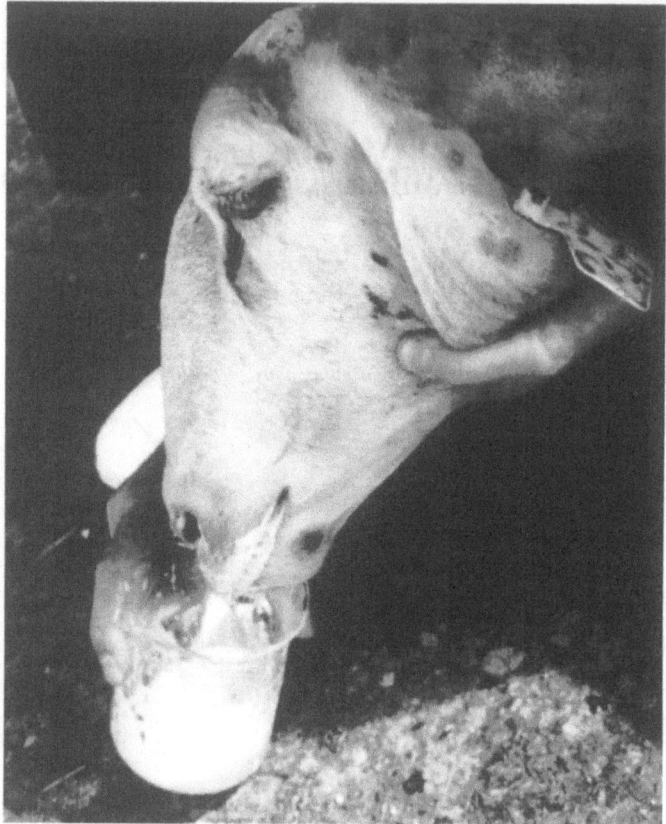

Figure 1. Clincical presentation of adenomatosis. Typical evacuation of mucoid fluid through the nostrils of an affected animal.

Symptoms are dyspnea on exercise, polypnea and weight loss. Death occurs usually from end stage lung failure, which may be due to *Pasteurella hemolytica* pneumonia. A typical sign is the running of abundant mucoid fluid from the nostrils when the rear of the animals is raised (Figure 1).

3. Pathology (reviewed in [4–6])

Lungs are enlarged and infiltrated with areas of tumor, varying from small nodules to lobar consolidation. The disease is bilateral (Figure 2) and the airways are filled with fluid. Pleural effusion is frequent in some series but without histological involvement [5]. Histologically, the normal alveolar cells are replaced by cuboidal or columnar cells with some intrabronchiolar proliferation (Figure 3). At early stages the disease appears as nodules

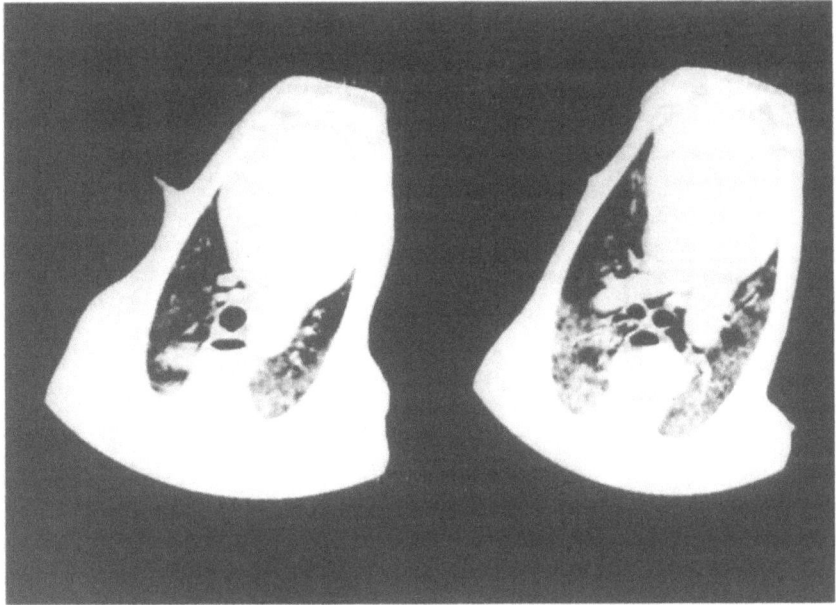

Figure 2. CT scan of adenomatosis. 1 mm slices were taken at different levels and show bilateral diffuse infiltrative lung disease.

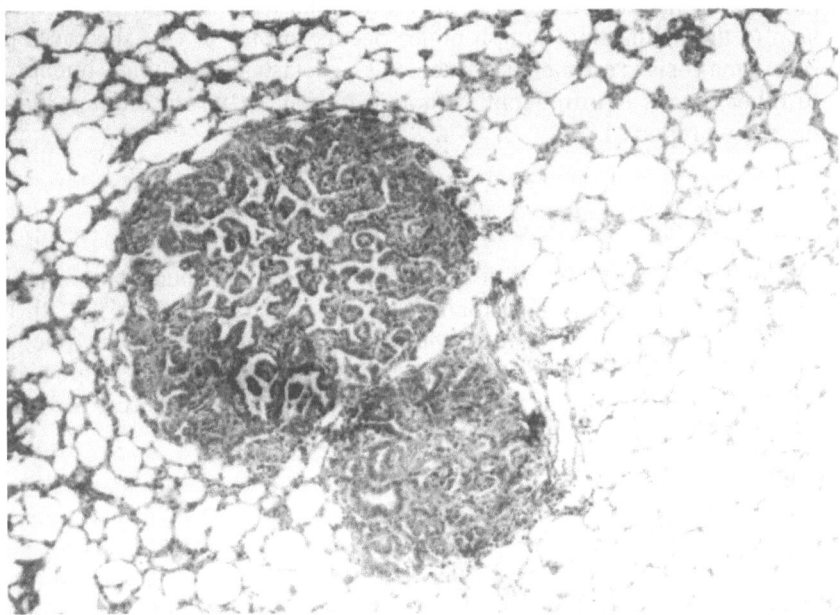

Figure 3. Pathology of adenomatosis. 3A: Isolated nodules of adenomatosis within a normal lung parenchyma (hematoxylin, safran, floxin; magnification: ×100).

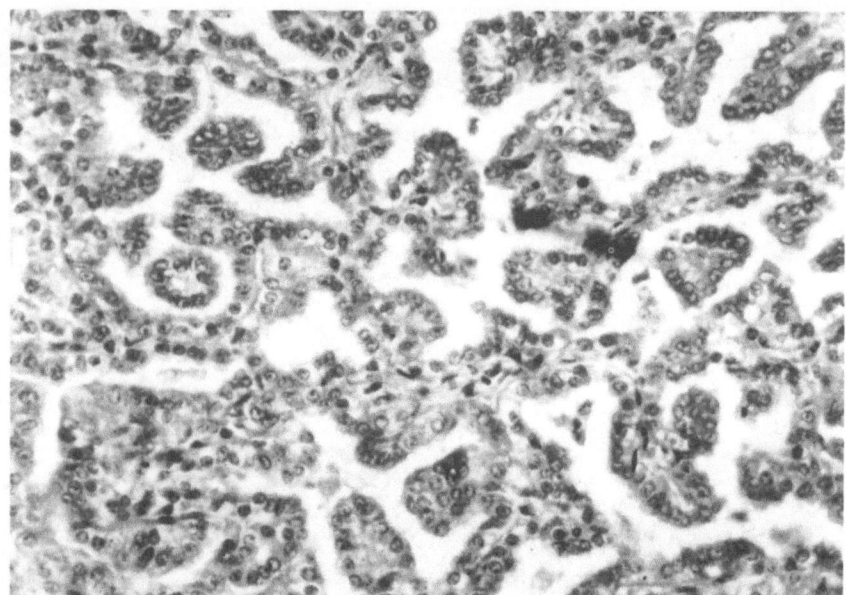

B

Figure 3 B. Enlarged view of typical aspect of adenomatosis (hematoxylin, safran, floxin; magnification: ×250).

within a normal lung parenchyma [5]. Cells forming the alveolar lesions are type II pneumocytes and, in the bronchiolar lesions, Clara cells. Extension to the mediastinal lymph nodes occurs in only 5% of the cases [5]. Adenoma-tosis is erroneously quoted as a metastasizing tumor, but spread to other organs is infrequent (although metastasis in muscle and kidney have been reported [7]).

3.1 Adenomatosis and Maedi Can Be Associated

Maedi is an interstitial lung disease associated with the persistant infection of alveolar macrophages by small ruminant lentiviruses (SRLV) [8, 9]. The association between maedi and adenomatosis has been apparent since the initial descriptions [3, 4] and has been widely described [10]. Up to 60% of the animals from flocks with adenomatosis are seropositive for SRLV [11, 12].

3.2 Adenomatosis Is Transmissible

It can be experimentally reproduced by intratracheal inoculation of tumor tissue into newborn lambs [13, 14], bronchial secretions [15] or cultured malignant epithelial cells (JS 15.4 cell line) [16]. It can even be reproduced by subcellular fractions of those cells [17].

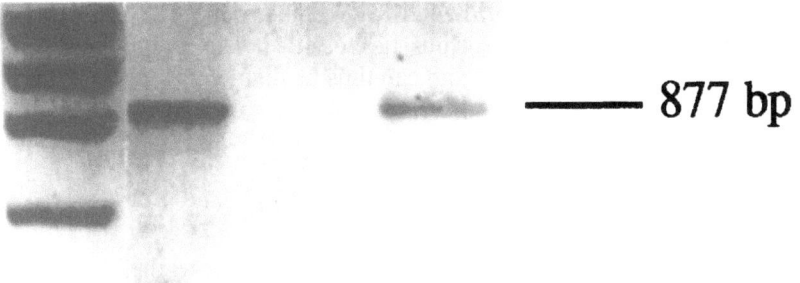

MW 9502 neg JS382

Figure 4. Viral RNA can be detected in bronchial secretions of animals with adenomatosis. RNA was extracted from bronchial secretions of an animal with adenomatosis (95.02), transcribed and amplified using primers directed to the protease gene of JSRV. Positive control is DNA from the molecular clone JS 382 (for methods see [19]). MW = molecular weight markers.

3.3 Adenomatosis Is Associated with a Retrovirus

Jaagsiekte sheep retrovirus (JSRV) has been obtained from bronchial secretions, cloned and sequenced [18]. Viral RNA can be detected in tumors and bronchial secretions (Figure 4). It copurifies with small ruminant lentiviruses. The two retroviruses SRLV and JSRV are distinct but can be isolated together. Intratracheal inoculation of both viruses induces both types of pathology [20]. JSRV seems to be a hybrid virus with capsid proteins related to type D retroviruses and an envelope related to type B retroviruses [18, 21]. It is endogenous [18, 22] (Figure 5): the sheep genome contains

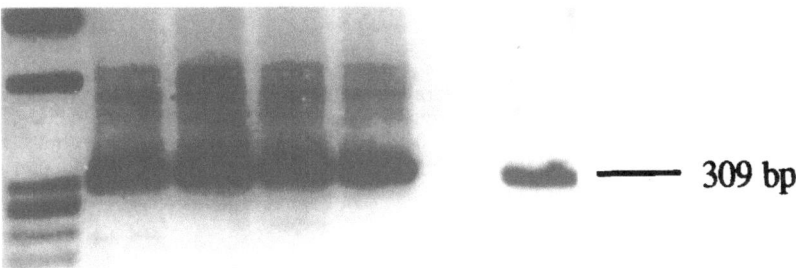

MW 683 684 685 687 neg JS382

Figure 5. Detection of Jaagsiekte related sequences in DNA of normal animals. DNA was extracted from alveolar macrophages (683, 684, 685, 687) and nested PCR used to amplify the same region as in Figure 4, the JS82 molecular clone being used as a positive control (for methods see [19]). MW = molecular weight markers.

15 to 20 copies of loci that hybridize to JSRV DNA probes [23]. The endogenous virus is expressed in various tissues [24]. The exogenous virus differs in its LTR sequences [25] and can thus be distinguish, although it is still clearly associated with adenomatosis [24].

3.4 The Pathogenesis of Adenomatosis Is Unknown

The development of adenocarcinoma may be due either to the exogenous form or to a reactivation of the endogenous virus. If the latter is true, reactivation could be caused by alveolar macrophages, infected by small ruminant lentiviruses releasing active mediators to their surroundings [9]. Adenomatosis cells do release mediators that can attract macrophages [26].

3.5 Sheep Adenomatosis is Similar to Bronchioloalveolar Cell Carcinoma

Although the existence of bronchioloalveolar cell carcinoma in humans is disputed, similarities between both disease were noted as early as 1939 [27–29]. Understanding the clinical presentation and molecular pathogenesis of adenomatosis could carry implications for the management of humans with bronchioloalveolar carcinoma.

4. Conclusion

Sheep adenomatosis is a model of virally induced lung cancer. Interactions between retroviruses seem to play a role in the pathogenesis of this disease.

Acknowledglements

This work was supported in part by grants form Agence Nationale de Recherche sur le SIDA. C. Leroux was the recipient of a fellowship from the Fondation pour la Recherche Médicale.

We wish to acknowledge the help of François Guiguen, Jean-Luc Cadoré, Patrice Bolland, Pierre Loubeyre and Didier Revel in generating data from animals and Gilles Quérat for providing us with the JSRV molecular clone.

References

1. Wandera JG (1971) Sheep pulmonary adenomatosis (Jaagsiekte). In: Brandly CA, Cornelius CE (eds): Advances in veterinary science and comparative medicine. Academic Press New York, pp 251–283.
2. DeMartini JC, Rosadio RH, Lairmore MD (1988) The etiology and pathogenesis of ovine pulmonary carcinoma (sheep pulmonary adenomatosis). Vet Microbiol 17: 219–236.

3. Cowdry EV (1925) Studies on the etiology of Jagziekte. I. The primary lesions. *J Exp Med* 17: 323–333.
4. Cowdry EV (1925) Studies on the etiology of Jagziekte. II. Origin of the epithelial proliferations, and the subsequent changes. *J Exp Med* 17: 335–345.
5. Cuba-Caparo A, Vega E, Copaira M (1961) Pulmonary adenomatosis of sheep. Metastasizing bronchiolar tumors. *Am J Vet Res* 22: 673–682.
6. Perk K, Hod I, Presentey B, Nobel TA (1971) Lung carcinoma of sheep (Jaagsiekte). II. Histogenesis of the tumor. *J Natl Cancer Inst* 47: 197–205.
7. Nobel TA, Neumann F, Klopfer U (1969) Histological patterns of the metastases in pulmonary adenomatosis of sheep (Jaagsiekte). *J Comp Pathol* 79: 537–540.
8. Mornex JF, Lena P, Loire R, Cozon G, Greenland T, Guiguen F, Jacquier MF, Cordier G (1994) Lentivirus-induced interstitial lung disease: pulmonary pathology in sheep spontaneously infected by the visna-maedi virus. *Vet Res* 25: 478–488.
9. Cadoré JL, Greenland T, Cordier G, Guiguen F, Mornex JF (1996) Histogenesis of the pulmonary lesions in the course of visna-maedi virus induced pneumonia. *Vet Res* 27: 419–426.
10. Snyder BP, DeMartini JC, Ameghino E, Caletti E (1983) Co-existence of pulmonary adenomatosis and progressive pneumonia in sheep in the central sierra of Peru. *Am J Vet Res* 44: 1334–1338.
11. Pritchart GC, Done SH (1990) Concurrent maedi-visna virus infection and pulmonary adenomatosis in a commercial breeding flock in East Anglia. *Vet Record* 127: 197–200.
12. Gonzales L, Juste RA, Cuervo LA, Idigoras I, Saez De Ocaritz C (1993) Pathological and epidemiological aspects of the coexistence of maedi-visna and sheep pulmonary adenomatosis. *Res Vet Sci* 54: 140–146.
13. Wandera JG (1970) Clinical pulmonary adenomatosis of sheep produced experimentally. *Br Vet J* 126: 185–193.
14. Rosadio RH, Lairmore MD, Russell HI, DeMartini JC (1988) Retrovirus-associated ovine pulmonary carcinoma (sheep pulmonary adenomatosis) and lymphoid interstitial pneumonia. I. Lesion development and age susceptibility. *Vet Pathol* 25: 475–483.
15. Sharp JM, Angus KW, Gray EW, Scott FMM (1983) Rapid transmission of sheep pulmonary adenomatosis (Jaaksiekte) in young lambs. *Arch Virol* 78: 89–95.
16. Coetzee S, Els HJ, Verwoerd DW (1976) Transmission of Jaagsiekte (ovine pulmonary adenomatosis) by means of a permanent epithelial cell line established from affected lungs. *Onderstepoort J Vet Res* 43: 133–142.
17. Verwoerd DW, Williamson AL, DeVilliers EM (1980) Aetiology of Jaagsiekte: transmission by means of subcellular fractions and evidence for the involvement of a retrovirus. *Onderstepoort J Vet Res* 47: 275–280.
18. York DF, Vigne R, Verwoerd DW, Querat G (1992) Nucleotide sequence of the Jaagsiekte retrovirus, and exogenous and endogenous type D and B retrovirus of sheep and goats. *J Virol* 66: 4930–4939.
19. Leroux C, Vuillermoz S, Mornex JF, Greenland T (1995) Genomic heterogeneity in the *pol* region of ovine lentiviruses obtained from bronchoalveolar cells of infected sheep from France. *J Gen Virol* 76: 1533–1537.
20. DeMartini JC, Rosadio RH, Sharp JM, Russell HI, Lairmore MD (1987) Experimental coinduction of type D retrovirus-associated pulmonary carcinoma and lentivirus-associated lymphoid interstitial pneumonia in lambs. *J Natl Cancer Inst* 79: 167–177.
21. York DF, Vigne R, Verwoerd DW, Querat G (1991) Isolation, identification, and partial cDNA cloning of genomic RNA of Jaagsiekte retrovirus, the etiological agent of sheep pulmonary adenomatosis. *J Virol* 65: 5061–5067.
22. Hecht SJ, Carlson JO, DeMartini JC (1994) Analysis of a type D retroviral capsid gene expressed in ovine pulmonary carcinoma and present in both affected and unaffected sheep genomes. *Virology* 202: 480–484.
23. Hecht SJ, Stedman KE, Carlson JO, DeMartini JC (1996) Distribution of endogenous type B and type D sheep retrovirus sequences in ungulates and other mammals. *Proc Natl Acad Sci USA* 93: 3297–3302.
24. Palmarini M, Cousens C, Dalziel RG, Bai J, Stedman K, DeMartini JC, Sharp JM (1996) The exogenous form of Jaagsiekte retrovirus is specifically associated with a contagious lung cancer of sheep. *J Virol* 70: 1618–1623.

25. Bai J, Zhu RY, Stedman K, Cousens C, Carlson J, Sharp JM (1996) Unique long terminal repeat U3 sequences distinguish exogenous Jaagsiekte sheep retroviruses associated with ovine pulmonary carcinoma from endogenous loci in the sheep genome. *J Virol* 70: 3159–3168.
26. Myer MS, Verwoerd DW, Garnett HM (1987) Production of a macrophage chemotactic factor by cultured Jaagsiekte tumor cells. *Onderstepoort J Vet Res* 54: 9–15.
27. Bonne C (1939) Morphological resemblance of pulmonary adenomatosis (Jaagsiekte) in sheep and certain cases of cancer of the lung in man. *Am J Cancer* 35: 491–501.
28. Nobel AT, Perk K (1978) Animal model of human disease. Bronchioloalveolar cell carcinoma. *Am J Pathol* 90: 783–786.
29. Perk K, Hod I (1982) Sheep lung carcinoma: an endemic analogue of a sporadic human neoplasm. *J Natl Cancer Inst* 69: 747–749.

Clinical and Biological Basis of Lung Cancer Prevention
ed. by Y. Martinet, F. R. Hirsch, N. Martinet, J.-M. Vignaud
and J. L. Mulshine
© 1998 Birkhäuser Verlag Basel/Switzerland

CHAPTER 16
Retinoic Acid Receptor β: An Exploration of its Role in Lung Cancer Suppression and its Potential in Cancer Prevention

André Toulouse [1], Johane Morin [1], Ying Ying [1], Joseph Ayoub [1, 2]
and W. Edward C. Bradley [1, 2]

[1] *Institut du cancer de Montréal and Centre de Recherche Louis-Charles Simard,*
Hôpital Notre-Dame, Montréal, Québec, Canada
[2] *Dépt. de Médecine, Université de Montréal, Montréal, Québec, Canada*

1   Introduction
1.1 The search for Lung Tumour Suppressor Genes on Chromosome 3
1.2 Retinoic Acid (RA) and its Nuclear Receptors
1.3 RARβ as a Tumour Suppressor
2   Recent Results
2.1 RNA Fingerprinting
2.2 Candidate Downstream Targets of RARβ2
2.3 Towards Clinical Applications and an Understanding of the Role of RARβ in Field Cancerization
3   Perspectives and Challenges
References

1. Introduction

Lung cancer is a group of very lethal diseases, accounting for more deaths than any other tumour type in Western societies [1]. It is made up of various histological types, mainly small cell lung cancer (SCLC), epidermoid (or squamous), adenocarcinoma and large cell. The latter three are sufficiently different from the first, both clinically and biologically, that they are frequently grouped together as non-small cell lung cancer (NSCLC). However, the classification of tumours is not perfectly exclusive, and NSCLC tumours are frequently found to have some cells with SCLC characteristics. Similarly, epidermoid and adenocarcinomas frequently have a minority of the other NSCLC type present. All lung cancer types are highly aggressive, with an overall five year survival of $\simeq 15\%$.

1.1. The Search for Lung Tumour Suppressor Genes on Chromosome 3

In 1982, Whang-Peng et al. [2] published the observation that a large deletion was detectable on the short arm of chromosome 3 (3p14−23) in essen-

tially all cultured cell lines established from small cell lung cancers
(SCLC). This now classic work suggested the presence of a tumour suppressor gene in this region, and as molecular tools became available, an
intensive search for it was initiated by many groups. Molecular definition
of the deletion (i.e. detection of loss of heterozygosity (LOH)) showed that
it usually extends from 3p14 or 3p21 to the telomere [3, 4; other work,
reviewed in ref. 1]; it often extends proximally to 3p13 [5]. Although the
SCLC LOH pattern is the most striking with respect to length and incidence, NSCLC also exhibit LOH on 3p. The pattern is interesting: roughly
half of adenocarcinomas have LOH in the proximal (3p21) but not distal
(3p24–26) part of this long chromosomal region, whereas epidermoid
tumours almost all show LOH at the distal end, 3p24-telomere, with a lower
frequency of proximal loss [6, 7]. This suggests that a suppressor gene in
3p21 may be important in adenocarcinoma, but in 3p24-ter in epidermoid.
Perhaps both are important in SCLC. In addition to the small region of 3p13
where homozygous loss was found in SCLC, a 2mb sequence in 3p21
was shown by DNA transfer to carry a candidate suppressor [8]. Thus, even
in the proximal region of 3p there are probably at least two important genes.
Several candidate cDNAs have been cloned from this and other regions
[4, 9–11].

Among these possible suppressor genes on 3p, one of the most interesting is the nuclear retinoic acid receptor β (*RARβ*), located in 3p24, the
region of near 100% LOH in epidermoid lung cancer. This has been the
subject of our laboratory's research for several years, and many groups are
now showing that this gene has a pivotal role to play in cancer progression
not only in lung, but in head and neck and breast cancer as well.

1.2. Retinoic Acid (RA) and its Nuclear Receptors

Vitamin A (the metabolic precursor of RA) is a powerful morphogen and
inducer of differentiation; it has also been shown by many epidemiological
studies to have anticancer activity, particularly for lung tissue [12]. It and
other retinoids are used successfully in many clinical settings, but not yet
on a routine basis for lung cancer, partly because at pharmacological doses,
retinoids are toxic. The nuclear receptors of RA, of which RARβ is one, comprise two retinoid receptor families, RARs and RXRs. Between them they are
thought to be the principal mediators of the effects of RA. Each of these families has three member genes (α, β and γ) and each of these genes can be
expressed as a variety of isoforms by use of two promoters and alternative
splicing at the 5′ end [13–15]. It is through this molecular diversity that RA
can exert its wideranging and sometimes contradictory effects. The main
isoform of RARβ which is expressed in human lung [16], breast [17] and
other tissues [our unpublished data] is RARβ2. We have found that RARβ1
is expressed very little or not at all in adult tissues, and RARβ3 appears

not to have a human homologue [16, 41]. We have also shown that RARβ1 is expressed in fetal tissue and in many SCLC [16].

1.3. RARβ as a Tumour Suppressor

A vast literature exists indicating that vitamin A and RA have tumour suppressive effects. About 20 epidemiological studies show that dietary vitamin A intake is inversely proportional to lung cancer risk [reviewed in 12]. Interestingly, the lung cancers most closely associated are epidermoid and SCLC (i.e. those where *RARβ* is most often inactivated and deleted). Additionally, animal studies have also established a link between retinoids and tumour suppression [18]. In organ culture, trachea can be induced to undergo squamous differentiation (a precancerous state) by tobacco distillates, and this is reversed by RA. Several lines of evidence suggest that among the various RA receptors, that which is most involved in mediating the tumour suppressor effect of RA is RARβ2. First, as indicated above, LOH occurs most frequently on 3p (distal) in epidermoid and SCLC; none of the other sites where RARs or RXRs are located (17q21; 12q13; 9q34; 6p21 and 1q22–23) are frequently involved in lung cancer [19]. 9q, where *RXRα* is located, shows LOH more frequently than the other four sites, but this region also carries the suppressor gene *ABL*.

Further circumstantial evidence is the link between inactivation of (the remaining copy of) *RARβ* and epidermoid lung cancer [7, 20, 21]. More recently, it has been found that many cancers including breast [17, 22] and head and neck cancers [23] (which are also inversely associated with dietary retinoids) are characterized by lack of RARβ expression in spite of the presence of RARβ message in the corresponding normal tissue.

The first direct demonstration that RARβ has tumour suppressor activity was accomplished by introducing *RARβ2* into two epidermoid lung cancer lines and analysing many RARβ-expressing derivatives and control nonexpressing clones [24]. In *all* RARβ^+ derivatives, tumorigenicity was reduced, in some cases to zero. Furthermore, 6/7 tumours which *did* appear in nude mice had near zero or much reduced RARβ2 expression. In addition, we showed that *RARβ2* conferred sensitivity to inhibition of growth by RA [24]. *RARα* transfected into the same cells had no significant effect on tumorigenicity, and there was no RA-mediated inhibition of growth [Toulouse et al., in preparation].

We have also developed various transgenic mouse lines which further indicate that *RARβ* plays a role in tumour suppression. First, a form of RARβ, truncated at the N-terminal end, which closely resembles RARβ4, induces hyperplasia and adenocarcinomas in lung and mammary tissues when ectopically expressed in mice [25]. Expression patterns showed that endogenous *RARβ2* (which has a retinoic acid response element (RARE) in its promoter) was downregulated in tissues where RARβ4 was strongly expressed [25]. This is consistent with the hypothesized role of *RARβ2* as a tumour suppressor, and suggests a dominant negative type of role for the truncated RARβ4 isoform. When human pulmonary adenocarcinomas were analysed, we found overexpression of RARβ4 [25]. It has not yet been shown that RARβ4 has this sort of role in the natural system, but the importance of these results is that they show how perturbation of the ensemble of RARβ action may lead to loss of homeostasis, and that RARβ4 expression may be important in lung tumorigenesis, especially that of adenocarcinomas.

Finally, we have shown that mice expressing antisense (AS) *RARβ2* constructs in lung are predisposed to lung cancer [26]. Three transgenic lines expressing AS sequences were generated, and message levels of the endogenous RARβ2 (but *not* RARβ4) were reduced by up to 30% in AS RARβ2 mice compared to those in nontransgenic littermates. Of 36 animals, 21 developed a total of 43 lesions (all adenomas), with a two-fold higher incidence in homozygous than hemizygous AS mice. Endogenous RARβ expression was further reduced in the tumours and immunohistochemical staining revealed detectable RARβ in normal tissue, but none in tumour tissue. Among 23 nontransgenic littermates, one had a single lung tumour. We concluded that *RARβ2* plays an important role in suppression of murine lung tumorigenesis. The tumours observed were adenomas and adenocarcinomas, not epidermoid, so it appears once again that RARβ4 expression is associated with pulmonary adenocarcinomas. In this context it is interesting to recall that human adenocarcinomas are not associated with LOH of RARβ2.

Several groups have assessed the potential tumour suppressor role in other human tumour systems. The reason for this intense interest stems from the fact that the enormous cancer control potential of RA has been very difficult to realize, mainly because the molecular mechanism has been elusive. In attempting to establish the tumour suppressor activity of *RARβ*, several parameters which are thought to be associated with tumorigenicity have been measured: 1) The effect of RA on growth rate in culture. This has long been a preferred surrogate parameter, especially for those working on breast cancer [25 and references therein], since for years before the cloning of the RARs this was the most testable aspect of the tumour suppressive effect of RA. 2) Growth in semisolid medium, either in the presence or absence of RA. 3) Growth *in vivo* in immunodeficient mice, either nude or SCID. 4) Inhibition of oncogene-mediated focus formation in transfection assays. (This was performed with rodent, not human cells). With these assays, a consistent picture has emerged indicating that *RARβ* (specifically *RARβ2*) has suppressive effects. Thus, *RARβ2* transfected into a breast cancer line [27] rendered the cells sensitive to RA inhibition of growth rate and also inhibited colony formation in semisolid medium; however, there was no significant reduction of growth in SCID mice, so, only some parameters showed a tumour suppressor effect. *RARα* transfected into this line [28] conferred sensitivity to RA growth inhibition, but had no effect on anchorage independence. *RARβ* is the only *RAR* turned off in many buccal precancerous lesions (leukoplakia) [29, 30], but is expressed in normal tissue [29]. Administration of RA to patients with leukoplakia induces regression of most of the RARβ-deficient lesions and coincidentally, RARβ levels are increased. All tested cell lines derived from cervical cancer have no detectable RARβ expression [B. Houle, Ph.D. thesis] although normal tissue has yet to be analysed. However, transfection of *RARβ2* into the cervical cancer-derived HeLa cell line reduces growth rate in the presence of RA, and greatly inhibits colony formation in semisolid medium [31].

Finally, since RARβ expression is upregulated in senescent normal breast cell lines, Lee et al. [32] tested inducibility of RARβ in fibroblast cultures and found high inducibility in cultures of low proliferative capacity. This group also demonstrated a striking inhibitory effect of RARβ on focus forming ability of oncogenes in a rat fibroblast transfection assay; this inhibitory effect was equal to that of transfected wild-type p53.

In summary, *RARβ* is associated with regression of precancerous lesions, and when transfected into tumour-derived lines has the following effects: confers sensitivity to RA-mediated growth inhibition (lung, breast, HeLa); confers anchorage dependence (breast, HeLa); inhibits focus-forming potential of transfected oncogenes (rat fibroblasts); inhibits tumorigenicity in nude mice (lung). In addition, we can infer that *RARβ* can arrest growth, perhaps by triggering a senescence-related mechanism, as it is overexpressed (or becomes expressible) in senescent cells and it is frequently difficult to obtain viable transfectants.

2. Recent Results

2.1. RNA Fingerprinting

To begin to understand what characteristics of the RARβ2+ derivatives of Calu-1 and other epidermoid cancer lines are important in tumour suppression, we have analysed several series of cell lines which we have generated and characterized, and which differ only in that they express, or do not express, a particular isoform of RARβ. Analysis was performed by RNA fingerprinting (RAP-PCR, or RNA-arbitrarily primed PCR; reviewed in [33]. This is a powerful technique used to describe degrees of identity in genetic programmes of related cell lines; it is feasible to survey the transcriptional status of > 1000 genes in cell lines under several different conditions.

The principle of RAP-PCR is that any arbitrarily chosen primer or combination of two primers will amplify a reproducible set of cDNAs when the first cycle or two are ramped from 35 to 40° with a given primer set. Generally, reproducible profiles of between 5 and 100 bands are produced which can allow comparison between lines, but we have improved the procedure by labelling an oligo with Cy5 (Pharmacia) and using an automatic sequencer (ALF express) to generate reproducibly about 120–180 peaks per run. We have performed RAP-PCR with 14 different combinations of oligonucleotides. Since only one oligo was fluorescent, about one third of the peaks obtained with each of the different partner oligos were common to all runs, since a significant number of amplified bands are the product of the Cy5-labelled oligo partnering with itself.

Analyses of the tracings showed differences among perhaps 5% of the peaks, using three sets of oligos, whereas the other 11 oligo combinations gave very few variations. Within the three combinations with more variations, 7.2% of the peaks were substantially and reproducibly altered in intensity by RA, 4.8% increased and 2.5% decreased; most of these had similar behaviour whether the line was *Calu-1*, *RARβ1*$^+$, *RARβ2*$^+$ or *RARα*-transfected. Two and three peaks out of 330 were respectively upregulated and downregulated in both of the RARβ2$^+$ lines. Corresponding numbers were 7 and 5 out of 305 for *β1*$^+$ and 7 and 5 out of 235 for *α*-transfected lines.

2.2. Candidate Downstream Targets of RARβ2

We then attempted to clone some of the peaks which were altered in the RARβ$^+$ cells using oligos Cy-5 and BRA80, by repeating the RAP-PCR with ^{32}P and running the samples on a conventional gel. The bands were identified by autoradiography, eluted, reamplified and sequenced. One, identified as hCRMP2 [34], was upregulated by ~2-fold by RARβ2 (Figure 1A). *hCRMP2* is a neuronal terminal differentiation marker which is part of a G protein signalling cascade triggered by a secreted protein named collapsin, and which eventually generates a negative environmental cue for axon cones (the leading tip of axon outgrowth which seeks other neurons with which to establish contact). The finding that this gene (the expression of which was until now not suspected in lung tissue [34]) is upregulated in the RARβ$^+$ lines is intriguing, since the ultimate target of the signalling pathway is a change in intracellular Ca^{++} concentration. Given the control role that Ca^{++} plays in multiple cellular functions, it is easy to imagine how such a change could have a major impact on cell behaviour. Further, some members of the semaphorin family, of which collapsin is a member, as well as some G proteins themselves, are coded for by genes in a chromosomal region usually deleted in lung cancer, 3p21 [35, 36]. Although it is not yet known whether these semaphorins are part of the hCRMP2 pathway in normal lung epithelial cells, it is interesting to speculate that Ca^{++} balance could become deregulated by a combination of perturbations of expression levels of various constituents of this pathway: for the semaphorins and G proteins, this would occur simply by reduced gene

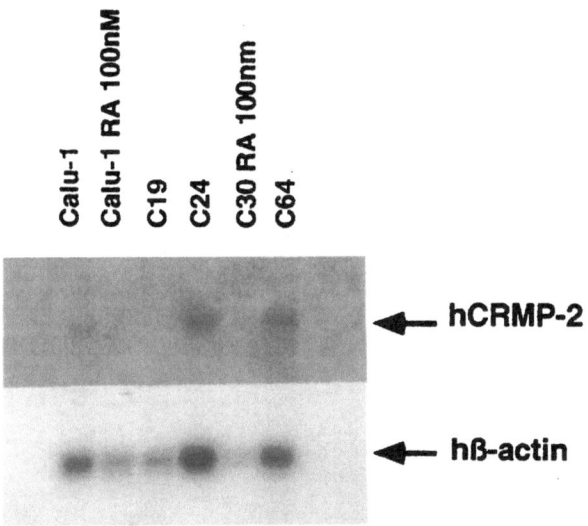

Figure 1A. Northern blot showing expression levels of two candidate genes whose message levels are influenced by RARβ2. Membranes were prepared using about 2 µg of polyA⁺ RNA from epidermoid tumour-derived cell lines which are RARβ⁻ (Calu-1 and its subclone, c30), grown in either the absence or present of added RA (10^{-7} M) or RARβ2⁺ (c19, c24 and c64, derived by transfected Calu-1 with RARβ2 in an expression vector) [16]. A: probed with hCRMP2.

dosage following LOH of 3p21, and for hCRMP2 because of reduced expression due to inactivation of *RARβ*.

A second sequence which was cloned based on differential expression in RARβ2⁺ vs RARβ2⁻ cells corresponded to mitochondrial cytochrome b. This gene was downregulated by RARβ2, judging by the intensities of Northern bands (Figure 1B). This is of interest, since a direct relationship is known to exist between oxidative phosphorylation state and tumorigenic status of cells [37]. Thus, if further work shows that RARβ2 consistently decreases levels of transcript of cytochrome b and perhaps other mitochondrial oxidative phosphorylation genes, this should suggest that one mechanism whereby RARβ exerts its tumour suppressive effect is through restricting the energy supply.

A third interesting gene, *ICAM-1*, has been identified by other researchers as being preferentially upregulated by *RARβ* via an RARE in its promoter [38]. The product of this gene is a member of a family of immunoglobulin-related cell surface proteins involved in intercellular adhesion, signalling and growth control. In particular ICAM-1 expression is necessary in tumour cells for their recognition by autologous T cells, natural killer cells and lymphokine-activated killer cells [38 and references therein], so the observation that *RARβ* is the *RAR* primarily involved in

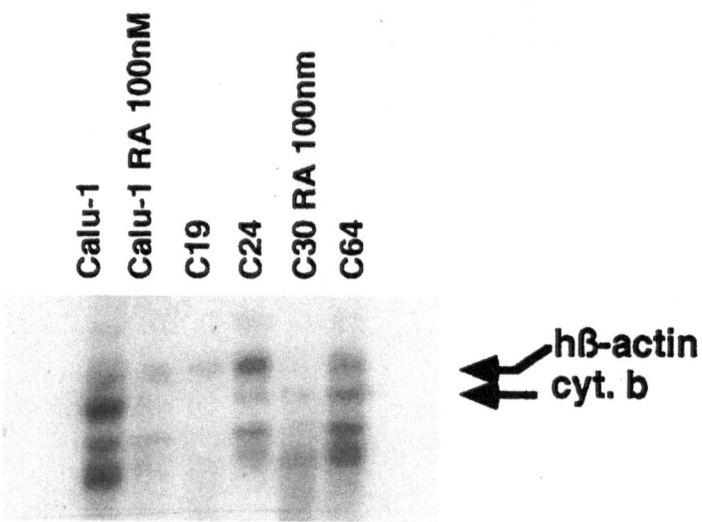

Figure 1 B. Probed with cytochrome b (this probe also detects additional transcripts of lower molecular weight). In each case, β actin was used as a control for RNA amounts.

transactivating *ICAM-1* expression immediately suggests that this gene may be an important downstream target of *RARβ*.

Thus, three genes are currently in hand for further exploration of the molecular mechanisms of cancer suppression by *RARβ*. In the case of hCRMP-2 and mitochondrial cytochrome b, we do not yet know if the control exerted by *RARβ* is direct (via a RARE in the promoters of the respective genes) or indirect, but even if the effect is indirect the genes may be biologically important members of the *RARβ* directed cascade.

2.3. Towards Clinical Applications and an Understanding of the Role of RARβ in Field Cancerization

Cancer of the respiratory tract is strongly correlated with smoking and can occur as a second primary tumour in individuals who have been cured of a first cancer like this. This fact led to the formulation of the concept of field cancerization (for review, see [39]), which postulates that continued exposure to the carcinogens present in tobacco smoke results in initiation of the tumorigenic process throughout the respiratory tract so that even before presentation for a first primary cancer a patient may have multiple preneoplastic lesions, which may be clinically detectable as dysplastic or metaplastic tissue, or may not be detectable at all. It is not yet known which early molecular changes preceding development of these lesions are important, but it is possible that such early events involve steps in the regulatory pathways controlled by retinoic acid (RA) (reviewed in [39]). If so, a logical possibility is that the early lesion(s) lie at the level of RARs, and particularly RARβ, for reasons described above.

To test whether reduced expression of RARβ could be an early marker for genetic damage characteristic of field cancerization in bronchi, we have analysed the level of expression of this gene in bronchial brushings of several normal nonsmoking individuals and a series of smokers, some of whom were diagnosed with chronic obstructive pulmonary disease (COPD), a condition which is associated with a further increase in the risk of lung cancer [40]. A subset of this patient population is currently entered in a randomized chemoprevention feasibility trial of 13 cis-RA, in which patients are given 30 mg RA per day for six months, after which a second bronchoscopy is performed. The final results will be available in spring 1997, but we have partial data for 38 patients so far.

Bronchoscopies were performed and brushings were taken from each patient, generally from two sites (designated A and B for the first bronchoscopy, A' and B' for the second). RNA was extracted and reverse transcription was performed by standard procedures, using random oligonucleotides as primer, and the cDNA was amplified for 35 cycles using RARβ2-specific primers generating a 719 bp fragment. These oligos also amplified a 365 bp fragment of the truncated RARβ4 isoform. As an internal control for RNA quality and quantity, we also amplified a 311 bp sequence of *RARα*. The expression of this gene in lung and other tissue has been shown to be unaffected during tumorigenesis [7, 29]. Amplified DNA was separated by electrophoresis, Southern blotted and probed with endlabelled oligonucleotides corresponding to sequences within the amplified fragments.

Representative results for four patients are shown in Figure 2. RARα was detected in 85 to 90% of the samples from >100 patients, and we assume that in the remainder, the RNA was degraded or in insufficient quantity. Of the RARα positive samples, 45% were RARβ negative, whereas the eleven healthy nonsmoking subjects all gave strong RARβ2 bands in samples from all sites brushed. Interestingly, the proportions of patients with at least one RARβ-deficient site was higher among those diagnosed with COPD than among other smokers. In all four cases, illustrated in Figure 2, the brushings obtained from the second bronchoscopy (A' and B' sites) yielded RARβ2/β4 levels which were not improved compared to the original samplings (indeed, in some cases RARβ levels went from detectable to nondetectable). However, among 23 patients who have undergone a second bronchoscopy to date, 11 have experienced an increase in RARβ. Once the accrual is complete we will determine whether there is a correlation between RA administration and increased RAR expression as has been found for preneoplastic lesions of the mouth [29].

What this study has already found is that reduced RARβ2 expression appears to be a frequent characteristic of the bronchial epithelium of

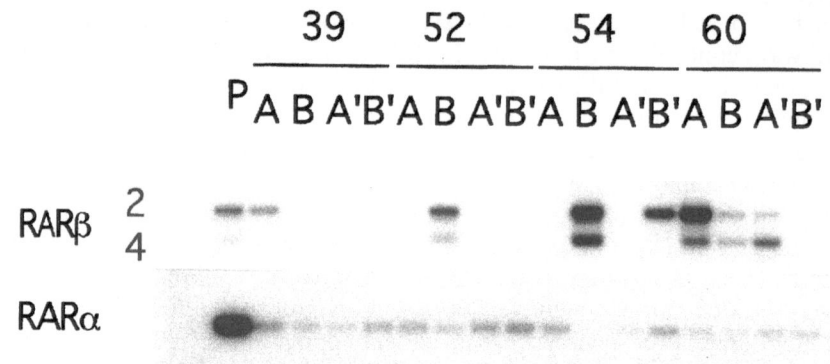

Figure 2. RT-PCR analyses of RARβ2 and RARβ4 expression levels in bronchial brushings. RNA was extracted (RN easy kit, Qiagen), reverse transcribed and aliquots were amplified with oligonucleotides specific for RARβ2/β4 and RARα, as described in the text. Results for four patients (numbered) are shown. P, positive control; A and B, two sites brushed before 6 month intervention with placebo or 13-*cis* RA; A′, B′ same sites brushed after intervention. The code will be opened in spring 1997.

smokers, and this deficiency is even more frequent among COPD patients. The fact that this reduction occurs even in apparently normal tissue suggests that this loss of expression represents a molecular marker for field cancerization. Modulation of the transcription of *RARβ* may therefore be an appropriate target for chemoprevention trials, such as the one currently underway, at Notre-Dame Hospital, Montréal.

3. Perspectives and Challenges

The overall goal of our research is to develop lung cancer prevention strategies based on an understanding of how the expression of RARβ is controlled and the role this gene plays in homeostasis. In our view the choice of *RARβ* as the focus of our attention is justified by the weight of evidence that the gene's product has tumour suppressive activity, and that it is underexpressed in respiratory epithelial tissues of patients at risk. It should nevertheless be noted that *RARβ* does not fulfill all the criteria of a classical tumour suppressor gene such as *RB1*, in that no point mutations or internal deletions have been found in tumours which could reflect a strong genetic selection against *RARβ* during tumorigenesis. How can this be explained? It is important to appreciate that *RARβ2* is unusual because there is an RARE in its promoter and occupation of this element by an activated (RA-bound) RAR-RXR dimer is essential for normal expression. Thus, a low RA concentration will tend to activate the gene less robustly. We also know that the highest incidence of lung cancer (especially epidermoid) occurs in smokers, and RA is probably highly labile in the presence of the oxidizing agents present in tobacco smoke. Furthermore, the highest cancer incidence is in individuals whose dietary intake of vitamin A is already in the lowest quintile [12], so it is logical to conclude that the breeding ground for epidermoid lung cancer, namely bronchial epithelium, is a tissue in which RA is low, and RARβ expression is already hampered. This has been shown to be the case for head and neck precancerous lesions: determination of RA levels by a specific monoclonal antibody has shown that the lesions in which RARβ expression is low have no reactivity with the antibody [30].

In this context, we know that physical loss of one copy of *RARβ* usually occurs at some point during tumour progression. RARβ2 expression is therefore abruptly reduced by half, and with low RA availability the remaining *RARβ2* allele is poorly transactivated and the cell is already partially capable of escaping whatever growth control *RARβ* exerts. From this point, other incremental mechanisms such as methylation of the CG-rich promoter may occur with relatively high frequency and they would be selected for under the driving force of the growth advantage of a RARβ⁻ phenotype. Thus, a point mutation would rarely be seen because it occurs at a lower frequency than that of the incremental events. If this scenario is correct, it offers hope that the chemoprevention trial which we describe above may yield useful results, since the intervention involves administration of the activating agent which may be deficient in the patients at highest risk, namely RA.

Alternative intervention strategies may suggest themselves as the molecular biology of the *RARβ*-controlled cascades becomes better understood. For example, if our preliminary result implicating *hCRMP2* leads to identification of Ca^{++} anomalies in bronchial tissues of patients at risk, a future trial could conceivably be designed to include and exploit this finding. Our findings so far, however, also point out the challenges ahead; the number of genes differentially expressed in RARβ⁺ vs RARβ⁻ cells is probably not very small, so there may be a real difficulty identifying which genes are important. A further complication is that conceivably there is no single gene of paramount importance among the repertoire selectively activated by *RARβ*, but rather, many genes may each contribute marginally to inhibiting tumorigenesis. It is noteworthy that of the first three candidate genes we and others have identified, all three potentially fall into this category. Thus, even though elucidating the molecular consequences of *RARβ* action is of interest at a fundamental level, more immediate clinical benefit may be derived from research on modulating expression of *RARβ* itself.

Acknowledgements

We are greatly indebted to Dr R. Jean-François and Dr Y. Cormier for furnishing bronchial epithelial brushings. Supported by Medical Research Council of Canada; Fonds de recherche en santé du Québec; FRSQ-Hydro-Québec; Mickey Stein Ski-O-thon.

References

1. Carney DN, Deleij L (1988) Lung Cancer Biology (Review). *Seminar Oncol* 15: 199–214.
2. Whang-Peng J, Bunn PA Jr, Kao-Shan CS, Lee EC, Carney DN, Gazdar A, Minna JD (1982) A nonrandom chromosomal abnormality, del 3p(14–23), in human small cell lung cancer (SCLC). *Cancer Genet Cytogenet* 6: 119–134.
3. Leduc F, Brauch H, Hajj C, Dobrovic A, Kaye F, Gazdar A, Harbour JW, Pettengill OS, Sorenson GD, van der Berg A, Kok K, Campling B, Paquin F, Bradley WEC, Zbar B, Minna J, Buys C, Ayoub J (1989) Loss of heterozygosity in a gene coding for a thyroid hormone receptor in lung cancers. *Am J Hum Genet* 44: 282–287.
4. Dobrovic A, Houle B, Belouchi A, Bradley WEC (1988) erb-A-related sequence coding for DNA-binding hormone receptor localized to chromosome 3p21–3p25 and deleted in small cell lung carcinoma. *Cancer Res* 48: 682–685.
5. Todd S, Franklin WA, Weissenbach J, Drabkin HA, Gemmill RM (1994) Proximal chromosome 3 harbors a DNA segment frequently deleted in small cell lung cancer. *Am J Hum Genet* 55, A72.
6. Yokoyama S, Yamakawa K, Tsuchiya E, Murata M, Sakiyama S, Nakamura Y (1992) Deletion mapping on the short arm of chromosome 3 in squamous cell carcinoma and adenocarcinoma of the lung. *Cancer Res* 52: 873–877.
7. Houle B, Leduc F, Bradley WEC (1991) Implication of RARβ in epidermoid (squamous) lung cancer. *Genes Chrom Cancer* 3: 358–366.
8. Killary AM, Wolf ME, Naylor SL (1992) Definition of a tumor suppressor locus within human chromosome 3p21–3p22. *Proc Natl Acad Sci* 89: 10877–10881.
9. Daly MC, Xiang RH, Hensel CH, Carlson HC, Killary AM, Kok K, Buys CH, Drabkin H, Naylor SL (1994) Characterization of a candidate suppressor gene on chromosome 3. *Am J Hum Genet* 55: A19.
10. Calabro V, Pengue G, Bartoli PC, Pagliuca A, Featherstone T, Lania L (1995) Positional cloning of cDNAs from the human chromosome 3p21–22 region identifies a clustered organization of zinc-finger genes. *Hum Genet* 95: 18–21.
11. Moscow JA, Schmidt L, Ingram DT, Gnarra J, Johnson B, Cowan KH (1994) Loss of heterozygosity of the human cytosolic glutathione peroxidase 1 gene in lung cancer. *Carcinogenesis* 15: 2769–2773.
12. Graham SJ (1984) Epidemiology of retinoids and cancer. *J Nat Canc Inst* 73: 1423–1428.
13. Chambon P (1996) A decade of molecular biology of retinoic acid receptors. *FASEB J* 10: 940–954.
14. Napgal S, Zelent A, Chambon P (1992) RARβ4 a retinoic acid receptor isoform is generated from RARβ2 by alternative splicing and usage of a CUG initiator codon. *Proc Natl Acad Sci* 89: 2718–2722.
15. Zelent A, Mendelson C, Kastner P, Krust A, Garnier J-M, Ruffenach F, Leroy P, Chambon P (1991) Differentially expressed isoforms of the mouse retinoic acid receptor β are generated by usage of two promoters and alternative splicing. *EMBO J* 10: 71–81.
16. Houle B, Pelletier M, Wu J, Goodyer C, Bradley WEC (1994) Fetal isoform of human retinoic acid receptor β expressed in small cell lung cancer lines. *Cancer Res* 54: 365–369.
17. Swisshelm K, Ryan K, Lee X, Tsou HC, Peacocke M, Sager R (1994) Down-regulation of retinoic acid receptor β in mammary carcinoma cell lines and its up-regulation in senescing normal mammary epithelial cells. *Cell Growth Diff* 5: 133.
18. Roberts A, Sporn M (1984) Cellular Biology and Biochemistry of the retinoids. *In:* Sporn M, Roberts A, Goodman D (eds): *The Retinoids*, Academic, Orlando, pp 210–286.
19. Almasan A, Mangelsdorf DJ, Ong ES, Wahl GM, Evans RM (1994) Chromosomal localization of the human retinoid X receptors. *Genomics* 20: 397–403.
20. Nervi C, Vollberg TM, George MD, Zelent A, Chambon P, Jetten AM (1991) Expression of nuclear retinoic acid receptors in normal tracheobronchial cells and in lung carcinoma cells. *Exp Cell Res* 195: 163–170.
21. Gerbert JF, Moghal N, Frangioni JV, Sugarbaker DJ, Neel BG (1991) High frequency of retinoic acid receptor β abnormalities in human lung cancer. *Oncogene* 6: 1859–1968.
22. Roman SD, Clarke CL, Hall RE, Alexander IE, Sutherland RL (1992) Expression and regulation of retinoic acid receptors in human breast cancer cells. *Cancer Res* 52: 2236–2242.

23. Hu L, Crowe DL, Rheinwald JG, Chambon P, Gudas LJ (1991) Abnormal expression of retinoic acid receptors and keratin 19 by human oral and epidermal squamous cell carcinoma cell lines. *Cancer Res* 51: 3972–3981.

24. Houle B, Rochette-Egly C, Bradley WEC (1993) Tumor-suppressive effect of the retinoic acid receptor β in human epidermoid lung cancer cells. *Proc Natl Acad Sci* 90: 985–989.

25. Bérard J, Gaboury L, Landers M, DeRepentigny Y, Houle B, Kothary R, Bradley WEC (1994) Hyperplasia and tumours in lung, breast and other tissues in mice carrying a RARβ4-like transgene. *EMBO J* 13: 5570–5580.

26. Bérard J, Laboune F, Mukuna M, Massé S, Kothary R, Bradley WEC (1996) Lung tumors in mice expressing an antisense RARβ2 transgene. *FASEB* 10:1091–1097.

27. Li X-S, Shao ZM, Sheikh MS, Eisemann JL, Sentz D, Jetten AM, Chen JC, Dawson MI, Aisner S, Rishi AK, et al. (1995) RARβ inhibits breast cancer anchorage independent growth. *J Cell Physiol* 165: 449–458.

28. Sheikh MS, Shao ZM, Li SX, Dawson M, Jetten AM, Wu S, Conley BA, Garcia M, Rochefort H, Fontana JA (1994) Retinoid-resistant ER negative human breast carcinoma cells transfected with RARα acquire sensitivity to growth inhibition by retinoids. *J Biol Chem* 269: 21440–21447.

29. Lotan R, Xu X-C, Lippman SM, Ro JY, Lee JS, Lee JJ, Hong WK (1995) Suppression of retinoic acid receptor-β in premalignant oral lesions and its upregulation by isotretinoin. *New Engl J Med* 332: 1405–1410.

30. Xu X-C, Zile M, Lippman S, Lee JS, Lee JJ, Hong WK, Lotan R (1995) RA antibody binding to human premalignant oral lesions, which occurs less frequently than binding to normal tissue, increases after RA treatment *in vivo* and is related to RARβ expression. *Cancer Res* 55: 5507–5511.

31. Si SP, Lee XL, Tsou HC, Buchsbaum R, Tibaduiza E, Peacoke M (1996) RARβ2-mediated growth inhibition in HeLa cells. *Exp Cell Res* 223: 102–111.

32. Lee X, Si SP, Tsou HC, Peacoke M (1995) Cellular aging and transformation suppression: a role for RARβ2. *Exp Cell Res* 218: 296–304.

33. McClelland M, Mathieu-Daude F, Welsh J (1995) *Trends in Genet* 11: 242–246.

34. Goshima Y, Nakamura F, Strittmatter P, Strittmatter S (1995) Collapsin-induced growth cone collapse mediated by an intracellular protein related to UNC-33. *Nature* 376: 509–514.

35. Xiang R-H, Hensel CH, Garcia DK, Carlson HC, Kok K, Daly MC, Kerbacher K, van den Berg A, Veldhuis P, Buys CH, Naylor SL (1996) Isolation of human SEMA3F at chromosome 3p21, a region deleted in lung cancer. *Genomics* 32: 39–48.

36. Sekido Y, Bader S, Latif F, Chen JY, Duh FM, Wei MH, Albanesi JP, Lee CC, Lerman MI, Minna JD (1996) Human Semaphorins A(V) and IV reside in the 3p21.3 SCLC deletion region and demonstrate distinct expression patterns. *Proc Natl Acad Sci USA* 93: 4120–4125.

37. Torroni A, Stepien G, Hodge JA, Wallace DC (1990) Neoplastic transformation is associated with coordinate induction of nuclear and cytoplasmic oxidative phosphorylation genes. *J Biol Chem* 265: 20589–20593.

38. Aoudjit F, Brochu N, Morin N, Poulin G, Stratowa C, Audette M (1995) Heterodimeric RARβ and RXRα complexes stimulate expression of the intercellular adhesion molecule-1 gene. *Cell Growth Diff* 6: 515–521.

39. Hong WK, Lippman SM, Hilleman WN, Lotan R (1995) Retinoid chemoprevention of aerodigestive cancer: from basic research to the clinic. *Clin Cancer Res* 1: 677–686.

40. Weiss W (1991) Chronic obstructive pulmonary disease and lung cancer. *In:* Cherniak, NS (ed): *Chronic obstructive pulmonary disease.* Philadelphia, Saunders, pp 344–347.

41. Toulouse A, Morin J, Pelletier M, Bradley WEC (1996) Structure of the human retinoic acid receptor β1 gene. *Biochim Biophys Acta* 1309: 1–4.

Clinical and Biological Basis of Lung Cancer Prevention
ed. by Y. Martinet, F. R. Hirsch, N. Martinet, J.-M. Vignaud
and J. L. Mulshine
© 1998 Birkhäuser Verlag Basel/Switzerland

CHAPTER 17
Cytochrome P450 Polymorphisms: Risk Factors for Lung Cancer?

Simone Benhamou and Catherine Bonaïti-Pellié

Unit of Cancer Epidemiology (INSERM U351), Institut Gustave-Roussy, Villejuif, France

1 Introduction
2 The CYP1A Polymorphisms and Lung Cancer
3 The CYP2D6 Polymorphism and Lung Cancer
4 Conclusion
References

1. Introduction

Lung cancer is a disease in which environmental factors play a major role, since 80 to 90% of cases of lung cancer in our countries may be attributable to tobacco [1]. However, the cumulative risk of lung cancer in a population of smokers remains largely lower than 1. There is no doubt that factors other than tobacco carcinogens are implied in its etiology and that some of them are probably genetic. Arguments for the role of genetic factors come from animal studies, family studies and studies on polymorphisms of enzymes implied in the metabolism of carcinogens, in particular the cytochrome P450 family.

Most family studies (reviewed in [2]) evidenced a significant excess of familial cases of lung cancer, when taking into account tobacco smoking. Sellers et al. [3] tested various models of inheritance from a family study of 337 lung cancer cases. Their data fit a codominant monogenic model, that is, heterozygous individuals for a predisposing gene have an inter-mediate risk between susceptible and normal homozygotes. The data also suggest some genotype-tobacco interaction.

2. The CYP1A Polymorphisms and Lung Cancer

Two forms of cytochrome P450, CYP1A1 and CYP1A2, are inducible by some carcinogens present in tobacco smoke. Both cytochromes convert procarcinogens into potent carcinogenic metabolites [4–7]. CYP1A1 cata-lyses the oxidation of polycyclic aromatic hydrocarbons (PAH) such as benzo(a)pyrene. CYP1A2 catalyses the metabolic activation of several primary arylamines and heterocyclic amines through N-oxidation [8].

Because of the type of inducers, the great majority of experimental studies have been performed in animals. In mice, the induction of these activities by upregulation of both genes is mediated via the *Ah* locus which encodes the cytosolic aryl hydrocarbon (Ah) receptor. The molecular mechanisms of induction of the *CYP1A1* gene have now been determined [9].

In most studies, aryl hydrocarbon hydroxylase (AHH) activity was measured as an expression of CYP1A1 and the extent of induction was used as an indicator of the phenotype at the Ah locus. This activity is measured by the overall production of some mono-oxygenated metabolites of benzo(a)pyrene following induction by 3-methylcholanthrene (3-MC). In the mouse, using this system, about half of all inbred strains studied responded with the induction of CYP1A1 (and have been called responsive) while the others failed to exhibit AHH induction (nonresponsive). Breeding experiments between responsive and nonresponsive inbred strains showed a single locus determinant of AHH induction, with the lack of responsiveness being an autosomal recessive trait. This genetic polymorphism has been showed to be associated with tumor development after intratracheal injection of 3-MC, with a higher number of tumors in responsive mice [10].

In humans, it was suggested that most of the variability of CYP1A1 and CYP1A2 induction level might be dependent on a regulatory gene such as the *Ah* gene (now called *Ahr*). *Ahr* polymorphism in the human population has been proposed to be similar to *Ahr* polymorphism in inbred mouse strains [11]. Kellermann et al. [12] exposed human peripheral blood lymphocytes to MC-type inducers and compared the resultant AHH activities. They claimed an important effect of a single gene on AHH activity. AHH inducibility in human lymphocytes exhibited a trimodal distribution in the white USA population, consistent with a hypothesis of two codominant allelic forms at a single genetic locus. The genetic transmission studied in nuclear families fitted this model. In addition, these authors compared AHH activity in lung cancer patients and controls and found a significant excess of high inducers in patients [13]. Some studies have been undertaken since this first one and have produced conflicting results (reviewed in [14]). More recently, Catteau et al. [15] studied 102 unrelated individuals and 57 nuclear families and measured the induced CYP1A1 activity by the ethoxyresorufin-O-deethylase (EROD) activity in lymphocytes. They found a clearly bimodal distribution due to a single gene with dominance of the high induction allele. The *Ahr* gene has now been cloned [16] and localized on chromosome 7 in humans [17]. Some polymorphisms have been described but are not associated with a higher susceptibility to lung cancer, which makes the hypothesis of the involvement of this gene somewhat unlikely.

Polymorphic changes in the DNA sequence of the *CYP1A1* gene located on chromosome 15 [18] could result in altered functional proteins modifying lung cancer risk. Two polymorphisms have been described: one is a RFLP (restriction fragment length polymorphism), *Msp*I, in strong linkage dis-equilibrium with the other, a substitution of the amino acid isoleucine for valine, which is possibly associated with differential activity of *CYP1A1* [19]. A Japanese study reported an association between *Msp*I and lung cancer [20] but several studies on European, American and African populations did not find such an association with any marker (reviewed in [14]). These differences could be due to the great variation of allele frequencies between populations [21].

There are fewer studies on CYP1A2, mainly expressed in liver, and thus noninducible *in vitro*. The level of urinary caffeine metabolites has been proposed as an indicator of CYP1A2 activity in humans [22]. Only induced activity in smokers (and not inducibility) can be measured. A plurimodality has been shown by two studies [23, 24], which do not, however control the use of oral contraceptives,which are known to decrease the metabolic ratio. Catteau et al. [25] found a unimodal distribution after adjusting for this factor and did not find any familial resemblance. Whether the metabolic ratio really measures CYP1A2 activity has been a matter of controversy [26]. Nevertheless, there are at present no arguments for the involvement of this cytochrome in lung cancer risk.

3. The CYP2D6 Polymorphism and Lung Cancer

CYP2D6 genetic polymorphism is responsible for the metabolism of the antihypertensive drug debrisoquine. This polymorphism is inherited as an autosomal recessive trait. Individuals can be divided into two groups: extensive metabolizers and poor metabolizers of debrisoquine. The poor metabolizer phenotype, accounting for 5 to 10% in Caucasian populations [27], is due to an absent CYP2D6 protein [28] or an altered protein [29]. The role of the CYP2D6 has been demonstrated in the metabolism of an important tobacco carcinogen, 4-(methylnitrosamino)-1-(3-pyridyl)-1-butanone [30].

The hypothesis of a decreased risk of lung cancer among individuals with a low capacity to metabolize debrisoquine (and therefore a decreased capacity for tobacco carcinogen activation), has been the subject of sever-al epidemiological studies during the last ten years (reviewed in [14]). The under-representation of extensive metabolizers among patients with lung cancer, reported in the pilot study [31], was not confirmed in any of the subsequent studies. Many differences in populations studied or in pheno-typing procedures could explain these divergent results. Moreover, the concomitant administration of drugs known to interfere with the debris-oquine metabolism was not systematically controlled.

The risk of cancer should depend both on the levels of tobacco expo-sure and or enzyme activity, and in the absence of tobacco exposure, no

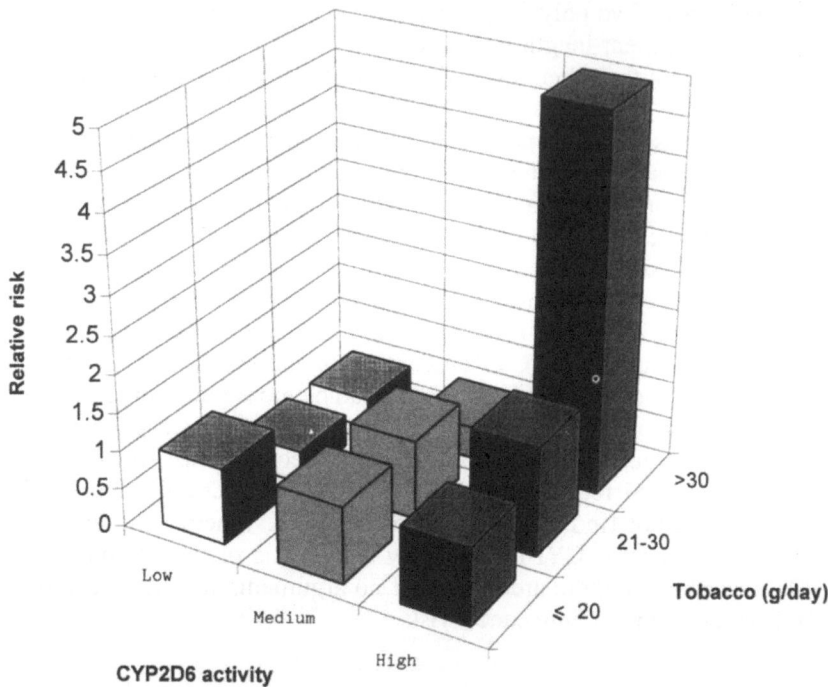

Figure 1. Lung cancer risks according to tobacco consumption and CYP2D6 activity. Adapted from [32].

difference in cancer risk should be observed between phenotypes. An inter-active effect of these two factors has recently been reported [32]. The lung cancer risk associated with increased levels of tobacco consumption was significantly increased among smokers having the highest CYP2D6 enzyme activity (Figure 1), and conversely the CYP2D6 activity was a risk factor only among heavy smokers.

Direct genotyping tests have recently been developed. These tests on DNA allow us to predict almost all the phenotypes, as around 95 % of the mutations on the *CYP2D6* gene responsible for the poor metabolizer phenotype have been identified. However, the results of epidemiological studies on lung cancer risk in relation to CYP2D6 genotypes are still difficult to interpret.

4. Conclusion

The different approaches described provide several arguments for the existence of interactions between environmental and genetic factors in lung cancer susceptibility. The combined effects of several genetic polymorphisms, particularly of *P4501A1* and glutathione S-transferase M1 (*GSTM1*), both involved in the metabolism of PAHs, have now been assessed. Of particular interest is a study of Japanese smokers showing that individuals null at the *GSTM1* locus, who also carried the *CYP1A1* polymorphism, are at very high risk for squamous cell carcinoma of the lung [33]. Moreover, this increase in risk has been related to low dose cigarette consumption [34]. Future studies on the joint effects of several polymorphisms should allow identification of subjects at very high risk of lung cancer.

References

1. Hill C (1993) Mortalité liée au tabagisme. *Rev Prat* 43: 1209–1213.
2. Economou P, Samet JM, Lechner JF (1994) Familial and genetic factors in the pathogenesis of lung cancer. *In:* Samet JM (ed): *Epidemiology of lung cancer Series: Lung biology in Health and Disease 74.* Dekker M Inc, New York, pp 353–396.
3. Sellers TA, Bailey-Wilson JE, Elston RC, Wilson AF, Elston GZ, Ooi WL, Rothschild H (1990) Evidence for Mendelian inheritance in the pathogenesis of lung cancer. *J Natl Cancer Inst* 82: 1272–1279.
4. Pelkonen O, Nebert D (1982) Metabolism of polycyclic aromatic hydrocarbons: etiologic role in carcinogenesis. *Pharmacological Rev* 34: 189–222.
5. Butler MA, Guengerich FP, Kadlubar FF (1989) Metabolic activation of the carcinogens 4-aminobiphenyl and 4,4′-methylene-bis(2-chloroaniline) by human hepatic microsomes and purified rat hepatic cytochrome P-450 monooxygenases. *Cancer Res* 49: 25–31.
6. Shimada T, Iwasaki M, Martin MW, Guengerich FP (1989) Human liver microsomal cytochrome P-450 enzymes involved in the bioactivation of procarcinogens detected by umu gene response in Salmonella Typhimurium TA 1535/pSK1002. *Cancer Res* 49: 3218–3228.
7. McManus ME, Burgess WM, Veronese ME, Huggett A, Quattrochi LC, Tukey RH (1990) Metabolism of 2-acetylaminofluorene and benzo(a)pyrene and activation of food-derived heterocyclic amine mutagens by human cytochromes P-450. *Cancer Res* 1: 3367–3375.
8. Guengerich FP, Shimada T (1991) Oxidation of toxic and carcinogenic chemicals by human cytochrome P-450 enzymes. *Chem Res Toxicol* 4: 391–407.
9. Fujii-Kuriyama Y, Ema M, Mimura J, Matsushita N, Sogawa K (1995) Polymorphic forms of the Ah receptor and induction of the CYP1A1 gene. *Pharmacogenetics* 5: S149–S153.
10. Kouri RE, Nebert DW (1991) Genetic regulation of susceptibility to polycyclic-hydrocarbon-induced tumors in the mouse. *In:* Hiatt HH, Watson JD, Winsten JA. *Origins of human cancer.* Cold Spring Harbor, New York, pp 811–835.
11. Nebert DW, Petersen DD, Puga A (1991) Human AH locus polymorphism and cancer: inducibility of CYP1A1 and other genes by combustion products and dioxin. *Pharmacogenetics* 1: 68–78.
12. Kellermann G, Luyten-Kellermann M, Shaw CR (1973) Genetic variation of aryl hydrocarbon hydroxylase in human lymphocytes. *Am J Hum Genet* 25: 327–331.
13. Kellermann G, Shaw CR, Luyten-Kellermann M (1973) Aryl hydrocarbon hydroxylase inducibility and bronchogenic carcinoma. *N Engl J Med* 289: 934–937.
14. Benhamou S, Bonaïti-Pellié C (1995) Susceptibilité au cancer bronchique: un exemple d'interaction génétique-environnement. *Ann Biol Clin* 53: 507–513.
15. Catteau A, Douriez E, Beaune P, Poisson N, Bonaïti-Pellié C, Laurent P (1995) Genetic polymorphism of induction of CYP1A1 (EROD) activity. *Pharmacogenetics* 5: 110–119.
16. Itoh S, Kamataki T (1993) Human Ah receptor cDNA: Analysis for highly conserved sequences. *Nucleic Acids Res* 21: 3578.
17. Le Beau MM, Carver LA, Espinosa III R, Schmidt JV, Bradfield CA (1994) Chromosomal localization of the human AHR locus encoding the structural gene for the Ah receptor to 7p21–p15. *Cytogenet Cell Genet* 66: 172–176.

18. Hildebrand CE, Gonzalez FJ, McBride OW, Nebert DW (1985) Assignment of the human 2,3,7,8-tetrachlorodibenzo-p-dioxin-inducible cytochrome P1-450 gene to chromosome 15. *Nucleic Acids Res* 13: 2009–2016.
19. Hayashi S, Watanabe J, Nakashi K, Kawajiri K (1991) Genetic linkage of lung cancer-associated MspI polymorphism with amino acid replacement in the heme binding region of the human cytochrome P450IA1 gene. *J Biochem* 110: 407–411.
20. Kawajiri K, Nakashi K, Imai K, Yoshii A, Shinoda N, Watanabe J (1990) Identification of genetically high risk individuals to lung cancer by DNA polymorphisms of the cytochrome P4501A1 gene. *FEBS Lett* 263: 131–133.
21. Cosma G, Crofts F, Taioli E, Toniolo P, Garte S (1993) Relationship between genotype and function of the human CYP1A1 gene. *J Toxicol Environ Health* 40: 309–316.
22. Grant DM, Tang BK, Kalow W (1983) Variability in caffeine metabolism. *Clin Pharmacol Ther* 33: 591–602.
23. Butler MA, Lang NP, Young JF, Caporaso NE, Vineis P, Hayes RB, Teitel CH, Massengill JP, Lawsen MF, Kadlubar FF (1992) Determination of CYP1A2 and NAT2 phenotypes in human populations by analysis of caffeine urinary metabolites. *Pharmacogenetics* 2: 116–127.
24. Bock KW, Schrenk D, Forster D, Griese E-U, Mörike K, Brockmeier D, Eichelbaum M (1994) The influence of environmental and genetic factors on CYP2D6, CYP1A2 and UDP-glucuronosyltransferases in man using sparteine, caffeine, and paracetamol as probes. *Pharmacogenetics* 4: 209–218.
25. Catteau A, Bechtel YC, Poisson N, Bechtel PR, Bonaïti-Pellié C (1995) A population and family study of CYP1A2 using caffeine urinary metabolites. *Eur J Clin Pharmacol* 47: 423–430.
26. Notarianni LJ, Oliver SE, Dobrocky P, Bennett PN, Silverman BW (1995) Caffeine as a metabolic probe: a comparison of the metabolic ratios used to assess CYP1A2 activity. *Br J Clin Pharmacol* 39: 65–69.
27. Price-Evans DAP, Maghoub A, Sloan TP, Idle JR, Smith RL (1980) A family and population study of the genetic polymorphism of debrisoquine oxidation in a white British population. *J Med Genet* 17: 102–105.
28. Gonzalez FJ, Skoda RC, Kimura S, Umeno M, Zanger UM, Nebert DW, Gelboin HV, Hardwick JP, Meyer UA (1988) Characterisation of the common genetic defect in humans deficient in debrisoquine metabolism. *Nature* 331: 442–446.
29. Broly F, Meyer UA (1993) Debrisoquine oxidation polymorphism: phenotypic consequences of a 3-base-pair deletion in exon 5 of the CYP2D6 gene. *Pharmacogenetics* 3: 123–130.
30. Crespi CL, Penman BW, Gelboin HV, Gonzalez FJA (1991) Tobacco smoke-derived nitrosamine, 4-(methylnitrosamino)-1-(3-pyridyl)-1-butanone, is activated by multiple human cytochrome P450s including the polymorphic human cytochrome P450 IID6. *Carcinogenesis* 12: 1197–1201.
31. Ayesh R, Idle JR, Ritchie JC, Crothers MJ, Hetzel MR (1984) Metabolic oxidation phenotypes as markers for susceptibility to lung cancer. *Nature* 312: 169–170.
32. Bouchardy C, Benhamou S, Dayer P (1996) The effect of tobacco on lung cancer risk depends on CYP2D6 activity. *Cancer Res* 56: 251–253.
33. Hayashi S-I, Watanabe J, Kawajiri K (1992) High susceptibility to lung cancer analyzed in terms of combined genotypes of P450IA1 and mu-class glutathione S-transferase genes. *Jpn J Cancer Res* 83: 866–870.
34. Nakachi K, Imai K, Hayashi S-I, Kawajiri K (1993) Polymorphisms of the CYP1A1 and glutathione S-transferase genes associated with susceptibility to lung cancer in relation to cigarette dose in a Japanese population. *Cancer Res* 53: 2994–2999.

Clinical and Biological Basis of Lung Cancer Prevention
ed. by Y. Martinet, F. R. Hirsch, N. Martinet, J.-M. Vignaud
and J. L. Mulshine
© 1998 Birkhäuser Verlag Basel/Switzerland

CHAPTER 18
Glutathione S-Transferases and Lung Cancer Risk

Janeric Seidegård

The Wallenberg Laboratory, University of Lund and Astra Draco AB, Lund, Sweden

1. Introduction

There is epidemiological evidence indicating that most human cancers are caused by environmental exposure to genotoxic agents. It is estimated that as many as two thirds of all human cancers originate from exposure to tobacco smoke and dietary components [1]. Tobacco use is a wellknown risk factor for multiple cancers including lung, oesophagus, and bladder cancers. It was estimated that there would be well over 150,000 deaths due to lung cancer in United States in 1995 [2]. It is therefore important to prevent lung cancer by reducing exposure to tobacco and possibly intervening in the carcinogenic process at an early stage. Despite the risks, most smokers do not develop lung cancer. Indeed, the lifetime risk of lung cancer in subjects smoking 20 cigarettes per day is still under 15% [3], suggesting that there may be important endogenous as well as exogenous factors that are likely to affect an individual lung cancer risk.

Environmental factors and the competing effect of other diseases, some of which are also smoking related, may be included here. For example, smokers may succumb to cardiovascular and pulmonary disease, thus leading to a reduction in the number of smokers who manifest lung cancer. The influence of malignancy may include a combination of total tobacco exposure (plus the influence of exposure to alcohol, dietary factors or viral infections) and genetic susceptibility. Several genetic polymorphisms and cancer genes have been investigated in case-control studies [4, 5]. Candidate polymorphisms have been sought among the DNA repair genes, oncogenes, tumour suppressor genes and Phase I and Phase II metabolic enzymes of detoxification.

Cigarette smoke contains more than 40 known or putative carcinogens [6]. Most chemical carcinogens require metabolic activation by Phase I enzymes, cytochrome P450s, to electrophilic intermediates, to generate DNA damage in smokers [7]. These reactive metabolites then become substrates for Phase II enzymes such as epoxide hydrolase, glutathione S-transferase (GST), N-acetyltransferase and sulfotransferase, resulting in detoxification of the reactive metabolites [7]. Thus, identifying inherited variant(s) of drug metabolizing enzyme activities, in their expression or regulation, may be an important factor in determining the relative risk of an individual's developing smoking-related lung cancer [8]. The allelism within certain GST loci may be associated with an altered risk of certain cancers.

GSTs are a complex multigene family of enzymes that can possess many biological functions, such as the important step in detoxification of a large number of electrophiles, many of which are carcinogenic [9, 10]. Mammalian GST can be classified according to substrate specificity, immunological identity, and protein and DNA sequence. Six classes of soluble GST have been identified in eukaryotes, Alpha, Mu, Pi, Theta, Sigma and Kappa (for the nomenclature of GSTs, see [11]). The structural similarity of the amino acid sequence identity among members within each class is >50% and there is less than 25% identity between members of different classes. The immunohistochemical localization of GSTs in human lung revealed that the Alpha class, GSTA1 and GSTA2, and the Pi class, GSTP1, are the most abundant GSTs in human lung, with varying intensity, and are present in the alveolar, the bronchial and the bronchiolar epithelium [12]. The Mu class, GSTM1, had a weak immunoreaction in lung tissue. GSTM2 was found in the epithelium of the terminal airways, and GSTM3 was observed in the ciliated airway epithelium and smooth muscle of the lung. Thus, the localization of the different GSTs in the bronchial wall suggests that they may contribute to susceptibility to lung cancer.

Within the Mu class GST, five genes have been identified: *GSTM1* to *GSTM5*. Of particular interest might be the gene encoding GSTM1 because of its polymorphic expression. Four different alleles of *GSTM1* have been described: *GSTM1*A*, *GSTM1*B*, *GSTM1*C*, and *GSTM1*0* [13]. GSTM1*A and GSTM1*B differ by only one amino acid with similar enzymatic activity towards substrates for GSTM1. GSTM1*C is rather rare and is still not fully characterized. The *GSTM1*0* allele consists of a deletion of the *GSTM1* gene; the expression of GSTM1 has been shown to be autosomal dominant inherited and to be expressed in about 40 to 60% of most populations [14]. Since GSTM1 catalyses the conjugation of a wide range of genotoxic and cytotoxic metabolites of tobacco smoke, and since the deficiency in GSTM1 increases the susceptibility to DNA-adduct formation [15] as well as cytogenetic damage [16], individuals with *GSTM1* deletion could potentially be at greater risk of developing smoking-related lung cancers.

2. Results and Discussion

2.1. GSTM1 Expression and Lung Cancer

Since the first published study in 1986 [17], suggesting that GSTM1 deficiency may constitute a risk factor for developing lung cancers among smokers, a large number of studies have been performed, comparing the frequency of GSTM1 deficiency in patients who have various forms of malignancies, with the frequency in control subjects. There have been studies confirming the association of GSTM1 deficiency with increased risk of lung cancer, and other studies in which no increased risk could be demonstrated. There are, however, several factors that may contribute to heterogeneity of the results among these studies. One major factor may be random variation due to limited power within individual studies. Another factor that merits consideration is the different study designs used. In a recent study by McWilliams et al. [18], a meta-analysis of published case-control studies of lung cancer risk and GSTM1 deficiency was done. Twelve of these studies included a total number of 1593 lung cancer patients and 2135 control subjects. An odds ratio of 1.41 (95% confidence interval [CI] = 1.23, 1.61; P <0.0001) was calculated, suggesting GSTM1 deficiency as a moderate risk factor for lung cancer development. When performing meta-analysis, we have to consider several potential biases, such as differences in racial distribution, variation in the distribution of histological types of lung cancer, misclassification of GSTM1, variation in gender and variation in smoking. However, most of these biases would not contribute to any significant level to the results. The meta-analysis performed confirmed that GSTM1 deficiency is one of several common genetic polymorphisms that confer a moderately high risk of developing lung cancer. An update of all case-control studies of the GSTM1 polymorphism are compiled in Table 1.

In this context, it has been revealed in recent studies [19] that two of the GSTM1 alleles, GSTM1*A and GSTM1*B, have different protective effects. The frequencies of GSTM1*B have been shown to be different in lung cancer patients compared with controls [19]. The mechanism for this effect is unclear but may be related to a linkage of GSTM1*A with GSTM3*B, a polymorphic variant at the Mu class GSTM3 locus that contains a recognition motif for the YY1 transcription factor [20], or because the expression of GSTM3 in lung is dependent on GSTM1 phenotype [21].

2.2. Smoking History and GSTM1 Genotype

By stratifying subjects according to smoking history, we might be able to see an elevated risk among the GSTM1-deficient individuals. However, conflicting data have arisen in this area. Most previous studies with con-

Table 1. Case-control studies of GSTM1 polymorphism and lung cancer risk

Ethnic group	No. of case patients (% null allele)	No. of control subjects (% null allele)	Investigator(s)
Caucasian	66 (65)	78 (41)	Seidegård et al. 1986 [17]
Caucasian	125 (62)	114 (42)	Seidegård et al. 1990 [41]
Caucasian	228 (43)	225 (42)	Zong et al. 1991 [42]
Japanese	212 (56)	358 (47)	Hayashi et al. 1992 [43]
Caucasian	66 (64)	120 (58)	Heckbert et al. 1992 [26]
Not given	35 (74)	43 (47)	Nazar-Stewart et al. 1993 [22]
Caucasian	117 (53)	155 (53)	Brockmöller et al. 1993 [44]
Caucasian	138 (53)	142 (44)	Hirvonen et al. 1993 [23]
Japanese	85 (59)	170 (49)	Nakachi et al. 1993 [25]
Caucasian	296 (56)	329 (53)	Alexandrie et al. 1994 [34]
Japanese	178 (61)	201 (45)	Kihara et al. 1994 [24]
Caucasian	184 (51)	465 (52)	London et al. 1995 [27]
Afro-American	158 (28)	251 (27)	London et al. 1995 [27]
Japanese	447 (56)	469 (49)	Kihara et al. 1995 [35]
Caucasian	106 (47)	577 (55)	Deakin et al. 1996 [19]
Caucasian	139 (57)	147 (46)	To-Figueras et al. 1996 [39]
Caucasian	58 (81)	67 (39)	Baranov et al. 1996 [45]

siderably lower numbers of lung cancer patients have given mixed results. For example, in four studies [17, 22–24] stronger associations were found among the heavier smokers (a pack-year (1 pack of cigarettes smoked per day for one year) cutoff between 30 to 54 pack-years). In contrast to these studies, some other previous studies supported a stronger association among light smokers [25, 26]. In a recent study by London et al. [27], including more than 300 lung cancer cases, a slightly elevated risk of lung cancer in relation to the GSTM1 null genotype was seen among smokers of less than 40 pack-years (OR = 1.77; CI = 1.11, 2.82) and not among those with a longer smoking history. Study design as well as limited power within individual studies may have influenced the heterogeneity of these study results.

2.3. Other GST Genes and GSTM1

Another GST gene family of interest is the recently identified Theta class. Two genes, GSTT1 and GSTT2 have been identified from human liver [28, 29]. The human GSTT1 isoenzyme has attracted recent interest since a null allele has been identified at this locus. Since the enzyme catalyses the detoxification of monohalomethanes and ethylene oxide in vitro, lymphocytes from expressors of the gene appear to be protected against the sister chromatid exchange (SCE) induced by these compounds. It is possible that, like individuals with GSTM1 null genotype, homozygotes for the GSTT1 null allele will have an altered cancer risk. The frequency of the null allele in a normal population has been reported to be 30 to 40% in one study from Germany [30] while in a Swedish population, only 10% expressed this null allele [31].

In a recent study where lung cancer patients and control subjects were compared, the frequencies of the putatively high risk *GSTT1* null genotype were not increased in the lung cancer cases compared with the controls. In the same study, the *GSTM1* genotype was also identified. However, no significant interactions between *GSTT1* and *GSTM1* null genotypes were seen in the lung cancer group in this study.

2.4. Combined Effect of Other Polymorphic Genes and GSTM1

Introducing examples of other common polymorphic genes that confer a moderately increased risk of lung cancer may increase our knowledge of the protective role *GSTM1* plays. A correlation of Phase I and Phase II enzymes with lung cancer susceptibility was first tested by Liu et al. [32], who showed that metabolic ratios of CYP1A1 to GST in lung tissue were significantly greater in lung cancer patients than in the corresponding control subjects. More recent studies using genotyping assays for *CYP1A1* and *GSTM1* further demonstrated that the combined genotype of *CYP1A1* mutant homozygote and *GSTM1* null genotype markedly increased the risk of smoking-related lung cancers among Japanese subjects [14]. These results were further supported by studies performed in Caucasian subjects where individuals expressing the *GSTM1* null genotype in combination with the *Msp*I variant allele of the gene tended to be over-represented in lung cancer patients [33, 34]. Further, it has been demonstrated that among 118 lung cancer patients and 331 control subjects, individuals having the *Msp*I variant allele combined with the *GSTM1* genotype are relatively resistant to tobacco-related lung cancers, whereas individuals with the combination of *Msp*I variant allele and the *GSTM1* null genotype are highly susceptible [35].

Other common genes are *p53* and K-*ras*, where it has been shown that mutation frequencies of the two target genes in lung cancer were affected significantly by *CYP1A1* and *GSTM1* genotypes. Thus, a synergistic increase in the mutation frequency of the *p53* gene among individuals with susceptibility genotypes in combination with *GSTM1* polymorphism is consistent with increased polycyclic aromatic hydrocarbon adduct formation [36], which may result in an increased probability of *p53* mutations. An alternative explanation is that deficient DNA repair or genomic instability, which might result from genotype-dependent initiation by cigarette smoking, may be included at an early stage in carcinogenesis [37, 38] and may influence the consequent genetic events. With an OR of 1.97 (CI = 1.03, 3.73) it has been suggested that the *Pro* allele of the p53 germline polymorphism may slightly increase the risk of the *GSTM1* null genotype among smokers [39].

3. Concluding Remarks

There is no clear understanding of the mechanisms of genetic predisposition to lung cancer. Lung carcinogenesis seems to start from a clonal expansion of the cells that gained a selective growth advantage by early genetic changes in the cells. Because the lungs are widely exposed to environmental carcinogens, including benzo(α)pyrene in cigarette smoke, early genetic lesions may be present in bronchial mucosa. Progression towards full tumorigenicity would then be acquired through accumulation of further genetic alterations. Thus genetic predisposing factors to smoking-induced lung cancer, such as *GSTM1* and *CYP1A1* polymorphism, may affect the mutation of target genes in early genetic alterations such as the somatic alteration of *p53* gene which seems to be a candidate in the precancerous genetic event [40]. However, future studies are needed to examine and quantitate the interactions between the excess lung cancer risk conferred by *GSTM1* deficiency and polymorphisms in the *CYP1A* and *p53* genes.

Acknowledgement

This work was supported by Nilsson's Foundation and the Medical Faculty, University of Lund, Sweden.

References

1. Doll R, Peto R (1981) The causes of cancer: quantitative estimates of avoidable risks of cancer in the United States today. *J Natl Cancer Inst* 66: 1191–1308.
2. Wingo PA, Tong T, Bolden S (1995) Cancer Statistics. *Cancer J Clin* 45: 8–30.
3. Law MR (1990) Genetic predisposition to lung cancer. *Br J Cancer* 61: 195–206.
4. Bell DA, Taylor JA, Paulson DF, Robertson CN, Mohler JL, Lucier GW (1993) Genetic risk and carcinogen exposure: a common inherited defect of carcinogen-metabolism gene glutathione S-transferase M1 (GSTM1) that increases susceptibility to bladder carcinoma. *J Natl Cancer Inst* 85: 1159–1164.
5. Kawajiri K, Nakachi K, Imai K, Watanabe J, Hayashi SI (1993) Germ line polymorphisms of *p53* and *CYP1A1* genes involved in human lung cancer. *Carcinogenesis* 14: 1085–1089.
6. United States Surgeon General. Reducing the Health Consequences of Smoking: 25 Years of Progress. Washington, DC: Office on Smoking and Health (1989).
7. Sipes IG, Gandolfi AJ (1991) Biotransformation of toxicants. *In:* Amdur MO, Doull J, Klaassen CD (ed): *Casarett and Doull's Toxicology*. Pergamon Press, New York, pp 172–174.
8. Caporaso NE, Landi MT, Vineis P (1991) Relevance of metabolic polymorphisms to human carcinogenesis: evaluation of epidemiological evidence. *Pharmacogenetics* 1:4–19.
9. Jakoby WB (1978) The glutathione S-transferases: A group of multifunctional detoxification proteins. *Adv Enzymol* 46: 383–413.
10. Mannervik B (1985) The isoenzymes of glutathione transferase. *Adv Enzymol Rel Areas Mol Biol* 57: 357–417.
11. Mannervik B, Awasthi YC, Board PG, Hayes JD, Di Ilio C, Ketterer B, Listowsky I, Morgenstern R, Muramatsu M, Pearson WR, Picket CB, Sato K, Widersten M, Wolf CR (1992) Nomenclature for human glutathione transferases. *Biochem J* 282: 305–306.
12. Antilla S, Hirvonen A, Vainio H, Husgafvel-Pursiainen K, Hayes JD, Ketterer B (1993) Immunohistochemical localization of glutathione S-transferases in human lung. *Cancer Res* 53: 5643–5648.

13. Fryer AA, Zhao L, Alldersea J, Boggild MD, Perret CW, Clayton RN, Jones PW, Strange RC (1993) The glutathione S-transferases: polymerase chain reaction studies on the frequency of the *GSTμ1 0* genotype in patients with pituitary adenomas. *Carcinogenesis* 14: 563–566.

14. Lin HJ, Han CY, Bernstein DA (1994) Ethnic distribution of the glutathione transferase μ 1-1 (GSTμ1) null genotype in 1473 individuals and application to bladder cancer susceptibility. *Carcinogenesis* 15: 1077–1081.

15. Liu YH, Taylor J, Linko P, Lucier GW, Thompson CL (1991) Glutathione S-transferase μ in lymphocyte and liver: role in modulating formation of carcinogen-derived DNA adducts. *Carcinogenesis* 12: 2269–2275.

16. Wiencke JK, Kelsey KT, Lamela RA, Toscano WA Jr (1990) Human glutathione S-transferase deficiency as a marker of susceptibility to epoxide-induced cytogenetic damage. *Cancer Res* 50: 1585–1590.

17. Seidegård J, Pero RW, Miller DG, Beattie EJ (1986) A glutathione transferase in human leukocytes as a marker for the susceptibility to lung cancer. *Carcinogenesis* 7: 751–753.

18. McWilliams JE, Sanderson BJS, Harris EL, Richert-Boe KE, Henner WD (1995) Glutathione S-transferase M1 (GST1) deficiency and lung cancer risk. *Cancer Epidemiol Biomarkers & Prevention* 4: 589–594.

19. Deakin M, Elder J, Hendrickse C, Peckham D, Baldwin D, Pantin C, Wild N, Leopard P, Bell DA, Jones P, Duncan H, Brannigan K, Alldersea J, Fryer AA, Strange RC (1996) Glutathione S-transferase GSTT1 genotype and susceptibility to cancer: studies of interactions with GSTM1 in lung, oral, gastric and colorectal cancers. *Carcinogenesis* 17: 881–884.

20. Inskip A, Elexperu-Camirugua J, Buxton N (1995) Identification of polymorphism at the glutathione S-transferase, GSTM3 locus: Evidence for linkage with *GSTM1*A*. *Biochem J* 312: 713–716.

21. Nakajima T, Elovaara E, Antilla S, Hirvonen A, Camus A-M, Hayes JD, Ketterer B, Vainio H (1995) Expression and polymorphism of glutathione S-transferase in human lungs: risk factors in smoking-related lung cancer. *Carcinogenesis* 16: 707–811.

22. Nazar-Stewart V, Motulsky AG, Eaton DL (1993) The glutathione S-transferase μ polymorphism as a marker for susceptibility to lung carcinoma. *Cancer Res* 53: 2313–2318.

23. Hirvonen A, Husgafel-Pursiainen K, Antilla S (1993) The GSTM1 null genotype as a potential risk modifier for squamous cell carcinoma of the lung. *Carcinogenesis* 14: 1479–1481.

24. Kihara M, Kihara M, Noda K (1994) Lung cancer risk of GSTM1 null genotype is dependent on the extent of tobacco smoke exposure. *Carcinogenesis* 15: 415–418.

25. Nakachi K, Imai K, Hayashi S (1993) Polymorphisms of the CYP1A1 and glutathione S-transferase genes associated with susceptibility of lung cancer in relation to cigarette dose in a Japanese population. *Cancer Res* 53: 2994–2999.

26. Heckbert SR, Weiss NS, Hornung SK (1992) Glutathione S-transferase and epoxide hydrolase activity in human leukocytes in relation to risk of lung cancer and other smoking-related cancers. *J Natl Cancer Inst* 84: 414–422.

27. London SJ, Daly AK, Navidi WC, Carpenter CL, Idle Jr (1995) Polymorphism of glutathione S-transferase M1 and lung cancer risk among African-Americans and Caucasians in Los Angeles county, California. *J Natl Cancer Inst* 87: 1246–1253.

28. Meyer DJ, Coles B, Pemble SE, Gilmore KS, Fraser GM, Ketterer B (1991) Theta, a new class of glutathione transferases purified from rat and man. *Biochem J* 274: 409–414.

29. Hussey AJ, Hayes JD (1992) Characterisation of a human class theta glutathione S-transferase with activity towards 1-menaphthyl sulphate. *Biochem J* 286: 929–935.

30. Peter H, Deutschmann S, Reichel D, Hallier E (1989) Metabolism of methyl chloride by human erythrocytes. *Arch Toxicol* 63: 351–355.

31. Warholm M, Rane A, Alexandrie A-K, Gemma M, Rannug A (1995) Genotypic and phenotypic determination of polymorphic glutathione transferase T1 in a Swedish population. *Pharmacogenetics* 5:252–254.

32. Liu L, Wang L (1988) Correlation between lung cancer prevalence and activities of aryl hydrocarbon hydroxylase and glutathione S-transferase in human lung tissues. *Biomed Environ Sci* 1: 283–287.

33. Antilla S, Hirvonen A, Husgafel-Pursiainen K, Karjalainen A, Nurminen T, Vainio H (1994) Combined effect of CYP1A1 inducibility and GSTM1 polymorphism on histological type of lung cancer. *Carcinogenesis* 15: 1133–1135.

34. Alexandrie A-K, Ingelman-Sundberg M, Seidegård J, Tornling G, Rannug A. (1994) Genetic susceptibility to lung cancer with special emphasis on *CYP1A1* and *GSTM1*: a study on host factors in relation to age at onset, gender and histological cancer types. *Carcinogenesis* 15: 1785–1790.

35. Kihara M, Kihara M, Noda K (1995) Risk of smoking for squamous and small cell carcinomas of the lung modulated by combinations of CYP1A1 and GSTM1 gene polymorphisms in a Japanese population. *Carcinogenesis* 16: 2331–2336.

36. Dickey CP, Bell DA, Santella R, Ottman R, Hemminki K, Savela K, Lucier G, Perera FP (1995) *GSTM1*, *CYP1A1*, *Msp*I, and DNA adducts in Workers exposed to PAH. *Proc Am Assoc Cancer Res* 36: 120.

37. Aaltonen LA, Peltomäki P, Leach FS, Sistonen P, Pylkkänen L, Mecklin J-P, Järvinen H, Powell SM, Jen J, Hamilton SR, Petersen GM, Kinzler KW, Vogelstein B, de la Chapelle A (1993) Clues to pathogenesis of familial colorectal cancer. *Science* 260: 812–816.

38. Ionov Y, Peinado MA, Malkhosyan S, Shibata D, Perucho M (1993) Ubiquitous somatic mutations in simple repeated sequences reveal a new mechanism for colonic carcinogenesis. *Nature* 363: 558–561.

39. To-Figueras J, Gené M, Gómez-Catalán J, Firvida J, Fuentes M, Rodamilans M, Huguet E, Estapé J, Corbella J (1996) Glutathione S-transferase M1 and codon 72 p53 polymorphisms in a Northwestern Mediterranean population and their relation to lung cancer susceptibility. *Cancer Epidemiol Biomarkers Prevention* 5: 337–342.

40. Sozzi G, Miozzo M, Donghi R, Pilotti S, Cariani CT, Pastorino U, Porta GP, Pierotti MA (1992) Deletion of 17p and *p53* mutations in preneoplastic lesions of the lung. *Cancer Res* 52: 6079–6082.

41. Seidegård J, Pero RW, Markowitz MM, Roush G, Miller DG, Beatti EJ (1990) Isoenzyme of glutathione transferase (class Mu) as a marker for the susceptibility to lung cancer: a follow up study. *Carcinogenesis* 11: 33–36.

42. Zhong S, Howie AF, Ketterer B, Taylor J, Hayes JD, Beckette GJ, Wathen CG, Wolf CR, Spurr NK (1991) Glutathione S-transferase mu locus: use of genotyping and phenotyping assays to assess association with lung cancer susceptibility. *Carcinogenesis* 12: 1533–1537.

43. Hayashi S-I, Watanabe J, Kawajiri K (1992) High susceptibility to lung cancer analyzed in terms of combined genotypes of *P450IA1* and μ-class glutathione S-transferase genes. *Jpn J Cancer Res* 83: 866–870.

44. Brockmöller J, Kerb R, Drakoulis N, Nitz M, Roots I (1993) Genotype and phenotype of glutathione S-transferase class mu isoenzymes mu and psi in lung cancer patients and controls. *Cancer Res* 53: 1004–1011.

45. Baranov VS, Ivaschenko T, Bakay B, Aseev M, Belotserkovskaya R, Baranova H, Malet P, Perriot J (1996) Proportion of the GSTM1 0/0 genotype in some Slavic populations and its correlation with cystic fibrosis and some multifactorial diseases. *Hum Genet* 97: 516–520.

Clinical and Biological Basis of Lung Cancer Prevention
ed. by Y. Martinet, F.R. Hirsch, N. Martinet, J.-M. Vignaud
and J.L. Mulshine

CHAPTER 19
The *p53* Tumor Suppressor Gene
in Lung Cancer: From Molecular to Serological
Diagnosis

Thierry Soussi[1,3], Jean Tredaniel[2], Richard Lubin[1,4], Gerard Zalcman[2]
and Albert Hirsh[2]

[1] *Unité 301 INSERM, Institut de Génétique Moléculaire, Paris, France*
[2] *Service de Pneumologie, Hôpital St Louis, Paris, France*
[3] *Present address: UMR218 CNRS, Institut Curie, Paris, France*
[4] *Present address: Pharmacell, Hôpital Saint-Louis, Paris, France*

1. Introduction

Alteration of *p53* is the most common alteration found in human cancer. It usually involves missense mutations that frequently stabilize the *p53* protein, which in turn accumulates to reach levels detectable by immunohistochemistry. Analysis of *p53* mutational events leads to significant conclusions concerning *p53* mutation and exposure to carcinogens. Although *p53* alteration does not seem to correlate with any clinical parameters, the observation that such mutations occur very early in lung tumorigenesis suggests that they can be used for early diagnosis.

2. Genetic Alterations in Lung Cancer

Lung cancer is the most frequently encountered tumor in the industrial world, with increasing incidence in both men and women linked to tobacco smoking epidemics [1]. Extensive analysis has revealed several types of genetic alterations that contribute to either small cell lung cancer (SCLC) or non-small cell lung cancer (NSCLC): *myc* gene activation, *ras* gene mutation and loss of heterozygosity (LOH) in chromosomes regions 3p,

13q and 17p [2]. The two first alterations result from amplification and/or mutation of dominant oncogenes. Allele loss is highly suggestive of the presence of a tumor suppressor gene at the deleted chromosomal site. Two well-known tumor suppressor genes, *Rb* and *p53*, have been identified in 13q14 and 17p13 respectively. More recently, alteration of a new gene named *FHIT* localized in 3p14.2, has been described in lung cancer [3] but due to the heterogeneity of the LOH on 3p, it is possible that more than one locus is the target for these deletions. Analysis of the timing of these molecular events indicates that 3p alteration is one of the earliest genetic changes detected in lung cancer. *p53* alterations have also been detected in early lung lesions such as mild dysplasia.

3. The *p53* Tumor Suppressor Gene

The tumor suppressor gene *p53* is a phosphoprotein expressed at such low levels in the nucleus of normal cells (half-life 20 minutes) that it is barely detectable [4]. Upon physical or chemical DNA damage, the functional *p53* can either arrest cell cycle progression in the late G1 phase [5, 6], thus allowing the DNA to be repaired before its replication, or else induce apoptosis leading to cell death [7, 8]. Growth arrest function is achieved by the transactivational properties of *p53*, which activate a series of genes involved in cell cycle arrest [9] whereas the apoptotic pathway of *p53* is undefined. In cells lacking functional *p53* (i.e. tumor cells), the various pathways described above are not functional, resulting in inefficient DNA repair and the emergence of genetically unstable cells [10, 11]. All these studies have led to the proposal that *p53* is a key element in the control of genome stability [12].

The most common change of *p53* in human cancers is a point mutation within the coding sequences of the gene which give rise to an altered protein [13, 14]. Mutations in the *p53* gene are found in all major histogenetic groups, including cancers of the colon, stomach, breast, lung, brain and esophagus. It is estimated that the *p53* mutation is the most frequent genetic event in human cancers, accounting for more than 50% of cases [15]. More than 90% of the point mutations reported so far are clustered between exons 4 and 9 and are localized in the DNA binding domain of the *p53* protein [13]. One of the most striking features of the inactive mutant *p53* protein is its increased stability. It has been found that mutant *p53* protein, which takes on an abnormal conformation, is more stable than the wildtype (half-life of several hours compared to 20 minutes for the wildtype *p53*), accumulates in the nucleus of neoplastic cells and thus becomes immunologically detectable. Therefore, positive immunostaining indicates abnormalities of the *p53* gene and its product [16].

There has been intensive investigation of *p53* alteration for the following reasons: *p53* mutations are the most common genetic alteration in human cancer; *p53* alteration can be easily detected by several approaches; the pattern of *p53* mutations in various tumor types establishes a clear link between cancer and carcinogen exposure; *p53* mutation is associated with the emergence of more aggressive tumors; loss or retention of *p53* function also appears to be a critical parameter in cancer treatment. Tumor cell death by radiation therapy or chemotherapeutic agents is probably due to the active process of apoptosis rather than the genotoxicity of the agents per se in many cases [8, 17]. As apoptosis is mediated by a functional *p53* in many cases, the effectiveness of a given therapy would seem to be correlated with the *p53* status of a given tumor [18].

4. Lung Cancers, Smoking and *p53* Mutations

Numerous investigations have consistently reported increased occurence of lung cancer among smokers. All investigations have shown a clear dose-response relationship between the amount of tobacco smoked daily and the subsequent risk of lung cancer [1]. It is now thought that cigarette smoking is responsible for 90% of lung cancers. In experimental animals, cigarette smoke induces tumors of the respiratory tract. This smoke is a complex mixture of several hundred different molecules, including well-characterized carcinogens such as polycyclic aromatic hydrocarbons (benzo(a)pyrene) and N-nitrosamines. Benzo(a)pyrene is a highly carcinogenic compound and was one of the molecules in coal tar that was found to be implicated in scrotal cancer during the nineteenth century. Exposure to coal tar is no longer a public health hazard, but benzo(a)pyrene from sources such as cigarette smoke and automobile exhaust fumes is highly prevalent in the environment.

p53 mutations are common in lung cancer and range from 33% in adenocarcinomas to 70% in SCLC [19, 20]. These mutations are mostly GC to TA transversions, with a rate of transition mutations lower than in other cancers (Figure 1). A strong correlation has been detected between the frequency of these GC to TA transversions and lifelong cigarette smoking. This high frequency of GC to TA transversions has not been detected for other cancers such as colon, breast, overian or brain cancer, which are not directly associated with smoking (Fig. 1). This observation is compatible with the role of exogenous carcinogens such as benzo(a)pyrene in lung cancer. It has been shown experimentally that after metabolic activation, one of the derivative products of benzo(a)pyrene binds predominantly to guanine and gives rise to specific GC to TA transversions. A recent study has shown that exposure of cells to benzo(a)pyrene can lead to the formation of adducts at codons 157, 248 and 273 in the *p53* gene [21]. These positions are the major mutational "hotspots" in human lung cancer. Thus, these studies clearly show that the *p53* gene is one of the targets of carcinogens found in tobacco.

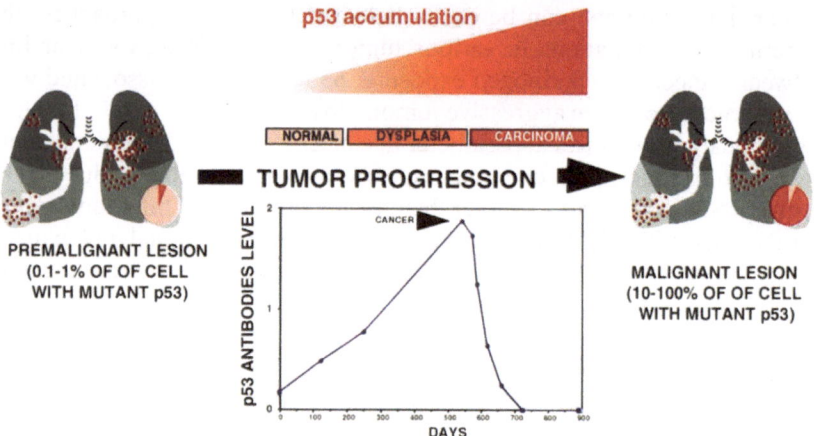

Figure 1. The spectrum of *p53* mutations in various types of tumours. All cancer types correspond to the 5800 mutations found in more than 40 types of cancer [54, 55]. GC to AT mutations at CpG dinucleotide are the consequence of spontaneous deamination of 5-methylcytosine, whereas GC to TA mutations are strongly indicative of exposure to exogenous carcinogens.

5. *p53* Gene Alteration and Clinical Parameters

Is it possible to correlate *p53* gene alterations with diagnostic or prognostic clinical parameters? How may this information contribute to the choice of treatment? In fact, since Cattoreti's study in 1988 [22], the analysis of *p53* accumulation in breast cancer shows that it occurs mainly in patients with a poor prognosis (absence of oestrogen receptors and high grade tumors). These findings in breast cancer have since been confirmed by molecular, immunohistochemical or serological approaches [23–27]. Thor et al. [28, 29] reported that *p53* alteration could be considered as a new, independent marker associated with lower patient survival.

Many similar studies have been conducted in other types of cancer, with results that are not as clear as in breast cancer. Overall, tumors with *p53* accumulation are generally high grade and more aggressive. For lung cancer, the results are not clear as to whether *p53* accumulation is related to poor patient prognosis (cf. letter by Mitsudomi and Passlick [30, 31]). As Mitsudomi indicates, it is important to establish some level of standardization so that studies of *p53* accumulation can be comparable from one series to another. Recent studies have suggested that *p53* abnormalities could have a prognostic value for adenocarcinomas, whereas there was no significant prognosis factor in NSCLC when all histological subtypes are combined [32, 33].

In lung cancer, it is now clear that *p53* alteration is an early event [34–36]. In a study of lung tissues containing preinvasive squamous neoplasms from patients with or without lung cancer, Bennet et al. [36]

detected *p53* protein accumulation in 0% of normal mucosas, 6.7% of squamous metaplasias, 29.5% of mild dysplasias, 26.9% of moderate dysplasias and 59.7% of severe dysplasias. More recently, Mao et al. [37] were able to detect *p53* mutations in patient sputum specimens obtained one year prior to clinical diagnosis of lung cancer (Figure 2).

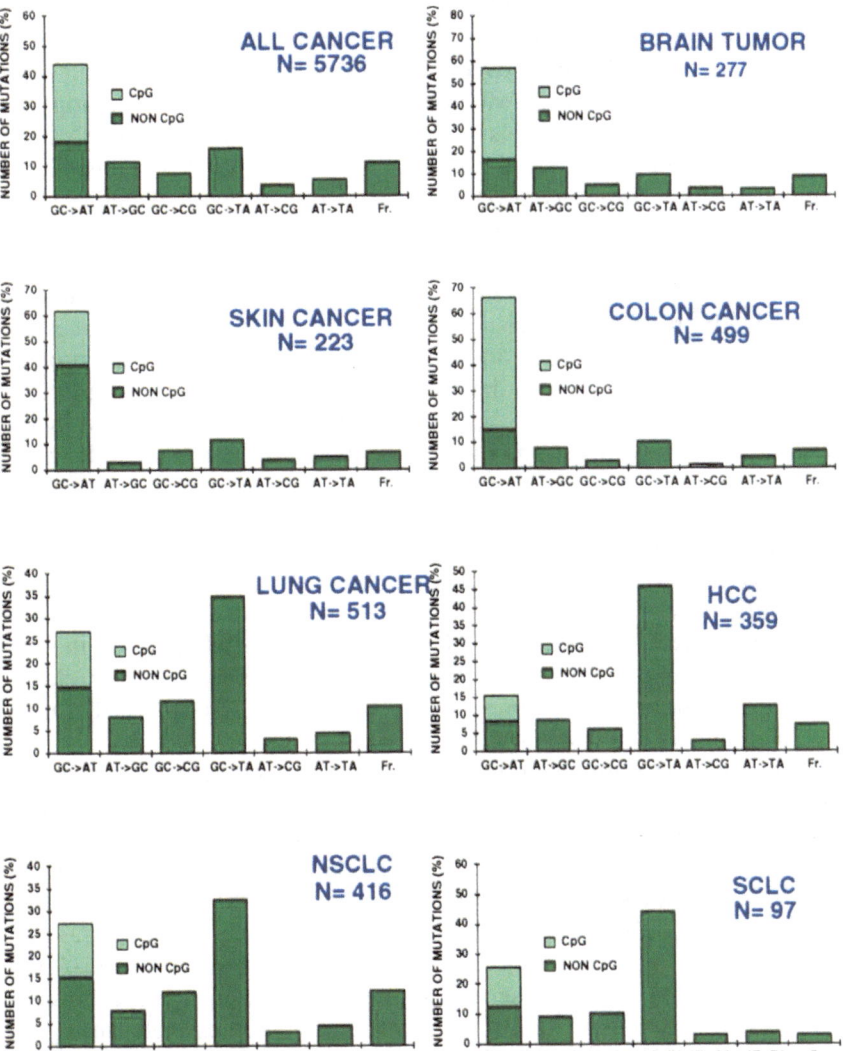

Figure 2. *p53* alteration in lung cancer. Using molecular analysis, several groups demonstrate that a small number of tumoral cells harbor a *p53* mutation in early neoplastic lesion of the lung [34, 35, 37]. During tumor progression, cells with *p53* mutations are selected and correspond to the majority of tumoral cells in the primary tumor. Immunohistochemistry identified the accumulation of mutant as early as dysplastic cells [36]. Serological analysis indicates that *p53*-Ab can be detected several years before the clinical diagnosis of the tumor.

6. *p53* Antibodies in Cancer Patients: Application to Lung Tumors

Ten percent of breast cancer patients have anti-*p53* antibodies (*p53*-Ab) in their serum [38]. This percentage reaches 20% in children with B lymphomas, while it is 0% in patients with T lymphomas [39]. These studies, conducted during a lull in scientific enthusiasm for *p53*, were reviewed more recently in light of new knowledge on *p53* inactivation and stabilization. *p53*-Ab have been found in most human cancers [24, 40, 43]. There is generally a good correlation between their frequency and that of *p53* gene alterations. In lung cancer, which has a high rate of *p53* mutation, the frequency of these *p53*-Ab is high (24%) [42, 44]. In prostate cancer where the *p53* mutation rate is low, or in mesotheliomas where it is nil, the incidence of seropositivity is very low. Several multifactorial studies show a very good correlation between the presence of *p53*-Ab, accumulation of the mutant protein in the tumor, and the presence of a mutation in the gene [40, 42, 45]. Detailed analysis of these antibodies indicates that they recognize both wildtype and mutant *p53* [24, 44–46]. The epitopes are mainly located in the amino and carboxy terminal regions of the protein, regions which are not in the „hotspot" areas [24, 44, 45]. These immunodominant epitopes have also been detected in the serum of mice hyperimmunized with wildtype *p53* [47]. Taken together, these studies show that accumulation of the *p53* protein in tumor cells is responsible for the appearance of autoantibodies.

Serological analysis has the following advantages: simplicity of analysis (ELISA); no need for tumor tissue; possibility of following the fate of the antibodies during treatment of the patient.

In lung cancer, the level of *p53*-Ab is closely correlated with the response to therapy, with a rapid diminution of antibody level correlating with a diminution of the tumor mass (T. Soussi, J. Tredaniel, R. Lubin, G. Zalcman and A. Hirsh, unpublished results).

One of the most promising future uses of *p53*-Ab is in the sera of people at high risk of lung cancer, of workers exposed to carcinogens. As stated above, *p53* alteration is an early event in lung cancer, several years before clinical diagnosis of a tumor (Figure 2). Recently, *p53*-Ab were detected in sera of two patients who were heavy smokers without diagnosed lung malignancy [48]. Both of these patients developed invasive squamous lung cancer 5 and 15 months, respectively, after detection of serum *p53*-Ab. In one patient, the level of serum antibodies directed against different epitopes of *p53* protein was shown to increase progressively during the 15 months of followup before the diagnosis (Figure 2). In this patient, *p53* accumulation was detected in tumoral cells from bronchial biopsy specimens. Since *p53* alterations represent an early genetic change in lung carcinogenesis, it is suggested that *p53*-Ab detection could be a new and sensitive tool for the identification of preneoplastic and microinvasive bronchial lesions in patients with a high risk of lung cancer (i.e. heavy smokers). This finding has been confirmed by Trivers et al. [49] using three types of assay to detect *p53*-Ab. They were able to find *p53*-Ab before diagnosis in several patients with Chronic Obstructive Pulmonary disease. This is also supported by the recent observation that *p53*-Ab can be detected in the sera of workers exposed to vinyl chloride who are highly susceptible to angiosarcoma of the liver [50].

It should be emphasized that assay of *p53*-Ab is a global approach to assessing *p53* alterations, and does not depend on sampling of the tumor, the composition of which may be very heterogenous. Molecular analysis of tumor tissue or biopsies corresponds to local analysis of *p53* status, and may be erroneous if the tumor is too heterogeneous or too highly contaminated by normal tissue. Furthermore, mutation is not necessary for *p53* accumulation [26, 51] and *p53* antibodies can be detected in such patients.

7. Conclusion

p53 alterations in lung cancer will have a very low, if any, clinical significance for prognosis. Nevertheless recent reports have shown that *p53* alterations could be correlated to resistance to cisplatine in NSCLC [52, 53]. Further work will be needed to see if such observations can be extended to other chemotherapeutic agents, and if they can be used for the choice of therapeutic regimen.

Serological analysis of *p53* alterations in human cancers is still in its infancy and will require some standardization before a clear picture can emerge concerning the true frequency of this *p53*-Ab. Commercial ELISA kits will soon be available and will enable large-scale analysis, with comparisons from various areas. Nevertheless, they should be an invaluable marker for clinical diagnosis of *p53* alterations and also a predictive marker for patients at high risk of lung cancer.

Acknowledgements

This work was supported by grants from the Association de Recherche sur le Cancer, the Ligue Nationale contre le Cancer (Comité de Paris and Comité National) and the MGEN.

References

1. IARC (1985) IARC monographs on the evaluation of the carcinogenic risk of chemicals to Human. Tobacco smoking 38: Lyon.
2. Minna JD (1993) The molecular biology of lung cancer pathogenesis. *Chest* 103: 449–456.
3. Sozzi G, Veronese ML, Negrini M, Baffa R, Cotticelli MG, Inoue H, Tornielli S, Pilotti S, Degregorio L, Pastorino U, et al. (1996) The FHIT gene at 3p14.2 is abnormal in lung cancer. *Cell* 85: 17–26.
4. Soussi T, May P (1996) Structural aspects of the p53 protein in relation to gene evolution: a second look. *J Mol Biol* 260: 623–637.

5. Kastan MB, Onyekwere O, Sidransky D, Vogelstein B, Craig RW (1991) Participation of p53 protein in the cellular response to DNA damage. *Cancer Res* 51: 6304–6311.
6. Smith ML, Chen IT, Zhan QM, Bae IS, Chen CY, Gilmer TM, Kastan MB, O'Connor PM, Fornace AJ (1994) Interaction of the p53-regulated protein gadd45 with proliferating cell nuclear antigen. *Science* 266: 1376–1380.
7. Yonish-Rouach E, Resnitzky D, Lotem J, Sachs L, Kimchi A, Oren M (1991) Wild-type p53 induces apoptosis of myeloid leukaemic cells that is inhibited by interleukin-6. *Nature* 352: 345–347.
8. Lowe SW, Ruley HE, Jacks T, Housman DE (1993) p53-dependent apoptosis modulates the cytotoxicity of anticancer agents. *Cell* 74: 957–967.
9. Pietenpol JA, Tokino T, Thiagalingam S, El-Deiry WS, Kinzler KW, Vogelstein B (1994) Sequence-specific transcriptional activation is essential for growth suppression by p53. *Proc Natl Acad Sci USA* 91: 1998–2002.
10. Livingstone LR, White A, Sprouse J, Livanos E, Jacks T, Tlsty TD (1992) Altered cell cycle arrest and gene amplification potential accompany loss of wild-type p53. *Cell* 70: 923–935.
11. Yin YX, Tainsky MA, Bischoff FZ, Strong LC, Wahl GM (1992) Wild-type p53 restores cell cycle control and inhibits gene emplification in cells with mutant p53 alleles. *Cell* 70: 937–948.
12. Lane D (1992) p53, guardian of the genome. *Nature* 358: 15–16.
13. Caron de Fromentel C, Soussi T (1992) Tumor suppressor gene: a model for investigating human mutagenesis. *Genes Chrom Cancer* 4: 1–15.
14. Soussi T, Legros Y, Lubin R, Ory K, Schlichtholz B (1994) Multifactorial analysis of p53 alteration in human cancer – a review. *Int J Cancer* 57: 1–9.
15. Greenblatt MS, Bennett WP, Hollstein M, Harris CC (1994) Mutations in the p53 tumor suppressor gene: clues to cancer etiology and molecular pathogenesis. *Cancer Res* 54: 4855–4878.
16. Dowell SP, Wilson POG, Derias NW, Lane DP, Hall PA (1994) Clinical utility of the immunocytochemical detection of p53 protein in cytological specimens. *Cancer Res* 54: 2914–2918.
17. Lowe SW, Bodis S, Mcclatchey A, Remington L, Ruley HE, Fisher DE, Housman DE, Jacks T (1994) p53 status and the efficacy of cancer therapy in vivo. *Science* 266: 807–810.
18. Fan SJ, El-Deiry WS, Bae I, Freeman J, Jondle D, Bhatia K, Fornace AJ, Magrath I, Kohn KW, O'Connor PM (1994) p53 gene mutations are associated with decreased sensitivity of human lymphoma cells to DNA damaging agents. *Cancer Res* 54: 5824–5830.
19. Takahashi T, Nau MM, Chiba I, Birrer MJ, Rosenberg RK, Vinocour M, Levitt M, Pass H, Gazdar AF, Minna JD (1989) p53 – a frequent target for genetic abnormalities in lung cancer. *Science* 246: 491–494.
20. Chiba I, Takahashi T, Nau MM, d'Amico D, Curiel DT, Mitsudomi T, Buchhagen DL, Carbon D, Piantadosi S, Koga H, et al. (1990) Mutations in the p53 gene are frequent in primary, resected non-small-cell lung cancer. *Oncogene* 5: 1603–1610.
21. Denissenko MF, Pao A, Tang MS, Pfeifer GP (1996) Preferential formation of benzo[a]pyrene adducts at lung cancer mutational hotspots in p53. *Science* 274: 430–432.
22. Cattoretti G, Rilke F, Andrealo S, D'amato L, Delia D (1988) p53 expression in breast cancer. *Int J Cancer* 41: 178–183.
23. Callahan R (1992) p53 mutations, another breast cancer prognostic factor. *J Natl Cancer Inst* 84: 826–827.
24. Schlichtholz B, Legros Y, Gillet D, Gaillard C, Marty M, Lane D, Calvo F, Soussi T (1992) The immune response to p53 in breast cancer patients is directed against immunodominant epitopes unrelated to the mutational hot spot. *Cancer Res* 52: 6380–6384.
25. Allred DC, Clark GM, Elledge R, Fuqua SAW, Brown RW, Chamness GC, Osborne CK, Mcguire WL (1993) Association of p53 protein expression with tumor cell proliferation rate and clinical outcome in Node-Negative breast cancer. *J Natl. Cancer Inst* 85: 200–206.
26. Andersen TI, Holm R, Nesland JM, Heimdal KR, Ottestad L, Borresen AL (1993) Prognostic significance of TP53 alterations in breast carcinoma. *Br J Cancer* 68: 540–548.
27. Thor AD, Yandell DW (1993) Prognostic significance of p53 overexpression in node-negative breast carcinoma – preliminary studies support cautious optimism. *J Nat Cancer Inst* 85: 176–177.

28. Thor AD, Moore DH, Edgerton SM, Kawasaki ES, Reihsaus E, Lynch HT, Marcus JN, Schwartz L, Chen LC, Mayall BH, et al. (1992) Accumulation of p53 tumor suppressor gene protein – an independent marker of prognosis in breast cancers. *J Natl Cancer Inst* 84: 845–855.

29. Barnes DM, Dublin EA, Fisher CJ, Levison DA, Millis RR (1993) Immunohistochemical detection of p53 protein in mammary carcinoma: an important new independent indicator of prognosis? *Hum Pathol* 24: 469–476.

30. Mitsudomi T (1994) *p53* in non-small-cell lung cancer – response. *J Natl. Cancer Inst* 86: 802–803.

31. Passlick B, Izbicki JR, Riethmuller G, Pantel K (1994) *p53* in non-small-cell lung cancer. *J Natl Cancer Inst* 86: 801–802.

32. Mitsudomi T, Oyama T, Nishida K, Ogami A, Osaki T, Nakanishi R, Sugio R, Yasumoto K, Sugimashi K (1995) p53 nuclear immunostaining and gene mutations in non-small-cell lung cancer and their effects on patients survival. *Annals of Oncology* 6 [Sup.]: S9–S13.

33. Nishio M, Koshikawa T, Kuroishi T, Suyama M, Uchida K, Takagi Y, Washimi O, Sugiura T, Ariyoshi Y, Takahashi T, et al. (1996) Prognostic significance of abnormal p53 accumulation in primary, resected non-small-cell lung cancers. *J Clin Oncol* 14: 497–502.

34. Sozzi G, Miozzo M, Donghi R, Pilotti S, Cariani CT, Pastorino U, Dellaporta G, Pierotti MA (1992) Deletions of 17p and p53 mutations in preneoplastic lesions of the lung. *Cancer Res* 52: 6079–6082.

35. Sundaresan V, Ganly P, Hasleton P, Rudd R, Sinha G, Bleehen NM, Rabbits P (1992) p53 and chromosome 3 abnormalities, characteristic of malignant lung tumours, are detectable in preinvasive lesions of the bronchus. *Oncogene* 7: 1989–1997.

36. Bennett WP, Colby TV, Travis WD, Borkowski A, Jones RT, Lane DP, Metcalf RA, Samet JM, Takeshima Y, Gu JR (1993) p53 protein accumulates frequently in early bronchial neoplasia. *Cancer Res* 53: 4817–4822.

37. Mao L, Hruban RH, Boyle JO, Tockman M, Sidransky D (1994) Detection of oncogene mutations in sputum precedes diagnosis of lung cancer. *Cancer Res* 54: 1634–1637.

38. Crawford LV, Pim DC, Bulbrook RD (1982) Detection of antobidies against the cellular protein p53 in sera from patients with breast cancer. *Int J Cancer* 30: 403–408.

39. Caron de Fromentel C, May-Levin F, Mouriesse H, Lemerle J, Chandrasekaran K, May P (1987) Presence of circulating antibodies against cellular protein p53 in a notable proportion of children with B-cell lymphoma. *Int J Cancer* 39: 185–189.

40. Davidoff AM, Iglehart JD, Marks JR (1992) Immune response to p53 is dependent upon p53/HSP70 complexes in breast cancers. *Proc Natl Acad Sci USA* 89: 3439–3442.

41. Hassapoglidoi S, Diamandis EP (1992) Antibodies to the p53 tumor suppressor gene product quantified in cancer patients serum with a time-resolved immunofluorometry technique. *Clin Biochem* 25: 445–449.

42. Winter SF, Minna JD, Johnson BE, Takahashi T, Gazdar AF, Carbone DP (1992) Development of antibodies against p53 in lung cancer patients appears to be dependent on the type of p53 mutation. *Cancer Res* 52: 4168–4174.

43. Angelopoulou K, Diamandis EP, Sutherland DJA, Kellen JA, Bunting PS (1994) Prevalence of serum antibodies against the p53 tumor suppressor gene protein in various cancers. *Int J Cancer* 58: 480–487.

44. Schlichtholz B, Tredaniel J, Lubin R, Zalcman G, Hirsch A, Soussi T (1994) Analyses of p53 antibodies in sera of patients with lung carcinoma define immunodominant regions in the p53 protein. *Br J Cancer* 69: 809–816.

45. Lubin R, Schlichtholz B, Bengoufa D, Zalcman G, Tredaniel J, Hirsch A, Caron de Fromentel C, Preudhomme C, Fenaux P, Fournier G, et al. (1993) Analysis of p53 antibodies in patients with various cancers define B-cell epitopes of human p53 – distribution on primary structure and exposure on protein surface. *Cancer Res* 53: 5872–5876.

46. Labrecque S, Naor N, Thomson D, Matlashewski G (1993) Analysis of the anti-p53 antibody response in cancer patients. *Cancer Res* 53: 3468–3471.

47. Legros Y, Lafon C, Soussi T (1994) Linear antigenic sites defined by the B-cell response to human p53 are localized predominantly in the amino and carboxy-termini of the protein. *Oncogene* 9: 2071–2076.

48. Lubin R, Zalcman G, Bouchet L, Trédaniel J, Legros Y, Cazals D, Hirsh A, Soussi T, (1995) Serum p53 antibodies as early markers of lung cancer. *Nature Med* 1: 701–702.

49. Trivers GE, De Benedetti VMG, Cawley HL, Caron G, Harrington AM, Bennet WP, Jett JR, Colby TV, Tazelaar H, Pairolero P, et al. (1996) Anti-p53 antibodies in sera from patients with chronic obstructive pulmonary disease can predate a diagnosis of cancer. *Clin Cancer Res* 2: 1767–1775.
50. Trivers GE, Cawley HL, Debenedetti VMG, Hollstein M, Marion MJ, Bennett WP, Hoover ML, Prives CC, Tamburro CC, Harris CC (1995) Anti-p53 antibodies in sera of workers occupationally exposed to vinyl chloride. *J Natl Cancer Inst* 87: 1400–1407.
51. Moll UM, Riou G, Levine AJ (1992) Two distinct mechanisms alter p53 in breast cancer – mutation and nuclear exclusion. *Proc Natl Acad Sci USA* 89: 7262–7266.
52. Rusch V, Klimstra D, Venkatraman E, Oliver J, Martini N, Gralla R, Kris M, Dmitrovsky E (1995) Aberrant p53 expression predicts clinical resistance to cisplatin-based chemotherapy in locally advanced non-small cell lung cancer. *Cancer Res* 55: 5038–5042.
53. Tsai CM, Chang KT, Wu LH, Chen JY, Gazdar AF, Mitsudomi T, Chen MH, Perngperng R (1996) Correlations between intrinsic chemoresistance and HER-2/neu gene expression, p53 gene mutations, and cell proliferation characteristics in non-small cell lung cancer cell lines. *Cancer Res* 56: 206–209.
54. Soussi T (1996) The p53 tumour suppressor gene: a model for molecular epidemiology of human cancer. *Mol Med Today* 2: 32–37.
55. Hainaut P, Soussi T, Shomer B, Hollstein M, Greenblatt M, Hovig E, Harris CC, Montesano R (1997) Database of p53 gene somatic mutations in human tumors and cell lines: Updated compilation and future prospects. *Nucleic Acids Res* 25: 151–157.

Clinical and Biological Basis of Lung Cancer Prevention
ed. by Y. Martinet, F. R. Hirsch, N. Martinet, J.-M. Vignaud
and J. L. Mulshine
© 1998 Birkhäuser Verlag Basel/Switzerland

CHAPTER 20
Endoscopic Localization of Preneoplastic Lung Lesions

Stephen Lam and Calum E. MacAulay

Cancer Imaging Department, British Columbia Cancer Agency and the University of British Columbia, Vancouver, B.C., Canada

1 Introduction
2 Pathogenesis of Lung Cancer
3 Morphometric Studies of Bronchial Biopsies
4 Fluorescence Bronchoscopy for Localization of Early Lung Cancer
5 Application of Fluorescence Bronchoscopy in Chemoprevention Studies
6 Summary
References

1. Introduction

Lung cancer is the most common cause of cancer death in North America. It is estimated that there will be approximately 200,000 new cases of lung cancer in Canada and the United States in 1996. The mortality rate has remained relatively unchanged over the last two decades and more than 85% of the patients with lung cancer will die of their disease. The lack of progress is due to the absence of an effective early diagnostic test and the unavailability of curative therapies for advanced disease. Although elimination of tobacco smoking is the best public health measure to reduce lung cancer incidence and mortality, longterm smokers who stop smoking retain a very high probability of developing lung cancer [1]. Thus, even if the target goal of the National Cancer Institute to reduce the fraction of smokers to 15% is reached by the year 2000, lung cancer incidence will continue to rise well into the next century. Therefore, the problem must be attacked on two fronts. We must deal with the population already at risk in addition to stopping the inflow of new people into the reservoir.

Currently, less than 15% of patients with invasive lung cancer can be cured of their disease. On the other hand, the potential for cure is over 90% for patients with early lung cancer discovered by sputum cytology examination [2]. In patients harboring preneoplastic lung lesions, chemopreventive agents can be used to revert or suppress the carcinogenic progression from premalignancy to fullblown malignancy [3].

There is precedence in other epithelial organs that detecting and treating pre-invasive neoplastic lesions will lead to a reduction in the incidence, and hence the mortality, of invasive cancer. An example is the well-established effectiveness of the cervical cytology screening program coupled with treatment of pre-invasive lesions with cryotherapy or carbon dioxide laser [4]. Recently, the National Polyp Study in the US also suggests that removal of colonic polyps may lead to a reduction of invasive colon cancer [5]. The success in these tumor sites offers hope that a similar strategy may also lead to a reduction in lung cancer mortality. The challenge for the implementation of such a strategy has been how to detect and localize pre-invasive lung lesions among individuals at risk of developing lung cancer.

2. Pathogenesis of Lung Cancer

In humans, lung cancer occurs after a prolonged latent period, encompassing several decades, during which the normal respiratory epithelium undergoes cellular alterations, consisting of squamous metaplasia with development of atypical changes, becoming gradually more severe with time and ultimately progressing to carcinoma in situ (CIS) and to invasive carcinoma [6–8]. The same steps have been extensively described in the uterine cervix, oral mucosa, colon [9] and to some degree in other anatomic sites. Similar modifications of the bronchial epithelium have been documented experimentally [10, 11]. The apparent reversibility of preneoplastic lesions [12, 13] and the long duration of the pre-invasive phase [14] has led to the prevailing conclusion that these lesions are benign and that there is no justification to detect or treat them. However, this dogma is based on scanty data on the natural history of pre-invasive lesions and lack of objective classification. When we consider that even with imperfect cytopathopathogical classification, 40 to 75% of individuals with severe atypia and approximately 10% of those with moderate atypia in their sputum samples will develop invasive lung cancer on followup [12, 13], it would be prudent to treat these lesions since the invasive phase of lung cancer is very short and the chance of survival is less than 15%.

3. Morphometric Studies of Bronchial Biopsies

Significant variation exists among pathologists in their interpretation of atypia/preneoplasia. A more reliable, consistent and quantitatively objective characterization of the pathology of bronchial preneoplasia is obviously required. There have been several attempts to produce accurate and reproducible grading systems using quantitative features. Most have focused on the quantitative grading of carcinoma or higher grade lesions. Extension of these studies to preinvasive lesions has been limited by the unavailability of specimens. Fluorescence bronchoscopy (discussed in the following section) allows harvesting of a large number of these lesions both from patients with lung cancer and from individuals who are at risk of developing lung cancer.

To illustrate this approach, high risk subjects (smokers or former smokers with a smoking history of 25 pack-years or more), over 45 years old, were selected for fluorescence bronchoscopy as part of an investigative trial using the LIFE system. The investigation consisted of a conventional white light bronchoscopy followed by fluorescence bronchoscopy. All areas suspicious for dysplasia or cancer under either examination were biopsied. The biopsies were fixed in formalin and embedded in paraffin blocks. Serial 5 μm sections were obtained. Sections numbered one and six were stained with haematoxylin and eosin (H and E) and cover-slipped. All H and E stained biopsy sections were systematically reviewed by at least two pathologists and all biopsies classified into one of nine groups; normal, metaplasia, hyperplasia, mild dysplasia, moderate dysplasia, severe dysplasia, CIS, microinvasive, and invasive carcinoma.

For this study, 206 bronchial biopsies were analysed. There were 23 normal biopsies, 4 with squamous metaplasia, 12 with hyperplasia, 43 with mild dysplasia, 48 with moderate dysplasia, 24 with severe dysplasia, 24 with CIS, 7 microinvasive, and 21 invasive cancers. For each biopsy a field covering the noted area of abnormality was imaged and the non-overlapping visually complete cells were imaged. For each of these cells, ~120 features were calculated describing the shape, size and DNA distribution in the nuclei. These features were then used to separate normal cells from those which exhibited the characteristics of cancer cells.

All the cells in the normal and invasive cancer biopsies which were outside the normal limits (mean IOD + 1.5 standard deviation and mean area + 1.5 standard deviation) were used to generate a discriminant function to differentiate between normal and cancer cells. Thus for each biopsy we could calculate the number of cells measured within normal limits and the number of cells classified by the discriminant function as cancer-like cells. These two numbers were used to calculate a morphometric index for each biopsy. This morphometric index was the number of cancer-like nuclei detected divided by the number of cancer-like nuclei and the number of nuclei within normal limits.

Figure 1 shows the distribution of the morphometric index across the nine pathological groups. The box represents the 25th to 75th percentile limits for each group, and the solid square boxes represent the mean morphometric index value for each group. The shaded area represents the central 50% pathway of the morphometric index as it progresses from normal through to invasive cancer. These studies demonstrate that the change in morphometric index is gradual until the stage of CIS, when there is a considerable rise in the index. Minimally invasive cancer and invasive cancer are accompanied by a further rise in the index. An objective classification system such as this may provide a more accurate basis in the decision-making process regarding intervention.

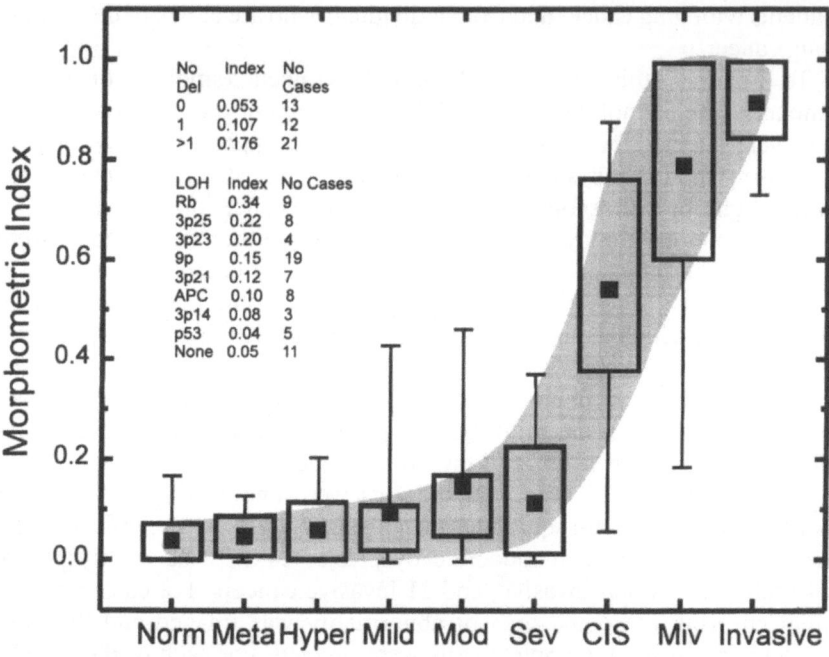

Figure 1. Relationship between histopathology and the morphometric index. The squares represent the mean values, the boxes represent the 25 to 75% confidence levels, and the bars the 95% confidence levels. Values for normal epithelium (norm), metaplasia (met), hyperplasia (hyp), mild, moderate (mod) and severe (sev) dysplasia, CIS, microinvasive (miv) and invasive (invas) cancer are illustrated.

4. Fluorescence Bronchoscopy for Localization of Early Lung Cancer

The flexible fiberoptic bronchoscope is extremely valuable for the diagnosis of lung cancer. Despite the advances and refinements in the technology of fiberoptics, localization of small radiologically occult lung cancers can be difficult using conventional white light examination. Only 30 to 40% of CIS are visible to an experienced endoscopist. To improve the detection rate, a device was developed at the British Columbia Research Centre based on the observation that when the bronchial surface is illuminated by a blue light (405 nm−442 nm) such as light from a krypton ion laser or a helium-cadmium laser, there is a progressive reduction in the fluorescence intensity as the tissue becomes more abnormal, especially in the green wavelength band of the autofluorescence spectrum [15]. The marked reduction in fluorescence intensity (up to 10-fold decrease in the green and about 5-fold in the red) in precancerous and cancerous tissue is thought to be due to a combination of an increase in the thickness of the bronchial epithelium, a very slight increase in blood content in the area of the sub-

Table 1. Localization of preneoplastic bronchial lesions by white-light and fluorescence bronchoscopy using the LIFE device

	White light	Fluorescence
Detection rate*	36% (25–42)	80% (67–96)
False positives*	17% (8–39)	28% (13–44)

* The mean value and range in ( ) are from several studies summarized in [18] and from unpublished data in the multicenter LIFE clinical trial in North America.

Table 2. Correlation between fluorescence bronchoscopy findings of "false-positive" lesions and LOH

	Number of sites of LOH		
	None	One	Two or more
Number of biopsies	66	24	33
Fluorescence positive	24	8	21
Fluorescence negative	42	16	12

mucosa of the lesion and a loss of fluorophore concentration or fluorescence quantum yield [16, 17]. Clinical experience worldwide involving over 600 patients showed that with this device, pre-invasive lesions (moderate/severe dysplasia or CIS) can be detected at more than twice the frequency of white light bronchoscopy ([18] and unpublished data) (Table 1). The specificity of fluorescence bronchoscopy appears to be lower. Some of the "false positive" biopsies were due to inexperience in interpretation of the image appearance, inflammation and trauma to the bronchial mucosa by the bronchoscope. However, correlation of "false positive" lesions (that is, lesions that were found to be normal), hyperplasia, metaplasia or mild dysplasia on biopsy with molecular studies of loss of heterozygosity (LOH) at one of five regions commonly deleted in lung cancers (3p, 5q, 9p, *Rb*, *p53*) indicates that at least half of the "false positives" represent lesions at the molecular level (Table 2) (Gazdar et al., unpublished data). The availability of fluorescence bronchoscopy allows *in vivo* sampling of these preinvasive lesions both for cross-sectional and for longitudinal studies to further our understanding of the pathogenesis of lung cancer [19].

5. Application of Fluorescence Bronchoscopy in Chemoprevention Studies

The areas of the bronchial tree accessible to the fiberoptic bronchoscope have been carefully named. Using this nomenclature and by reviewing

Table 3. Reversal of bronchial dysplasia in smokers by sialor treatment

Outcome 6 Months After Sialor	Number of Biopsies at Enrolment		
	Mild Dysplasia (N = 7)	Moderate Dysplasia (N = 5)	Severe Dysplasia (N = 2)
Regression	3	3	2
Stable	4	2	0
Progression	0	0	0
New lesions	0	0	0

digital images captured by the LIFE device, the same area can be revisited and precisely biopsied in subsequent examinations. Thus, the outcome of preneoplastic lesions with or without chemopreventive intervention can be studied on a lesion by lesion basis using this method. The biopsy material also provides a very valuable resource to study the effect of various chemopreventive agents. We have demonstrated the feasibility of this approach in a pilot study using Sialor (anetholtrithione). The study involved five women and five men with a mean age of 65 years (range 47–77 years). Five were current smokers and five were former smokers. The medication was well tolerated by the patients except one who had persistent diarrhea despite reducing the dose of the medication from 25 mg three times daily by mouth to twice and then once a day. This diarrhea resolved after the medication was stopped. Fluorescence bronchoscopy and precise rebiopsy of all areas found to have bronchial dysplasia were performed after 6 months of sialor (25 mg tid orally) in the remaining nine subjects. The results are summarized in Table 3. Fifty-seven percent of the dysplastic lesions regressed by two grades or more (e.g. moderate dysplasia to metaplasia). The remaining 43 % remained stable. There was no progression of any of the lesions. In addition, there were no new dysplastic lesions observed.

6. Summary

Fluorescence bronchoscopy using differences in autofluorescence between normal and preneoplastic tissues has been found to be useful in the localization of preneoplastic lung lesions. The ability to sample a large number of these lesions *in vivo* provides the material to establish a more precise classification of preneoplastic lesions using computer-assisted image analysis and molecular biomarker studies of the tissue sections from the biopsies which in turn will aid our decision-making process regarding intervention. As a research method, it offers the possibility of studying the pathogenesis of lung cancer and the effect of chemopreventive treatment.

Acknowledgements

The LIFE device for the study was provided by Xillix Technologies Corp., Vancouver, B.C., Canada. The study is supported in part by NIH-NCI-CN-45597-63 and the Medical Research Council of Canada.

References

1. Halpern M, Gillespie B, Warner K (1993) Patterns of absolute risk of lung cancer mortality in former smokers. *J Natl Cancer Inst* 85: 457–464.
2 Cortese DA, Pairolero PC, Bergstral H, et al. (1983) Roentgenographically occult lung cancer: A ten year experience. *J Thorac Cardiovasc Surg* 86: 373–380.
3. Greenwald P, Kelloff G, Burch-Whitman C, Kramer BS (1995) Chemoprevention. *CA Cancer J Clin* 45: 31–49.
4. Anderson GH, Boyes DA, Benedet JL, Le Riche JP, Matisie JP, Suen KC, Worth AJ, Millner A, Bennett OM, et al. (1988) Organization and results of the cervical cytology screening program in British Columbia, 1955–85. *Br Med J* 296: 975–978.
5. Winawer SJ, Zauber AG, Ho MN, O'Brien MJ, Gottlieb LS, Sternberg SS, Waye JD, et al. (1993) Prevention of colorectal cancer by colonoscopic polypectomy. *N Engl J Med* 329: 1977–1981.
6. Auerbach O, Stout AP, Hammond EC, Garfinkel L (1961) Changes in the bronchial epithelium in relation to smoking and cancer of the lung. *N Engl J Med* 265: 253–267.
7. Nasiell M (1966) Metaplasia and atypical metaplasia in the bronchial epithelium: A histopathologic and cytopathologic study. *Acta Cytol* 10: 421–427.
8. Saccomanno G, Archer VE, Auerbach O, Saunders RP, Brennan LM (1974) Development of carcinoma of the lung as reflected in exfoliated cells. *Cancer* 33: 256–270.
9. Volgelstein B, Kinzler KW (1993) The multistep nature of cancer. *Trends Genet* 9: 138–141.
10. Kato H, Konaka C, Hayata Y, Ono J, Imura I, Matsushima Y (1982) Lung cancer histogenesis following *in vivo* bronchial injections of 20-methycholanthrene in dogs. *Recent Results Cancer Res* 82: 69–86.
11. Schreiber H, Saccomanno G, Martin DH, Brennan L (1974) Sequential cytological changes during development of respiratory tract tumors induced in hamsters by benzo(a)pyrene-ferric oxide. *Cancer Res* 34: 689–698.
12. Band P, Feldstein M, Saccomanno G (1986) Reversibility of bronchial marked atypia: implication for chemoprevention. *Cancer Detection and Treatment* 9: 157–160.
13. Frost JK, Ball WC Jr, Levin MI, Tockman MS, Erozan YS, Gupta PK, Eggleston JC, Pressman NJ, Donitham MP, Kimball AW, et al. (1986) Sputum cytology: Use and potential in monitoring the workplace environment by screening for biological effects of exposure. *J Occup Med* 28: 692–703.
14. Saccomanno G (1982) Carcinoma in-situ of the lung: its development, detection, and treatment. *Semin Res Med* 4: 156–160.
15. Hung J, Lam S, LeRiche JC, MacAulay C, Palcic B (1991) Autofluorescence of normal and malignant bronchial tissue. *Lasers Surg Med* 11: 99–105.
16 Qu J, MacAulay C, Lam S, and Palcic B (1994) Optical properties of normal and carcinoma bronchial tissue. *Applied Optics* 33(31): 7397–7405.
17. Qu J, MacAulay C, Lam S, Palcic B (1995) Laser induced fluorescence spectroscopy at endoscopy: Tissue optics; Monte Carlo modeling and in-vivo measurements. *Optical Engineering* 34: 3334–3343.
18. Lam S, Becker HD (1996) Future diagnostic procedures. *Chest Surgery Clinics N America* 6: 363–380.
19. Thiberville L, Payne P, Vielkinds J, LeRiche J, Horsman D, Nouvet G, Palcic B, Lam S (1995) Evidence of cumulative gene losses with progression of premalignant epithelial lesions to carcinoma of the bronchus. *Cancer Res* 55: 5133–5139.

Clinical and Biological Basis of Lung Cancer Prevention
ed. by Y. Martinet, F. R. Hirsch, N. Martinet, J.-M. Vignaud
and J. L. Mulshine
© 1998 Birkhäuser Verlag Basel/Switzerland

CHAPTER 21
Antigen Retrieval Improves hnRNP A2/B1 Immunohistochemical Localization in Premalignant Lesions of the Lung

Melvyn S. Tockman[1], Tatyana A. Zhukov[1], Yener S. Erozan[1],
William H. Westra[1], Jun Zhou[2] and James L. Mulshine[2]

[1] *The H. Lee Maffitt Cancer Center & Research Institute, University of South Florida, Tampa, Florida, USA*
[2] *Cell and Cancer Biology Department, Medicine Branch, Division of Clinical Sciences, National Cancer Institute, Rockville, Maryland, USA*

1. Introduction

Monoclonal antibody 703D4 recognizes a 31 kD lung cancer associated antigen (p31) expressed both in resected lung tumor and in sputum cells shed from the bronchial epithelium in advance of clinical cancer [1, 2]. Originally developed by mouse immunization using a whole non-small cell lung cancer (NSCLC) tumor-cell extract, 703D4 recognizes a protein expressed by most NSCLC as well as small cell lung cancer (SCLC) cell lines [1, 3]. Recently, the 703D4 antigen has been purified by a seven-step chromatographic procedure, guided by Western blotting [4]. Sequencing of the principal immunostaining protein identified a heterogeneous nuclear ribonucleoprotein-A2 (hnRNP-A2). A splice variant, hnRNP-B1, was identified as a minor copurifying immunoreactive protein. Table 1 presents a summary of the advances in understanding of p31 expression in pulmonary tissues.

Messenger RNA transcripts of protein-coding genes are termed heterogeneous nuclear RNAs (hnRNAs), a term which describes their size heterogeneity and cellular location [9]. While in the nucleus, the hnRNA

Table 1. Chronology of 703D4 early detection development

1983	Antibody created	[3]
1985	Double-bridged ABC staining method	[5]
1988	703D4 validated as early detection marker in sputum/tumor archive	[1]
1993	Dual wavelength image cytometry	[6]
1994	LCEDWG prospective trial description	[7]
1996	Epitope characterized as hnRNP A2/B1	[4]
1996	Peripheral airway field mapping	[2]
1996	Clinical trials advance report	[8]

transcripts associate with binding proteins (hnRNPs) which facilitate hnRNA processing into mRNAs, and accompany their transport into the cytoplasm. Neither the cytoplasmic localization nor function of the hnRNPs is well understood.

Immunohistochemical mapping of hnRNP A2/B1 upregulation in resected formalin-fixed, paraffin-embedded tumor and adjacent normal lung cells has helped to understand the distribution and intensity of p31 expression in three lung compartments (bronchi, bronchioli, and alveoli) [2]. Recently, we have used heat-induced epitope retrieval prior to immunostaining to provide a clearer impression of hnRNP A2/B1 localization in resected lung tumors with adjacent, uninvolved lung.

2. Methods

2.1. Tissues

Formalin-fixed, paraffin-embedded sections from nine resected NSCLC from nine patients, sections of one SCLC and sections of one adenocarcinoma of the colon metastatic to the lung were obtained from the Surgical Pathology files of the Johns Hopkins Hospital. After pathologists reviewed hematoxylin and eosin stained sections (YSE, WHW), the tumors were diagnosed according to the WHO classification [10]. For each specimen, a representative immunostained section was chosen to record the hnRNP expression in tumor and three compartments (bronchi, bronchioli, alveoli) of the adjacent, uninvolved lung.

2.2. Immunohistochemistry

We optimized vendor protocols for hnRNP immunostaining with an automated, capillary-gap immunostaining machine, mildly acidic steam heat-induced epitope retrieval and staining reagents (HIER, Biotek Solutions/Ventana Medical Systems, Tucson, AZ). Following protocol optimization in our laboratory (TAZ), staining of histological sections was performed by the Clinical Immunopathology Laboratory of the Johns Hopkins Hospital. A single lot of monoclonal antibody to hnRNP (designated 703D4) had been purified from mouse ascites using a Protein A column and discontinuous glycine NaCl/citrate gradient (Pierce, Rockford, IL) [3] and was applied (10 µg/ml) to tissue sections. Overnight incubation at room temperature detected hnRNP upregulation in 4 µm formalin-fixed, paraffin-embedded tissue sections with minimal background staining. For simultaneously processed negative control sections, the primary antibody was replaced by Biotek dilution buffer. Immunostaining was considered positive or negative by comparison to background stromal staining on the same slide.

3. Preliminary Results

3.1. hnRNP Expression in SCLC and NSCLC

The simplified HIER technique maps weak hnRNP A2/B1 upregulation to all four major primary lung cancer cell types (epidermoid, adenocarcinoma, undifferentiated large cell as well as undifferentiated small cell lung cancer) in seven (70%) of ten primary cancers (Table 1; Figures 1a, 2a, 3a and 4a). We observed both focal (detected in solitary cells or small groups of tumor cells) and diffuse (≥ 50% of tumor cells positive) staining. Most often, both SCLC and NSCLC expressed weakly homogeneous cytoplasmic staining with an intensity equivalent to background. Occasional tumors demonstrating intraluminal vascular and lymphatic invasion were more intensely stained, possibly representing artefact. In moderately and well differentiated adenocarcinomas, intracytoplasmic mucin also showed intense, nonspecific staining.

3.2. hnRNP Expression in Non-neoplastic Lung

3.2.1. Bronchioli: Intensely staining perinuclear granules were found in the nuclear organizing region of bronchiolar ciliated cells in the uninvolved regions of SCLC and in five of nine NSCLC cases (Table 2; Figures 1b, 2b, 3b and 4b). This perinuclear, cytoplasmic granular staining of ciliated cells often accompanied basal cell proliferation. In the absence of basal cell proliferation, epithelial staining was usually either absent or weakly homogeneous throughout the cytoplasm. Nonspecifically stained intracellular mucus accompanied goblet cell hyperplasia. No perinuclear staining was seen in the bronchioles of the metastatic adenocarcinoma.

3.2.2. Alveoli: Reactive type II pneumocytes demonstrate similar perinuclear, granular cytoplasmic staining in SCLC and five of nine NSCLC

cases (Table 2; Figures 1 c, 2 c, 3 c and 4 c). In the presence of intense mononuclear cell infiltrate or fibrosis, we observed bronchiolization of the alveoli
with intense staining of the ciliated epithelial cells. Alveolar macrophages
within the air spaces were often nonspecifically stained. No perinuclear
staining was seen in alveolar cells of the metastatic adenocarcinoma.

4. Discussion

The hnRNP antigen is well preserved and easily immunostained when
exfoliated sputum epithelial cells are fixed in 50% alcohol [1]. However,
tissue fixation in formaldehyde (10% neutral buffered formalin as methylene glycol, $CH_2[OH]_2$) leads to methylene crosslinks between protein
hydrogen atoms [11]. Progressive crosslinking and loss of antigenicity is
associated with prolonged (8 to 24 hr) formalin fixation. Yet, these methylene linkages may be dissociated, and it is possible to "unmask" antigenic
determinants [11]. Previous studies of hnRNP A2/B1 expression did not
use any antigen recovery techniques [2, 3].

The original antigen retrieval technique, described by Shi et al., relies
upon high temperature heating of tissue sections in a microwave oven with
metal ion buffers [12]. Poor results with this technique in our laboratory
may be due to the introduction of morphological and antigenic artefacts
which have been associated with heating tissue sections to over 100 °C
[11]. We achieved excellent antigen retrieval using the proprietary Biotek
citrate buffer – steamer technique which heats, but does not boil the tissue
sections. Nevertheless, we observed areas of unsatisfactory staining within
sections possibly due to nonuniformity of formalin fixation, antigen retrieval
or stain distribution. Examples of hnRNP A2/B1 immunostained sections
from all four major lung cancer cell types is shown in Figures 1–4.

Observed with both NSCLC and SCLC, but not adenocarcinoma metastatic to the lung, perinuclear hnRNP A2/B1 staining often associated with
basal cell hyperplasia may indicate proliferative lung epithelium. Biamonti
et al. have reported that expression of hnRNP A1 mRNA, the product of a
closely related but distinct gene, is subject to proliferation-dependent regulation in normal fibroblasts and lymphocytes but is proliferation-indepen-
dent in transformed cell lines and tumors [13].

Zhou et al. have shown that hnRNP A2/B1 mRNA is proliferation-
dependent in normal bronchial epithelial cell primary cultures, but not in
transformed cell and tumor cell lines [4]. They observed that in normal
bronchial epithelial cell primary cultures, the levels of hnRNP A2/B1
mRNA fell after the cells leave log-phase growth, while mRNA levels do
not decline significantly after transformed cells and tumor cell lines leave
log phase growth. These *in vitro* findings parallel our observations in tissue
sections, and suggest different mechanisms of hnRNP overexpression in
transformed compared to nontransformed cells.

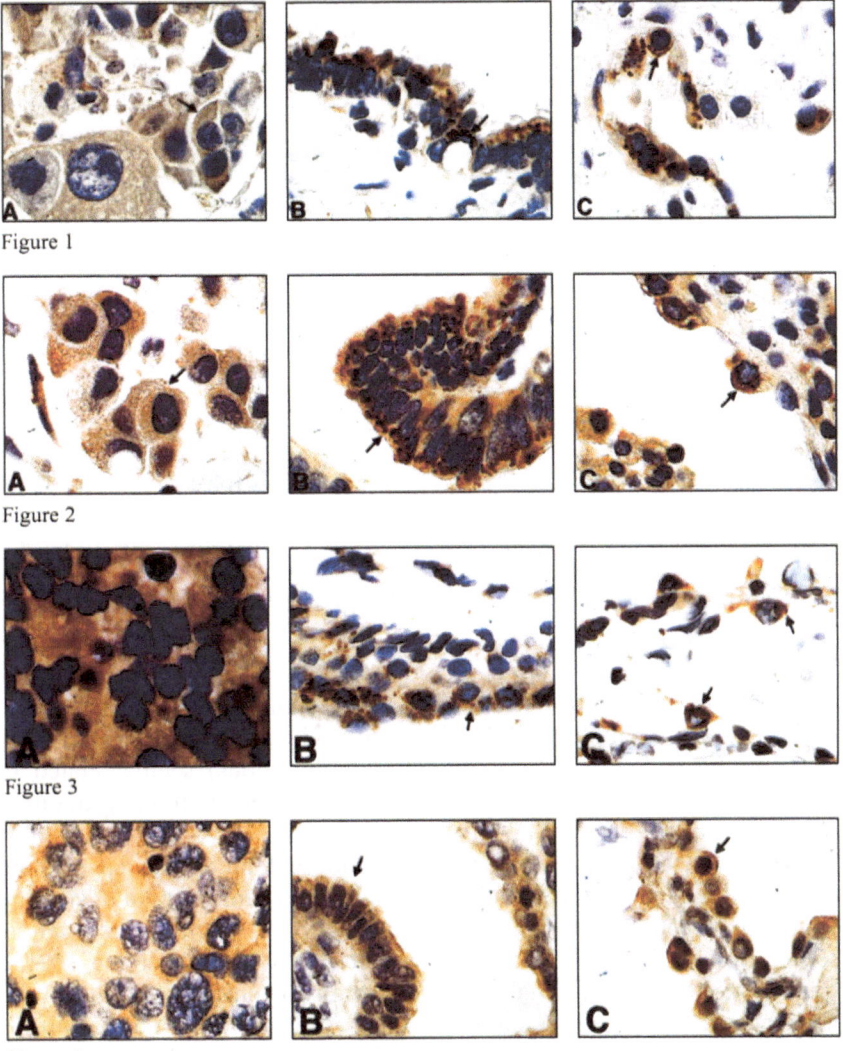

Figure 1

Figure 2

Figure 3

Figure 4

Figure 1. Adenocarcinoma of the lung, poor differentiation ($1000 \times$). A: Light, homogeneous staining in tumor section. B: Apical and perinuclear granular staining in ciliated cells of bronchiolar epithelium. C: Perinuclear granular staining in reactive alveolar type II pneumocyte.

Figure 2. Squamous cell carcinoma of the lung, poor differentiation ($1000 \times$). A: Negative staining in tumor section. B: Apical and perinuclear granular staining in ciliated cells of bronchiolar epithelium. C: Perinuclear granular staining in reactive alveolar Type II pneumocyte.

Figure 3. Large cell undifferentiated carcinoma of the lung ($1000 \times$). A: Light, homogeneous staining in tumor section. B: Light, homogeneous staining in ciliated cells of bronchiolar epithelium. C: Light, homogeneous staining in alveolar Type II pneumocytes.

Figure 4. Small cell undifferentiated carcinoma of the lung ($1000 \times$). A: Light, homogeneous staining in tumor section. B: Granular cytoplasmic staining in ciliated cells of bronchiolar epithelium. C: Granular cytoplasmic staining in reactive alveolar Type II pneumocytes.

Table 2. hnRNP immunostaining in resected tumor and adjacent lung

Homogenous or granular staining

Lung cancer			Adjacent, uninvolved lung		
Cell type	Stage	Tumor	Bronchus	Bronchiole	Alveolus
Adenocarcinoma					
Bronch-Alv	1	H	G	G	G
Bronch-Alv	1	–	H	H	H
Bronch-Alv	1	H	o	H	G
Poorly Dif	2	H	o	G	G
Mod Dif	3 a	H	–	H	H
Squamous Cell					
Poorly Dif	1	–	o	G	G
Mod Dif	1	H	G	G	G
Poorly Dif	3 a	–	G	G	G
Lg Cell Undif	1	H	H	H	H
Sm cell Undif	1	H	G	G	G
Met Colon Adeno		H	o	H	H

H = Homogenous staining; G = Granular staining; – = Negative; o = Structure not present.

The cytoplasm of most NSCLC and SCLC tumors immunostain homogeneously with an intensity comparable to background. Neither the intensity nor the staining pattern (granular/homogeneous) seems related to tumor cell type or stage (Table 2), nor to patient age or smoking duration (data not shown).

In contrast, bronchioles in uninvolved lung exhibit a granular staining pattern associated with basal cell proliferation and similar granular staining is seen in reactive alveolar Type II pneumocytes. Whether this contrast results from differential regulation associated with transformation, altered transcription or altered localization (function) of hnRNP A2/B1 in fully transformed tumor cells remains unknown. Perhaps under normal proliferative stimulation, high levels of hnRNP are associated with granular organelles (e.g. ribosomes). In transformed cells, unregulated hnRNP overexpression may lose this association with normal cellular organelles and appear homogeneously distributed in the cytoplasm.

Additional features remain to be clarified. First, the granular pattern of hnRNP immunostaining seen in formalin-fixed, paraffin-embedded bronchiolar and alveolar epithelial cells is not seen in exfoliated, alcohol-fixed sputum cells which exhibit a homogeneous, cytoplasmic staining. Comparison of immunostained tissue sections with formalin-fixed sputum specimens must be undertaken to determine whether the different staining pattern is the result of a fixative effect. It is also possible that the exfoliated cells are more fully transformed than the epithelial cells which remain.

In their experiments, Zhou et al., found uninvolved peripheral lung hnRNP immunostaining most commonly in reactive, hyperplastic type II cells [2]. This finding is particularly relevant since some pulmonary adeno-carcinomas are thought to arise from Clara cells and type II pneumocytes. Similarly, we have observed that reactive type II pneumocytes are the most frequently stained cell in the adjacent, uninvolved lung.

Zhou and colleagues describe a statistically significant increase in p31 expression in both bronchioli and alveoli of older individuals and in bronchioli of patients with the most extensive smoking exposure [2]. This contrasts with the absence of p31 immunoreactivity in histologically normal epithelium obtained from young, nonsmoking trauma victims [3]. No association of age or smoking duration is observed in the present series, although the numbers are too small to draw any relevant associations.

These observations in the uninvolved lung are consistent with a role of hnRNP in epithelial cell proliferation. Although the mechanism of hnRNP A2/B1 upregulation may differ from uninvolved lung to transformed cells, detection of overexpression of hnRNP A2/B1 may signal an early event which precedes cytomorphological change in the conducting airways. Further studies of hnRNP A2/B1 expression may benefit from improved signal: noise detection by utilization of citrate buffer-steamer antigen recovery.

References

1. Tockman MS, Gupta PK, Myers JD, Frost JK, Baylin SB, Hold E, Chase AM, Wilkinson PH, Mulshine J, et al. (1988) Sensitive and specific monoclonal antibody recognition of human lung cancer antigen on preserved sputum cells: a new approach to early lung cancer detection. *J Clin Oncol* 6: 1685–1693.
2. Zhou J, Jensen SM, Steinberg SM, Mulshine JL, Linnoila RI (1996) Expression of early lung cancer detection marker p31 in neoplastic and non-neoplastic respiratory epithelium. *Lung Cancer* 14: 85–97.
3. Mulshine JL, Cuttitta F, Bibro M, Fedorko J, Fargion S, Little C, Carney DN, Gazdar AF, Minna JD (1983) Monoclonal antibodies that distinguish non-small cell from small cell lung cancer. *J Immunol* 131: 497–502.
4. Zhou J, Mulshine JL, Unsworth EJ, Avis I, Cuttitta F, Treston A (1996) Purification and characterization of a protein that permits early detection of lung cancer. Identification of the heterogeneous nuclear ribonucleoprotein-A2/B1 as the antigen for monoclonal antibody 703D4. *J Biol Chem* 271: 10760–10766.
5. Gupta PK, Myers JD, Baylin SB, Mulshine JL, Cuttitta F, Gazdar AF (1985) Improved antigen detection in ethanol-fixed cytologic specimens. A modified avidin-biotin-peroxidase complex (ABC) method. *Diagn Cytopathol* 1: 133–136.
6. Tockman MS, Gupta PK, Pressman NJ, Mulshine JL (1993) Cytometric validation of immunocytochemical observations in developing lung cancer. *Diagn Cytopathol* 9(6): 615–622.
7. Tockman MS, Erozan YS, Gupta PK, Piantadosi S, Mulshine JL, Ruckdeschel JC, and the LCEDWG Investigators (1994) The early detection of second primary lung cancers by sputum immunostaining. *Chest* 106: 385s–390s.
8. Tockman MS, Mulshine JL, Piantadosi S, Erozan YS, Gupta PK, Ruckdeschel JC, Taylor PR, Zhukov T, Zhou WH, Qiao YL, Yao SX, for the LCEDWG Inverstigators and the YTC Investigators (1997) Prospective Detection of Preclinical Lung Cancer: Results from Two Studies of hnRNP Overexpression. *Clin Cancer Res* (in press)

9. Dreyfuss G, Matunis MJ, Pinol-Roma S, Burd CG (1993) HnRNP proteins and the bio-genesis of mRNA. *Annu Rev Biochem* 62: 289–321.
10. World Health Organization (1982) The World Health Organization histological typing of lung tumors. *Am J Clin Pathol* 77: 123–36.
11. Taylor CR, Shi SR (1994) Fixation, processing, special applications. *In:* Taylor CR, Cote RJ (eds): *Immunomicroscopy: A diagnostic tool for the surgical pathologist,* W.B. Saunders co, Philadelphia, pp 42–70.
12. Shi SR, Key ME, Kalra KL (1991) Antigen retrieval in formalin-fixed, paraffin-embedded tissues: an enhancement method for immunohistochemical staining based on microwave oven heating of tissue sections. *J Histochem Cytochem* 39: 741–748.
13. Biamonti G, Bassi MT, Cartegni L, Mechta F, Buvoli M, Cobianchi F, Riva S (1993) Human hnRNP protein A1 gene expression. Structural and functional characterization of the promoter. *J Molec Biol* 230: 77–79.

Clinical and Biological Basis of Lung Cancer Prevention
ed. by Y. Martinet, F.R. Hirsch, N. Martinet, J.-M. Vignaud
and J.L. Mulshine

CHAPTER 22
Molecular Pathological Mechanisms in NSCLC and the Assessment of Individuals with a High Risk of Developing Lung Cancer

J.K. Field[1,2], H. Ross[1,2], T. Liloglou[1,2], F. Scott[1,2], W. Prime[1,2],
J.R. Gosney[3], J. Youngson[1,2] and R.J. Donnelly[4]

[1] *Molecular Genetics and Oncology Group, Clinical Dental Sciences, The University of Liverpool, Liverpool, UK*
[2] *Roy Castle International Centre for Lung Cancer Research, Liverpool, UK*
[3] *Department of Pathology, The University of Liverpool, Liverpool, UK*
[4] *Cardiothoracic Centre, Liverpool, UK*

1. Introduction

Lung cancer is responsible for more deaths than any other cancer, accounting for 785,000 deaths per year world wide [1]. It is the most common malignancy in males the UK. The highest incidence rates of lung cancer for both men and women are found in the Merseyside region of North West England. In the Liverpool area the cumulative rate (0–74 years) in 1989–1993 was 12.5% for males and 6.0% for females compared with a national average of 7.3% for males and 3.0% for females in 1991 [2, 3]. Furthermore, the incidence rate for females is increasing faster than the national rate and has also exceeded the incidence rate for breast cancer in Liverpool. Incidence of lung cancer in males is also not declining in line with the national trend. Detection of lung cancer usually occurs late in the disease when it is beyond effective treatment, and consequently there is a high mortality rate and a five year overall survival rate of 6% in Merseyside. Increased attention for earlier detection and intervention management is therefore imperative. The Liverpool Lung Project (LLP), funded by the Roy Castle Foundation, UK, is a 10-year longitudinal study which will use risk factors identified by molecular genetics and epidemiology to define populations and individuals who are most at risk of developing lung cancer.

In conjunction with the early detection programme an intervention strategy will be developed since there is currently a need to develop a noninvasive intervention therapy appropriate to the preneoplastic stage at which the diagnosis was made.

Carcinogenesis in the lung is a multistep process involving multiple genetic changes that may include genetic instability due to DNA mismatch repair defects, activation or overexpression of oncogenes and loss or inactivation of tumour suppressor genes. Our current understanding of the molecular pathological mechanisms involved in the development of lung cancer will be discussed in this chapter, and it is from our understanding of these mechanisms that we will select the most powerful and informative molecular markers for the identification of high risk individuals in the LLP.

1.1. Loss of Heterozygosity Analysis

A range of genetic changes at the chromosomal level has been identified in lung tumour specimens and in cell lines derived from human lung tumours using allelic imbalance or loss of heterozygosity (LOH) analysis. This technique has been used primarily to identify regions on specific chromosomes that contain putative tumour suppressor genes. LOH studies on non-small cell lung cancer (NSCLC) tumours have demonstrated that certain chromosomal regions, in particular 3p, 5p, 9p and 17p, are involved in the development of these tumours [4−9]. In addition to confirming the role of a number of previously identified tumour suppressor genes, this type of analysis may reveal the existence and location of previously unknown tumour suppressor genes.

1.2. Genetic Instability in NSCLC

A number of allelotype analyses have been undertaken in lung and in head and neck cancers [10−14]. Recently an in-depth study of (NSCLC) was undertaken [9] in order to measure the degree of genetic instability in each tumour, and thus provide a useful molecular parameter with which to assess NSCLC.

1.3. p53 Tumour Suppressor Gene

Tobacco smoking is responsible for more than 80% of lung cancer [15]. Cigarette smoke contains a large number of carcinogens (including benzo(a)pyrene), which act in the initiation and/or promotion stages of carcinogenesis [16]. The majority of carcinogens are also mutagens and thus it may be possible to identify the carcinogenic exposure which gave rise to the tumour by analysing the spectrum of mutations in a gene. Recently, the similarity between the mutation spectrum of benzo(a)pyrene and the mutation spectrum in lung cancer tissue has been cited as a causative link between tobacco carcinogens and lung cancer [17].

The *p53* gene has been found to be mutated in a large range of human tumours and, as might be expected, its 53 kD nuclear phosphoprotein product has an important role in transcription, regulation of the cell cycle and DNA damage management [18–20]. Lung tumours have been shown to contain a variety of genetic changes in the *p53* gene including point mutations, insertions, deletions and LOH at the *TP53* locus. Point mutations in smokers are most commonly GC to TA transversions, which may arise from exposure to polycyclic aromatic hydrocarbons (PAH) such as benzo(a)pyrene [21–23]. However, in the Merseyside region of the UK, GC to AT transitions are the most common form of point mutations. This altered mutation spectrum may reflect exposure of this population to carcinogens in addition to those found in cigarette smoke.

1.4. ras Oncogene Family

In lung cancer, members of the *ras* oncogene family are considered to be candidate target genes. In a study of *ras* mutations in 141 adenocarcinomas from smokers, 41 tested positive for a point mutation in codon 12 for K-*ras*, whereas only two of 40 nonsmokers had a mutation at this site [24]. In the publications by Rodenhius and coworkers, most of the mutations have been found in codon 12 of K-*ras* and mainly in adenocarcinomas. In a study of *ras* mutations in 66 NSCLC, 20% were found to have K-*ras* mutations in codons 12 or 61 and *ras* mutations were more common in squamous cell carcinomas (8/38) than adenocarcinomas (3/22). The most common substitution was from glycine to valine. Several groups have found a correlation between K-*ras* point mutations and a poor clinical outcome [25–27]. Li et al. [28] have suggested that K-*ras* mutations are an early event in the development of adenocarcinomas. However, Sugio et al. [26] found few K-*ras* mutations in dysplastic lesions.

1.5. Microsatellite Alterations

Recently, another type of cancer-associated gene has been discovered, in addition to oncogenes and tumour suppressor genes. This group of genes is involved in DNA mismatch repair and its discovery arose from work on hereditary non-polyposis colorectal cancer (HNPCC). It was observed that microsatellite DNA sequences from colonic tumours were also unstable, which implies that instability was due to errors in mismatch repair [29]. Furthermore, tumour DNA had a different number of repeats than DNA from adjacent normal tissue [29]. Analysis of HNPCC-associated colon cancers showed that 86% of tumours demonstrated this phenomenon, later described as microsatellite instability (MI), compared to only 16% of sporadic colon cancer [29, 30]. Using the extensive homology between the yeast mismatch repair gene *Mut S* and its human counterpart, Fishel et al. [31] and later Leach et al. [32] cloned *hMSH2*, the first human mismatch repair gene. Bronner et al. [33] and later Papodopoulos et al. [34] identified *hMLH1*, the *Mut L* homologue and localised it to 3p21. Many tumours with microsatellite instability do not contain mutations within these genes, which would suggest that there are other as yet unidentified mismatch repair genes.

1.6. hnRNP Overexpression

HnRNP A2/B1 is a 31 kd protein which has been characterised as homologous to the pre-mRNA binding heterogeneous nuclear ribonuclear protein [35]. These RNA binding proteins are responsible for the post-transcriptional regulation of gene expression by capping, splicing, polyadenylation and cytoplasmic transport of mRNAs [36].

A particularly informative lung cancer screening trial was undertaken by Tockman et al. [37, 38]. Sputum samples underwent immunohistochemical analysis using an antibody to the p31 kD protein antigen of NSCLC. Immunostained specimens from patients with known clinical outcomes was 90% accurate in predicting those that would develop lung cancer. The earliest epitope expression was detected among serial specimens that were collected approximately two years before the clinical appearance of the disease. These results have been replicated in exfoliated sputum specimens from Chinese tin miners who subsequently developed lung cancer (Tockman et al., unpublished data).

1.7 Analysis of Peptide Growth Factors and Peptide Amidating Enzymes (PAM)

Peptide amidating enzyme (PAM) activity is involved in the production of a range of biologically active amidated peptides. PAM activity has been measured in lung cancer cell lines of all histologies [39] and was found to be at highest levels in small cell lung cancer cell lines. The presence of PAM in premalignant lesions adjacent to lung tumours has also been demonstrated by immunohistochemical techniques [40]. PAM activity is therefore of potential use as an indicator for the presence of malignant cells, and also as an indicator of the extent of differentiation in lung epithelium. PAM activity has been detected in bronchial lavage fluid from patients at risk of a second primary [41].

2. *Ras* Mutations in Lung Cancer

We have recently investigated mutations of the K-*ras* gene in bronchial carcinomas using a PCR-RFLP detection system and a PCR based ARMS assay (Amplification Refractory Mutation System) [42]. The ARMS assay allows the specific detection of rare mutant sequences against a background of normal DNA (i.e. 1 in 1000–2000). ARMS employs the powerful discriminatory potential of PCR amplification from primers modified at the 3' end such that extension from nonmatched templates is essentially eliminated under appropriate conditions. ARMS analysis can be used for K-*ras* mutation detection and, since the relevant mutation spectrum is limited, the procedure requires either a general PCR multiplex for 'broad' K-*ras* mutations, or relatively few single tests to pinpoint exactly which mutation may be present. We have detected mutations in 25% of our current database of adenocarcinomas using both PCR-RFLP and the ARMS assay and although both techniques detected mutations in the same group of tumours, the ARMS assay specified the actual K-*ras* 12 mutations [43]. Other K-*ras* mutation assays under development such as the PCR/ligase chain reaction assay [44] have the advantage of potential multiplex assay of multiple base changes in a single codon. However, adaptation of these assays to a nonradioactive format is needed to be economically competitive with the ARMS assay.

3. *p53* Gene Alterations in Lung Cancer

p53 gene activation by mutation or allelic loss has been implicated in the development of lung cancer [21]. In our recent study of the *p53* mutational profile of patients with NSCLC on Merseyside, 28% of tumours contained mutations in the *p53* gene [45]. This is significantly lower ($p < 0.0002$) than the mutation frequency of 56% in the *p53* gene of lung cancer patients, recently reported in a major review [18]. However, Suzuki et al. [46] reported a mutation frequency of 47% in 30 NSCLC, which is statistically not significantly different from the Merseyside study ($p = 0.82$).

On analysing the *p53* mutation profile in these NSCLC specimens, more than half the base substitutions were found to occur at guanine residues. However, in contrast to previous reports, in which GC to TA transversions were the most common mutations, there is a prevalence of GC to AT transitions (37.5% of all mutations). In our study GC to TA transversions accounted for only 12.5% of all mutations. A comparison of the GC to TA: GC to AT ratio in this study and in the Greenblatt review [21] found a statistically significant difference (p = 0.04). Findings similar to our own have been reported in NSCLC patients from Taiwan where GC to TA transversions comprised only 6% of all *p53* mutations [47].

Strikingly, in our study, all four C to T and one out of three G to A mutations (5/7 GC to AT in total) occur at non-CpG dinucleotides (in this case, in CpC/GpG dinucleotides). CpG sites can account for mutations due to spontaneous deamination of 5-me-cytosine residues but the reason for the occurrence of GC to AT transitions at non-CpG sites is unclear. Currently, little is known about methylation at non-CpG sites in mammalian cells [48]. It is uncertain whether GC to AT transitions at non-CpG sites represent induced or spontaneous mutations [49].

It is hoped that differences in mutation spectra arising from the differing chemical selectivities of carcinogens may ultimately provide clues as to the cause of lung cancer "hotspots".

3.1. WAF1/CIP1 Gene

The human *WAF1/CIP1* gene was simultaneously identified by a number of research groups as a mediator of p53, a cyclin-dependent kinase (CDK) interacting protein and inhibitor of CDKs [50–54]. p21^{wafl} binds and inhibits cyclin/CDK complexes causing G1 arrest but it does not seem to participate directly in apoptosis [55]. p21^{wafl} expression is induced by wild-type p53 and by p53-independent signals such as TGFβ [56] and the gene's promoter region contains response elements for p53 [50, 57] as well as TGFβ, Sp-1 and Sp-3 [58]. Liloglou et al. [59] analysed the part of the promoter region that contains the p53 binding sites (nucleotides −1280 to −2230) for mutations in 50 matched normaltumour cases of lung carcinomas and 11 individuals with no history of cancer. The results showed no mutations in any of the three p53 binding sites, but two polymorphic sites were found, one at nucleotide −2203 and the second including nucleotides −1463, −1526, −1533 and −1594. These results, together with previously reported polymorphisms in the coding or noncoding regions of *WAF1/CIP1*, suggest that the *WAF1/CIP1* gene is probably highly polymorphic.

The effect of these polymorphisms on the promoter region of the *WAF1/CIP1* gene and on gene expression is still unclear. A computer-aided search indicated that these regions are potential binding sites of transcription factors, and that the polymorphism in one fragment occurs four nucleotides upstream from one of the p53 binding sites, but the significance of this is unclear. The fact that these polymorphisms were found to have the same incidence in a noncancerous population, suggests that they may not be tumour-specific.

4. Allelotype of NSCLC

We have undertaken an allelotype analysis of NSCLC and have provided evidence of genetic instability on most of the chromosome arms [9]. This finding is in agreement with the previous allelotype analysis using RFLP analysis by Tsuchiya et al. [10] and Sato et al. [11], particularly on 3p, 9p and 17p. The role of allelic imbalance on the short arms of chromosomes 3, 9, and 17 in NSCLC has received a great deal of attention and it has been proposed that these events are associated with the early stages of pathogenesis of these tumours [4–8]. Hibi et al. [60] described three distinct regions involved in lung cancer on 3p at 3p25, 3p21.3 and 3p14-cen. and other researchers have shown that these regions are frequently lost in lung tumours. The recently discovered gene, fragile histidine triad gene (*FHIT*) [61] located at 3p14.2, has been considered to be involved in the control of tumorigenic phenotype in a wide variety of human neoplasias including NSCLC.

LOH on chromosome 9 has been reported to be a frequent event in lung, bladder, head and neck and other tumours [62–69]. Deletion mapping has identified a critical region on 9p21 where a tumour suppressor gene (TSG) may be present [70, 63, 68, 69]. Recently, several publications have indicated other novel sites on 9p, which include 9p1-p22 [62], a site telomeric to IFNA [69], and a site distal to IFNA including the markers DS162-D9S157 [68].

A high frequency of loss on chromosome 9p21-p23 has been demonstrated in a range of lung tumours [71–73]. The cyclin-dependent kinase-4 inhibitor genes, *p15* and *p16*, whose products inhibit progression through the G_1 phase of the cell cycle, both map to 9p21. Deletions and mutations of these putative TSGs have been reported recently in NSCLC [74, 75]. However *p16* sequence analysis in other tumours with loss on chromosome 9p has demonstrated that point mutations are infrequent [64, 76]. This does not exclude *p16* as a target gene in tumourigenesis. Hayashi et al. [77] reported *p16* mutations in 30% of the Japanese NSCLC investigated. Okamoto et al. [78] however found no *p16* mutations in primary NSCLC but did find that six of 22 metastatic NSCLC contained mutations in the *p16* gene. No *p16* mutations were found in SCLC primary, metastatic tissues or in SCLC cell lines, or in *p15* or *p16* genes from primary or metastatic NSCLC or SCLC tissues. Recently *p16* inactivation has been shown to occur by promoter methylation in some human cancers. Merlo et al. [79] have shown that the 5' CpG island methylation of *p16* may be considered as an alternative pathway by which this gene is inactivated in certain tumours.

We have recently analysed NSCLC with a panel of highly polymorphic microsatellite markers on chromosome 9. Our results indicate that loss on 9p is concentrated within the D9S156–D9S161 region. In lung tumours, however, the locus with minimal loss was found at D9S157 (9p23), with 50% LOH (11/22), whereas loss at the IFNA locus was found in only 6% (2/34) of tumours [71]. Six of the lung tumours in the study which demonstrated LOH at D9S157 retained heterozygosity at the adjacent informative markers lying centromeric and telomeric to D9S157. These results indicate the presence of a further putative TSG on 9p at the D9S157 locus (9p23).

Allelic deletion on 5q of the tumour suppressor gene *APC* (5q21) has been frequently reported in NSCLC [80] and correlates with poor prognosis. In addition 5q33–35 is another region considered to contain a novel region in NSCLC [81]. A del-27 locus on chromosome 5 has been described by Wieland et al. [82;83]. This locus is found at 5p13–12, proximal to the *MCC/APC* gene and represents a new TSG site in lung cancer. Wieland et al. [82] have clearly demonstrated that del-27 is a distinct locus from the *APC* gene, as they have shown two distinct LOH regions using a range of polymorphic markers.

LOH on 17p has been reported by a number of investigators. Fong et al. [80] have shown that 17q may be equally important, with 42% LOH on 17p and 59% LOH on 17q. Their results indicated a correlation between 17q loss and late stage disease (T_3, T_4) as well as with a poor prognosis. Neville et al. [9] found LOH on 17q to be significantly lower (18%) than that found on 17p (38%) but that LOH on the 17q arm was more frequent in squamous cell carcinomas.

4.1. Accumulated Genetic Damage in NSCLC Assessed by FAL

In the allelotype analysis of 45 NSCLC, Neville et al. [9] calculated a median fractional allele loss (FAL) value of 0.09 (range 0.00–0.45). FAL is the number of chromosome arms showing LOH divided by the number of informative chromosome arms. In this analysis no correlation was found between FAL (greater than or less than the median value) with any of the clinicopathological parameters. As these patients have so far been followed for less than 18 months, no survival calculations have yet been undertaken. No correlation was found between *p53* or *ras* mutations in the NSCLC specimens we have investigated from the Merseyside region [43, 45] and their FAL values. Accumulated genetic damage, as provided by this allelotype analysis, thus provides a useful molecular parameter by which to assess NSCLC and may in time assist in the determination of the clinical behaviour and outcome of these tumours.

4.2. Distinct Genetic Populations in NSCLC

Allelic imbalance on the short arms of chromosomes 3, 9, and 17 in NSCLC has received a great deal of attention and it has been argued that these events are associated with the early stages of tumour pathogenesis [4–8]. Investigators have studied a number of dysplastic and neoplastic tissues from the same patient in great detail by performing microdissection of the specimens. All of the six paired dysplastic and tumour tissue specimens investigated by Sundaresan et al. [4] showed allelic imbalance on 3p. Similarly, Hung et al. [6] found that six of the seven patients examined with paired preneoplastic and neoplastic lesions showed loss on 3p. Kishimoto et al. [7] have also reported similar findings of LOH on 9p in the same specimens. Thiberville et al. [8] have investigated LOH with a number of microsatellite markers on 3p, 5q and 9p in 13 patients who demonstrated progressive stages of bronchial carcinoma. Their results indicate that the corresponding genetic alterations in the dysplastic samples are often also found in the invasive carcinomas of the same patients. These results raise the question of whether all NSCLC have allelic imbalance on 3p and 9p as their initiating events.

A FAL value has been calculated for each of the 45 NSCLC reported by Neville et al. [9] (median 0.09, range 0.0–0.45). The LOH data were examined on the following basis: low FAL (LFAL) (0.00–0.04), medium FAL (MFAL) (0.05–0.13) and high FAL (HFAL) (0.14–0.45) based symmetrically around the median FAL value of 0.09. Tumours with HFAL values showed a very clear polarization of the LOH data on chromosome arms 3p, 9p and 17p, such that 80% showed loss on 3p, 80% on 9p and 73% on 17p. These incidences of LOH were significantly higher than would be expected since overall genetic instability in these HFAL tumours ranged from 14% to 45% LOH. However, nine of the 14 patients in the LFAL group were found to have no LOH on 3p, 9p or 17p, but five of these had LOH at other sites: i.e. LOH on 5p, 5q, 8p, 13q, 16q and 19q. These results indicate that LFAL patients form a new subset of NSCLC tumours with distinct molecular initiating events, and may represent a discrete genetic population [84].

4.3. Microsatellite Alterations

Microsatellite instability is important in studies on lung cancer since it is believed to be a very early event in carcinogenesis. It is hypothesised that MI results from a mutation giving the cell a "mutator phenotype" [85]. Thus, there is a reduced fidelity for replication, leading to an accumulation of other mutations in the cell over time. Detection of the cells with this mutator phenotype might lead to earlier detection before mutations have arisen.

Four investigations have been undertaken for MI in NSCLC. Peltomaki et al. [86] found no instability (eight different microsatellites in 86 tumours); whereas in another analysis, [87] 34% of tumours (13 of 38) demonstrated microsatellite instability.

We have investigated 45 NSCLC with 92 polymorphic microsatellite markers and have found 42% of these samples to contain RER defects, whereas Mao et al. [88] found only 9% that contained RER defects. Only 13 of the 92 markers we used demonstrated RER defects, and when seven of these markers were selected, we still observed a 31% level of RER defects in 45 NSCLC. This represents 75% of all the RER defects seen with the 92 markers used in the allelotype analysis (Field et al. unpublished). We are currently using these seven markers to investigate RER defects in the bronchial lavage specimens for high risk individuals.

5. Liverpool Lung Project

The highest incidence of lung cancer in England and Wales is in the Mersey region, particularly among women. The purpose of the Liverpool Lung Project is to compare the timing, sensitivity and specificity of certain markers for detection of lung cancer at a reversible stage. We are proposing a ten year prospective cohort study of 7000 people to investigate specific high risk groups of patients. Individuals who have been recruited into the Liverpool Lung Project will have up to ten years follow-up with sputum sampling every 6 to 24 months. An epidemiological assessment will be undertaken of all the individuals who are recruited into this project using an interview-based questionnaire which will assess their smoking, diet, occupation, residence and family cancer history. Thus the results of this study will provide a very valuable molecular genetics and epidemiological assessment of all the high risk individuals which will form the basis of our future thinking in the field of lung cancer chemoprevention.

The challenge will be to design clinical trials for successfully evaluating intervention strategies in these high risk cohorts. The molecular/epidemiological techniques used to assess their high risk status may also be used as intermediate endpoints for chemoprevention. Chemoprevention trials should be undertaken on former smokers who are considered to be at a high risk of developing lung cancer, based on the molecular/epidemiological criteria.

New molecular pathological techniques have identified sputum specimens with evidence of progression to lung cancer well in advance of clinical malignancy. Genetic abnormalities identified in lung tumour specimens such as K-*ras* and *p53* mutations, have been associated with the patients' smoking histories. It is of particular relevance that *ras* and/or *p53* mutations and microsatellite alterations have been identified in the archived sputum of patients, one year prior to their clinical diagnosis of lung cancer. Furthermore, a monoclonal antibody (Mab) with a specificity for a heterogeneous nuclear ribonuclear protein (hnRNP, A2/B1) (703D4) has been shown to have very high sensitivity and specificity for the recognition of neoplastic antigens in sputum two years in advance of a clinical cancer [89].

In order to translate these important new molecular markers into a clinical setting, research must be carried out in a large prospective study with stringent quality control. This research will then provide an accurate risk assessment of direct relevance to the planning of future health care strategy.

References

1. Pisani P, Parkin DM, Ferlay J (1993) Estimates of the worldwide mortality from eighteen major cancers in 1985. Implications for prevention and projections of future burden. *Int J Cancer* 55: 891–903.
2. Williams EMI, Youngson J, Ashby D, Donnelly RJ (eds) (1992) *Lung Cancer Bulletin – A framework for action.* Liverpool: Merseyside and Cheshire cancer registry.
3. Registration of cancer diagnosed in 1991 England and Wales. Monitor MBI 96/1, London ONS. 1996.
4. Sundaresan V, Ganly P, Hasleton P, Rudd R, Sinha G, Bleehen NM, Rabbitts P (1992) p53 and chromosome 3 abnormalities, characteristic of malignant lung tumours, are detectable in preinvasive lesions of the bronchus. *Oncogene* 7: 1989–1997.
5. Gazdar AF, Bader S, Hung J, Kishimoto Y, Sekido Y, Sugio K, Virmani A, Fleming J, Carbone DP, Minna JD (1994) Molecular genetic changes found in human lung cancer and its precursor lesions. *Cold Spring Harb Symp Quant Biol* 59: 565–572.
6. Hung J, Kishimoto Y, Sugio K, Virmani A, McIntire DD, Minnna JD, Gazdar AF (1995) Allele-specific chromosome 3p deletions occur at an early-stage in the pathogenesis of lung carcinoma. *JAMA* 273: 558–563.
7. Kishimoto Y, Sugio K, Hung JY, Virmani AK, McIntire DD, Minna JD, Gazdar AF (1995) Allele-specific loss in chromosome 9p loci in preneoplastic lesions accompanying non-small-cell lung cancers [see comments]. *J Natl Cancer Inst* 87: 1224–1229.
8. Thiberville L, Bourguignon J, Metayer J, Bost F, Diarra-Mehrpour M, Bignon J, Lam S, Martin JP, Nouvet G (1995) Frequency and prognostic evaluation of 3p21–22 allelic losses in non-small-cell lung cancer. *Int J Cancer* 64: 371–377.
9. Neville EM, Stewart MP, Swift A, Risk JM, Liloglou T, Ross H, Gosney JR, Donnelly RJ, Field JK (1996) Allelotype of non-small cell lung cancer. *Int J Oncol* 1996; 9: 533–539.
10. Tsuchiya E, Nakamura Y, Weng SY, Nakagawa K, Tsuchiya S, Sugand H, Kitagawa T (1992) Allelotype of non-small cell carcinoma: comparison between loss of heterozygosity in squamous cell carcinoma and adenocarcinoma. *Cancer Res* 52: 2478–2481.
11. Sato S, Nakamura Y, Tsuchiya E (1994) Difference of allelotype between squamous-cell carcinoma and adenocarcinoma of the lung. *Cancer Res* 54: 5652–5655.
12. Ah-See KW, Cooke TG, Pickford IR, Soutar D, Balmain A (1994) An allelotype of squamous carcinoma of the head and neck using microsatellite markers. *Cancer Res* 54: 1617–1621.
13. Nawroz H, Vanderriet P, Hruban RH, Koch W, Ruppert JM, Sidransky D (1994) Allelotype of head and neck squamous cell carcinoma. *Cancer Res* 54: 1152–1155.
14. Field JK, Kiaris H, Risk JM, Tsiriyotis C, Adamson R, Zoumpourlis V, Rowley H, Taylor K, Whittaker J, Howard P (1995) Allelotype of squamous cell carcinoma of the head and neck: fractional allele loss correlates with survival. *Br J Cancer* 72: 1180–1188.
15. Shopland DR, Eyre, HJ and Pechacek TF (1991) Smoking-attributable cancer mortality in 1991: Is lung cancer the leading cause of death among smokers in the United States? *J Natl Cancer Inst* 83: 1142–1148.

16. DeMarini DM (1983) Genotoxicity of tobacco-smoke and tobacco-smoke condensate. *Mutation Res* 114: 59–89.
17. Denissenko MF, Pao A, Tang MS, Pfeifer GP (1996) Preferential formation of benzo[a]pyrene adducts at lung cancer mutational hotspots in p53. *Science* 274 (5286): 430–432.
18. Lane DP (1992) p53, guardian of the genome. *Nature* 358: 15–16.
19. Levine AJ, Momand J, Finlay CA (1991) The p53 tumour suppressor gene. *Nature* 351: 453–456.
20. Yin Y, Tainsky MA, Bischoff FZ, Strong LC, Wahl GM (1992) Wild-type p53 restores cell cycle control and inhibits gene amplification in cells with mutant p53 alleles. *Cell* 70: 937–948.
21. Greenblatt MS, Bennett WP, Hollstein M, Harris CC (1994) Mutations in the p53 tumor suppressor gene: clues to cancer etiology and molecular pathogenesis. *Cancer Res* 54: 4855–4878.
22. Husgafvel-Pursiainen K, Ridanpaa M, Anttila S, Vainio H (1995) p53 and ras gene mutations in lung cancer: implications for smoking and occupational exposures. *J Occup Environ Med* 37: 69–76.
23. Ramet M, Castren K, Jarvinsen K, Pekkala K, Turpeenniemi-Hujanen T, Soini Y, Paakko P, Vahakangas K (1995) p53 protein expression correlated with benzoapyrene-DNA adducts in carcinoma cell lines. *Carcinogenesis* 16: 2117–2124.
24. Rodenhuis S, Slebos RJC (1992) Clinical significance of *ras* oncogene activation in human lung cancer. *Cancer Res* 52: 2665s–2669s.
25. Slebos RJC, Kibbelaar RE, Dalesio O, Kooistra A, Stam J, Meijer CJLM, Wagenaar SS, Vanderschueren RGJRA, Van Zandwijk N, Moot WJ (1990) K-Ras oncogene activation as a prognostic marker in adenocarcinoma of the lung. *N Eng J Med* 323: 561–565.
26. Sugio K, Inoue T, Inoue K, Yaita H, Inuzuka S, Ishida T, Sugimachi K (1993) Different site mutation of the K-ras gene in a patient with metachronous double lung cancers. *Anticancer Res* 13: 2469–2471.
27. Rosell R, Li S, Skacel Z, Mate JL, Maestre J, Canela M, Tolosa E, Armengol P, Barnadas A, Ariza A (1993) Prognostic impact of mutated K-ras gene in surgically resected non-small cell lung cancer patients. *Oncogene* 8: 2407–2412.
28. Li EE, Heflich RH, Bucci TJ, Manjanatha MG, Blaydes BS, Delclos KB (1994) Relationships of DNA adduct formation, K-ras activating mutations and tumorigenic activities of 6-nitrochrysene and its metabolites in the lungs of CD-1 mice. *Carcinogenesis* 15: 1377–1385.
29. Aaltonen LA, Peltomaki P, Leach FS, Sistonen P, Pylkkanen L, Mecklin J-P, Jarvinen H, Powell SM, Jen J, Hamilton SR (1993) Clues to the pathogenesis of familial colorectal cancer. *Science* 260: 812–816.
30. Aaltonen LA, Peltomaki P, Mecklin J-P, Jarvinen H, Jass JR, Green JS, et al. (1994) Replication errors in benign and malignant tumours from hereditary nonpolyposis colorectal cancer patients. *Cancer Res* 54: 1645–1648.
31. Fishel R, Lescoe MK, Rao MRS, Copeland NG, Jenkins NA, Garber J, Kane M, Kolodner R (1993) The human mutator gene homolog MSH2 and its association with hereditary nonpolyposis colon cancer. *Cell* 75: 1027–1038.
32. Leach FS, Nicolaides NC, Papadopoulos N, Liu B, Jen J, Parsons R, Peltomaki P, Sistonen P, Aaltonen LA, Nystom-Lahti M (1993) Mutations of a Mut S homolog in HNPCC. *Cell* 75: 1215–1225.
33. Bronner CE, Baker SM, Morrison PT, Warren G, Smith LG, Lescoe MK, Kane M, Earabino C, Lipford J, Lindblom A (1994) Mutation in the DNA mismatch repair gene homlogue hMLH1 is associated with hereditary non-polyposis colon cancer. *Nature* 368: 258–261.
34. Papadopoulos N, Nicolaides NC, Wei Y-F, Ruben SM, Carter KC, Rosen CA, Haseltine WA, Fleischmann RD, Fraser CM, Adams MD (1994) Mutation of a MutL homolog in hereditary colon cancer. *Science* 263: 1625–1629.
35. Zhou JN, Linder S (1996) Expression of CDK inhibitor genes in immortalized and carcinoma derived breast cell lines. *Anticancer Res* 16: 1931–1935.
36. Burd CG, Dreyfuss G (1994) Conserved structures and diversity of functions of RNA-binding proteins. *Science* 265: 615–621.
37. Tockman MS, Prabodh KG, Pressman NJ, Mulshine JL (1992) Considerations in bringing a cancer biomarker to clinical application. *Cancer Res* 52: 2711–2718.

38. Tockman MS, Erozan YS, Prabodh KG, Piantadosi S, Mulshine JL, Ruckdeschel JC (1994) The early detection of second primary lung cancers by sputum immunostaining. *Chest* 106: 385–390.

39. Treston AM, Scott FM, Vos M, Iwai N, Mains RE, Eipper BA, Cuttitta F, Mulshine JL (1993) Biochemical characterization of peptide a-amidating enzyme activities of human neuroendocrine lung cancer cell lines. *Cell Growth Diff* 4: 911–920.

40. Saldise L, Martinez A, Montuenga LM, Treston A, Springall DR, Polak JM, Vazquez JJ (1996) Distribution of peptidyl-glycine alpha-amidating mono-oxygenase (PAM) enzymes in normal human lung and in lung epithelial tumors. *J Histochem Cytochem* 44: 3–12.

41. Scott FM, Treston AM, Shaw GL, Avis I, Sorenson J, Kelly K, Dempsey E, Cantor AB, Tockman M, Mulshine JL (1996) Peptide amidating activity in human bronchoalveolar lavage fluid. *Lung Cancer* 14: 230–251.

42. Newton CR, Graham A, Heptinstall LE, Powell SJ, Summers C, Kalsheker N, Smith JC, Markham AF (1989) Analysis of any point mutation in DNA- the amplification refractory mutation system (ARMS). *Nucl Acids Res* 17: 2503–2516.

43. Neville EM, Ellison G, Kiaris H, Stewart MP, Spandidos DA, Fox JC, Field JK (1995) Detection of K-ras mutations in non-small cell lung carcinoma. *Int J Oncol* 7: 511–514.

44. Lehman TA, Scott F, Seddon M, Kelly K, Dempsy EC, Wilson VL, Mulshine JL, Modali R. Detaction of K-ras oncogene mutations by polymerase chain reaction-based ligase chain reaction. *Analyt Biochem.* In press.

45. Liloglou, T, Ross, H, Prime, W, Donnelly, RJ, Spandidos, DA, Gosney, JR, Field, JK (1997) p53 gene aberrations in non-small cell lung carcinomas from a smoking population. *B J Cancer.* 75: 1119–1124.

46. Suzuki H, Takahashi T, Kuroishi T, Suyama M, Ariyoshi Y, Takahashi T, Ueda R (1992) p53 Mutations in Non-Small Cell Lung Cancer in Japan: Association between Mutations and Smoking. *Cancer Res* 52: 734–736.

47. Lee LN, Shew JY, Sheu JC, Lee YC, Lee WC, Fang MT, Chang HF, Yu CJ, Yang PC, Luh KT (1994) Exon 8 mutations of the p53-heat shock 70 protein complexes in human lung carcinoma cell lines. *Am J Respir Crit Care Med* 150: 1667–1671.

48. Tasheva ES, Roufa DJ (1994) Densely methylated DNA islands in mammalian chromosomal replication origins. *Molec Cell Biol* 14: 5636–5644.

49. Yang AS, Gonzalgo ML, Zingg JM, Millar RP, Buckley JD, Jones PA (1996) The rate of CpG mutation in Alu repetitive elements within the p53 tumor suppressor gene in the primate germline. *J Molec Biol* 258: 240–250.

50. El-Deiry WS, Tokino T, Velculescu V, Levy DB, Parsons R, Trent JM, Lin D, Mercer E, Kinzler KW, Vogelstein B (1993) WAF1, a potentional mediator of p53 tumor suppression. *Cell* 75: 817–825.

51. Harper JW, Adami GR, Wei N, Keyomarsi K, Elledge SJ (1993) The p21 Cdk-interacting protein Cip1 is a potent inhibitor of G1 cyclin-dependent kinases. *Cell* 75: 805–816.

52. Xiong Y, Hannon GJ, Zhang H, Casso D, Kobayashi R, Beach D (1993) p21 is a universal inhibitor of cyclin dependent kinase. *Nature* 366: 701–704.

53. Gu Y, Turck CW, Morgan DO (1993) Inhibition of CDK2 activity by an associated 20 K regulatory subunit. *Nature* 366: 707–710.

54. Noda A, Ning Y, Venable SF, Pereirasmith OM, Smith JR (1994) Cloning of senescent cell derived inhibitors of DNA-synthesis. *Exp Cell Res* 211: 90–98.

55. Wang Y, Okan I, Szekely L, Klein G, Wiman KG (1995) bcl-2 inhibids wild-type p53-triggered apoptosis but not G1 cell cycle arrest and transactivation of WAF1 and bax. *Cell Growth Diff* 6: 1071–1075.

56. Datto MB, Yu Y, Wang X-F (1995) Functinal analysis of the transforming growth factor b responsive elements in the WAF1/Cip1/p21 promoter. *J Biol Chem* 270: 28623–28628.

57. El-Diery WS, Tokino T, Waldman T, Oliner JD, Velculescu VE, Burrell M, Hill DE, Healy E, Rees JL, Hamilton SR (1995) Topological control of p21WAF1/CIP1 expression in normal and neoplastic tissues. *Cancer Res* 55: 2910–2919.

58. Datto MB, Li Y, Panus JP, Howe DJ, Xiong Y, Wang X-F (1995) Transforming growthfactor b induces the cyclin-dependent kinase inhibitor p21 through a p53-independent mechanism. *Proc Natl Acad Sci USA* 92: 5545–5549.

59. Liloglou, T, Risk, JM and Field, JK (1996) Polymorphisms in the promoter region of the WAF1/CIP1 gene. *Int J Oncol* 9: 559–562.

60. Hibi K, Takahashi T, Yamakawa K, Ueda R, Sekido Y, Ariyoshi Y, Suyama M, Tagaki H, Naka-muran Y, Takahashi T (1992) Three distinct regions involved in 3p deletion in human lung cancer. *Oncogene* 7: 445–449.

61. Sozzi G, Veronese ML, Negrini M, Baffa R, Cotticelli MG, Inoue H, Tornieili S, Pilotti S, Degregorio L, Pastorino U (1996) The FHIT gene at 3p14.2 is abnormal in lung cancer. *Cell* 85: 17–26.

62. Center R, Lukeis R, Dietzsch E, Gillespie M, Garson MO (1993) Molecular Deletions of 9p Sequences in Non-Small Cell Lung Cancer and Malignant Mesothelioma. *Genes Chromosomes and Cancer* 7: 47–53.

63. Merlo A, Mabry M, Gabrielson E, Vollmer R, Baylin SB, Sidransky D (1994) Frequent microsatellite instability in primary small cell lung cancer. *Cancer Res* 54: 2098–2101.

64. Cairns P, Shaw ME, Knowles MA (1993) Preliminary mapping of the deleted region of chromosome 9 in bladder cancer. *Cancer Res* 53: 1230–1232.

65. Coleman A, Fountain JW, Nobori T, Olopade OI, Robertson G, Houseman DE, Lugo TG (1994) Distinct Deletions of Chromosome 9p Associated with Melanoma versus Glioma, Lung Cancer, and Leukemia. *Cancer Res* 54: 344–348.

66. Orlow I, Lianes P, Lacombe L, Dalbagni G, Reuter VE, Cordon-Cardo C (1994) Chromo-some 9 allelic losses and microsatellite alterations in human bladder tumors. *Cancer Res* 54: 2848–2851.

67. van der Riet P, Nawroz H, Hruban RH, Corio R, Tokino K, Koch W, Sidransky D (1994) Frequent loss of chromosome 9p21–22 early in head and neck cancer progression. *Cancer Res* 54: 1156–1158.

68. Holland EA, Beaton SC, Edwards BG, Kefford RF, Mann GJ (1994) Loss of heterozygosity and homozygous deletions on 9p21–22 in melanoma. *Oncogene* 9: 1361–1365.

69. Keen AJ, Knowles MA (1994) Definition of two regions of deletion on chromosome 9 in carcinoma of the bladder. *Oncogene* 9: 2083–2088.

70. Wiest JS, Franklin WA, Otstot JT, Forbey K, VarellaGarcia M, Rao K, Drabkin H, Gemmill R, Ahrent S, Sidransky D, et al. (1997) Identification of a novel region of homozygous deletion on chromosome 9p in squamous cell carcinoma of the lung: The location of a putative tumor suppressor gene. *Cancer Res* 57: 1–6.

71. Neville EM, Stewart M, Myskow M, Donnelly RJ, Field JK (1995) Loss of heterozygosity at 9p23 defines a novel locus in non-small cell lung cancer. *Oncogene* 11: 581–585.

72. Mead LJ, Gillespie MT, Irving LB, Campbell LJ (1994) Homozygous and hemizygous dele-tions of 9p centromeric to the interferon genes in lung cancer. *Cancer Res* 54: 2307–2309.

73. Nobori T, Miura K, Wu DJ, Lois A, Takabayashi K, Carson DA (1994) Deletions of the cyclin-dependent kinase-4 inhibitor gene in multiple human cancers. *Nature* 368: 753–756.

74. Washimi O, Nagatake M, Osada H, Ueda R, Koshikawa T, Seki T, Takahashi T (1995) In vivo occurrence of p16 (MTS1) and p15 (MTS2) alterations preferentially in non-small cell lung cancers. *Cancer Res* 55: 514–517.

75. Xiao S, Li D, Corson JM, Vijg J, Fletcher JA (1995) Codeletion of p15 and p16 genes in primary non-small cell lung carcinoma. *Cancer Res* 55: 2968–2971.

76. Zhang PL, Calaf G, Russo J (1994) Allele loss and point mutation in codons 12 and 61 of the c-Ha-ras oncogene in carcinogen-transformed human breast epithelial cells. *Molecular Carcinogenesis* 9: 46–56.

77. Hayashi N, Sugimoto Y, Tsuchiya E, Ogawa M, Nakamura Y (1994) Somatic mutations of the MTS (multiple tumor suppressor)1/CDK41 (cyclin-dependent kinase-4 inhibitor) gene in human primary non small cell lung carcinoma. *Biochem Biophys Res Commun* 202: 1426–1430.

78. Okamoto A, Hussain SP, Hagiwara K, Spillare EA, Marek RR, Demetrick DJ, et al. (1995) Mutations in the p16INK4/MTS/CDKN2, p15INK4B/MTS2, and p18 genes in primary and metastatic lung cancer. *Cancer Res* 55: 1448–1451.

79. Merlo A, Herman JG, Mao L, Lee DJ, Gabrielson E, Burger PC, Baylin SB, Sidransky D (1995) 5′ CpG island methylation is associated with transcriptional silencing of the tumour suppressor p16/CDKN2/MTS1 in human cancers. *Nature Med* 1: 686–692.

80. Fong KM, Zimmerman PV, Smith PJ (1995) Microsatellite instability and other molecular abnormalities in non-small cell lung cancer. *Cancer Res* 55: 28–30.

81. Hosoe S, Ueno K, Shigedo Y, Tachibana I, Osaki T, Kumagai T, Tanio Y, Kawase I, Naka-mura Y, Kishimoto T (1994) A frequent deletion of chromosome-5q21 in advanced small-cell and non-small-cell carcinoma of the lung. *Cancer Res* 54: 1787–1790.

82. Wieland I, Bohm M (1994) Frequent allelic deletion at a novel locus on chromosome 5 in human lung cancer. *Cancer Res* 54: 1772–1774.
83. Wieland I, Bohm M, Arden KC, Ammermuller T, Bogatz S, Viars CS, Rajewsky MF (1996) Allelic deletion mapping on chromosome 5 in human carcinomas. *Oncogene* 12: 97–102.
84. Field JK, Neville EM, Stewart MP, Swift A, Liloglou T, Risk JM, Ross H, Gosney JR, Donnelly RJ (1996) Fractional allele loss data indicate distinct genetic populations in the development of non-small cell lung cancer. *Br J Cancer* 74: 1968–1974.
85. Loeb LA (1994) Microsatellite instability: marker of a mutator phenotype in cancer. *Cancer Res* 54: 5059–5063.
86. Peltomaki P, Lothe RA, Aaltonen LA, Pylkkanen L, Nystrom-Lahti M, Seruca R, David L, Holm R, Ryberg D, Haugen A et al. (1993) Microsatellite instability is associated with tumors that characterize the hereditary non-polyposis colorectal carcinoma syndrome. *Cancer Res* 53: 5853–5835.
87. Shridhar V, Siegfried J, Hunt J, Alonso MM, Smith DI (1994) Genetic instability of micro-satellite sequences in many non-small cell lung carcinomas. *Cancer Res* 54: 2084–2087.
88. Mao L, Hruban RH, Boyle JO, Tockman M, Sidransky D (1994) Detection of oncogene mutations in sputum precedes diagnosis of lung cancer. *Cancer Res* 54: 1634–1637.
89. Zhou J, Mulshine JL, Unsworth EJ, Scott FM, Avis IM, Vos MD, Treston AM (1996) Purification and characterization of a protein that permits early detection of lung cancer. *J Biol Chem* 271: 10760–10766.

Clinical and Biological Basis of Lung Cancer Prevention
ed. by Y. Martinet, F.R. Hirsch, N. Martinet, J.-M. Vignaud
and J.L. Mulshine
© 1998 Birkhäuser Verlag Basel/Switzerland

CHAPTER 23
Chemoprevention of Lung Cancer

Ugo Pastorino

Royal Brompton Hospital, Thoracic Surgery, London, UK

1. Introduction

Research into cancer prevention has provided better comprehension of the mechanisms of human carcinogenesis and has improved the selectivity and efficacy of intervention. Lung cancer prevention covers different areas of experimental and clinical research: primary prevention, aimed at eliminating or reducing the environmental exposure to known carcinogens; secondary prevention, including early diagnosis and treatment of preneoplastic or pre-invasive lesions; and pharmacological prevention or chemoprevention, aimed at inhibiting the process of carcinogenesis by the administration of drugs, or other natural substances which are present in human physiology or a normal diet.

Widespread control of tobacco consumption and reduction of environmental exposure to known carcinogens are the main targets of lung cancer prevention. Chemoprevention should never be considered a substitute for primary prevention, but only a potential complement. In fact, with the success of tobacco-control policies, an expanding cohort of ex-smokers will remain at high risk of lung cancer for 15 to 20 years, and there is an objective need for strategies aimed at reducing cancer mortality in individuals who have stopped smoking.

A large body of experimental data has proved that chemoprevention of upper aerodigestive tract cancer is feasible but the evidence of a beneficial effect in humans is still limited and controversial. Selection of high risk individuals and identification of more effective preventive agents remain the most critical aspects of chemoprevention [1]. Despite all the difficulties encountered so far, research into prevention has a indisputable priority in a disease that is so common and barely curable.

2. Dietary Factors in Lung Cancer

Based on the evidence of geographic and historical trends in cancer incidence, human epidemiological studies have correlated the risk of lung cancer with environmental factors other than tobacco consumption. Among these, dietary deficiency of vitamins, micronutrients, or specific foods has emerged as a potential modifier of lung cancer risk. A relative protection against lung cancer has been hypothesized for β-carotene and other substances belonging to the group of antioxidants, such as selenium or vitamin E (α-tocopherol), both in terms of dietary consumption and serum levels.

A major limit in defining individual habits is represented by the low accuracy of dietary questionnaires, and the poor specificity of epidemiological instruments with respect to the individual substance with biological anticancer activity.

Overall, the epidemiological data support the hypothesis that a different intake of common dietary components could modulate the risk of lung cancer, but unequivocal confirmation can only be provided by prospective trials testing the effect of specific dietary measures [2].

3. Latency and Intervention

Human epidemiology and experimental data on multistep carcinogenesis indicate that the development of invasive lung cancer requires a complex sequence of critical events. In fact, most descriptive epidemiological studies of time trends and human cohorts, as well as analytical case-control studies, have consistently demonstrated that the interval between the beginning of the exposure to known carcinogens and the occurrence of lung cancer ranges from 10 to 30 years. Such a long phase of latency suggests a large potential space for intervention.

Theoretically, we could hypothesize a combination of selective chemopreventive agents aimed at the various phases of carcinogenesis: from the inhibition of early induction (metabolic activation, formation of DNA adducts, DNA repair) to the antagonism of tumour promotion and the reversal of progression to invasive cancer.

Biological and clinical research related to chemoprevention is now trying to identify the preclinical steps of lung carcinogenesis and the genetic basis of individual susceptibility to tobacco exposure, with ultimate benefits in the collateral fields of screening of precancerous lesions and early diagnosis of invasive cancer.

4. Experimental Evidence

Experimental data have demonstrated that lung cancer can be pharmacologically prevented or inhibited. Substances with potential chemopreventive properties, such as retinoids and antioxidants, have been investigated using nearly all the available systems for testing anticarcinogenic activity, *in vitro* and *in vivo* [3]. Retinoids exert a strong regulatory effect upon the physiological mechanisms of cell proliferation and differentiation, as they are able to inhibit malignant transformation and suppress tumour promotion, particularly in the presence of indirect carcinogens such as benzopyrene or methylcholanthrene [4]. The antipromotion effect of retinoids is of great interest in human lung cancer chemoprevention, for the possibility of interfering with the late stages of tumour progression. Upregulation or downregulation of specific nuclear retinoic acid receptors (RARα, β, γ) may explain how retinoids can interfere with epithelial cell growth, or inhibit progression of premalignant cells to cancer [5].

Antioxidants, including selenium, β-carotene, α-tocopherol (vitamin E) and N-acetyl-cysteine, may inhibit the process of carcinogenesis at various steps: from metabolic inactivation or detoxification of chemical carcinogens, to prevention of DNA damage by free radicals scavenging. New interest has been aroused in N-acetyl-cysteine (NAC), an aminothiol and synthetic precursor of intracellular cysteine and glutathione (GSH), widely used in the past as a mucolytic drug and antidote against acetaminophen-induced hypatotoxicity. NAC has proven effective in decreasing the direct mutagenicity of several chemical compounds, inhibiting the *in vivo* formation of carcinogen-DNA adducts and DNA damage, as well as inhibiting urethane-induced lung tumours in mice [6].

Further promising agents with preclinical and early clinical data include folate, B12, tea polyphenols, selenium and NSAIDs.

5. Clinical Development of Preventive Agents

Retinoids have been extensively investigated as potential chemopreventive agents, in view of the experimental data and of proven clinical activity against skin cancer [7]. Of the hundreds of compounds tested in the laboratory, only a few ultimately entered thorough clinical investigation: retinyl esters (palmitate, acetate), all-*trans*-retinoic acid (ATRA), 13-*cis*-retinoic acid (13-CRA), etretinate, and fenretinide (4-HPR). This is a highly heterogeneous group of substances, with peculiar properties in terms of resorption, metabolism, pharmacokinetics, bioavailability, and toxicity.

Significant interest and expectations were generated by the studies in oral leukoplakia as a model for upper aerodigestive tract carcinogenesis. Randomized placebo-controlled trials proved that 13-*cis*-retinoic acid could achieve clinical and pathological regression of premalignancy in a high proportion of patients. Unfortunately, most patients did not tolerate the treatment for more than 6 months, and relapse occurred in most cases after the interruption of treatment. Overall, the toxicological profile of synthetic retinoids has been less favourable than expected, and the degree of toxicity (dry skin, itching, flaking, xerostomia, and cheilitis) observed in patients receiving 13-*cis*-retinoic acid at full dosage was a limiting factor for chemoprevention studies. In the group of antioxidants, the ongoing clinical trials include natural substances such as β-carotene and α-tocopherol and N-acetyl-cysteine (NAC), a promising compound with excellent longterm tolerability.

In the United States, the National Cancer Institute (NCI) has invested considerable resources to identify and test specific dietary components and drugs for chemoprevention purposes, through a comprehensive programme covering preclinical screening of new agents, assessment of efficacy and safety, and conduct of clinical trials in humans [8]. The results of such a large effort may not be fully established before the next decade.

6. Primary Chemoprevention Trials in Healthy Individuals

Table 1 summarizes the randomized trials on lung cancer chemoprevention in high-risk individuals, funded by the National Cancer Institute [1].

Table 1. Randomized clinical trials on lung cancer chemoprevention

Investigator	Population	Agent	Dose	No. subjects	Endpoint
Hennekens, Harvard (PHS)	Male physicians 40–84 yr	β-Carotene	50 mg/alt. days	22,071	Epithelial cancer, mortality
Albanes, Finland (ATBC)	Smokers 50–69 yr	β-Carotene Vitamin E	20 mg qd 50 mg qd	29,133	Lung cancer, mortality
Omenn (Seattle) (CARET)	Smokers, 50–69 yr; Asbestos workers	β-Carotene Retinol	30 mg qd 25,000 IU qd	18,314	Lung cancer
Intergroup (USA)	NSCLC stage I	13-CRA	30 mg qd	600	Second primary tumours
EUROSCAN (Europe)	NSCLC stage I–III	Retinyl palmitate N-acetyl-cysteine	300,000 IU qd 600 mg qd	2,595*	Second primary tumours, survival
Hong (Houston)	Bronchial metaplasia + prior cancer	4-HPR	200 mg qd	100	Metaplasia, dysplasia, intermediate markers

NSCLC = non-small cell lung cancer; * including head and neck cancer patients.

Table 2. Results of NCI trials on primary chemoprevention: incidence and mortality per 10,000 person per year

ATBC Trial	β-Carotene	No β-Carotene	Difference %
Lung cancer incidence	56	47	+ 18
Cancer mortality	69	63	+ 9
Total mortality	218	201	+ 8
CARET Trial	β-Carotene + Retinol	Placebo	Difference %
Lung cancer incidence	59	46	+ 28
Total mortality	144	119	+ 21
PHS trial	β-Carotene	Placebo	Difference %
Lung cancer incidence	6	6	0
Cancer mortality	29	29	0
Total mortality	74	73	0

Three of these trials have been recently completed and their results published (Table 2) [9–11]. The Finnish trial (ATBC) was conducted in cooperation with the National Public Health Institute of Finland, to test the effects of dietary supplementation of β-carotene (20 mg/day) and α-tocopherol (Vitamin E, 50 mg/day) in a population of heavy smokers. The study accrued 29,133 men, aged 50 to 69, randomized with a 2 by 2 factorial design into four separate treatment groups, to receive either β-carotene or vitamin E, or both. Against all the expectations, this trial did not show any protective effect of either α-tocopherol or β-carotene [9]. On the contrary, β-carotene supplementation was associated with a statistically significant increase of lung cancer incidence (56.3% vs 47.5%) and mortality (35.6% vs 30.8%). Mortality for ischaemic heart disease was also higher in the group receiving β-carotene, thus contributing to the overall excess in mortality of 8%. This study enrolled only active smokers, and the vast majority of them (79%) continued to smoke throughout the intervention. The detrimental effect of β-carotene has been recently confirmed by the other large trial on heavy smokers (CARET) which showed a 28% increase of lung cancer incidence in the treated group compared to the placebo group [10]. However an opposite effect was noted in the subgroup of former smokers. The third trial (PHS), that enrolled only a small minority of current smokers (11%) could not demonstrate any effect of β-carotene administration [11]. These data suggest a possible unfavourable interaction between current smoking and β-carotene treatment. A residual confounding effect of the quantity and duration of smoking during trial can be hypothesized taking into account the huge difference in lung cancer incidence (6 versus 47) and overall mortality (73 versus 201) among the control arms of the three studies, much larger than the one observed within each trial (Table 2).

While a definitive judgement of these findings will be possible only after a more extensive publication of the results, and perhaps a longer followup, it is clear that vitamin supplementation cannot replace primary prevention. Therefore, it appears reasonable to concentrate future chemoprevention programmes on former smokers as part of a wider tobacco-control policy.

7. Treatment of Precancerous Lesions

Two randomized trials have been conducted on heavy-smoker volunteers with the aim of reverting bronchial metaplasia and dysplasia with retinoids. Both studies were negative.

The first study tested the efficacy of etretinate on sputum cytology of heavy smokers. After 6 months of treatment, the degree of atypia measured in the sputum of etretinate-treated subjects was similar to that observed in the placebo group [12]. The second trial tested the effect of 13-*cis*-retinoic acid versus placebo on 87 chronic smokers with bronchial dysplasia and/or metaplasia index greater than 15%, as assessed by multiple bronchoscopic biopsies. A new bronchoscopy, performed after 6 months of treatment, showed a significant decrease in the frequency of squamous metaplasia in those patients who had stopped smoking, but no difference between the two treatment arms (55 vs 59%) [13].

Although negative, these experiments have provided a methodological setup for prospective investigation of bronchial premalignancy with intermediate biomarkers, and new research prospects are now being generated by innovative endoscopic instruments using spontaneous fluorescence to detect dysplastic areas and carcinoma in situ on macroscopically normal bronchial mucosa.

8. Trials on Chemoprevention of Second Primary Tumours

The potential benefit of retinoids as adjuvant treatment, to reduce the occurrence of second primary tumours, has been demonstrated by two independent randomized trials. The first study was conducted on 103 patients with previously treated head and neck cancer, randomized to receive either isotretinoin or placebo for 12 months [14]. The incidence of second primary tumours was significantly lower in the treatment arm after a median followup of 32 months (4% versus 24%), and persisted at a later analysis with 54 months median followup (14% versus 31%).

The second trial was conducted on 307 patients with early stage lung cancer, randomized after complete surgical resection to receive high dose retinol palmitate for 12 to 24 months or no further treatment. The rationale for such a treatment schedule has been discussed extensively in the first report of the trial [15]. In summary, natural retinol was chosen due to its peculiar properties in human embryology and adult physiology, including development and maintenance of highly differentiated epithelia responsible for vision, reproduction and mucus secretion, that were not shared by other synthetic retinoids. The dose of 300,000 I.U./day for a minimum of 12 months was then selected on the basis of two elements: the highest therapeutic effect achieved in the treatment of dermatological diseases (like ichthyosis, psoriasis and oral leukoplakia), and maximum tolerance in toxicological studies (4,000 I.U./kg./day). The emulsified preparation of retinol palmitate was chosen in consideration of its absorption properties, resulting in a 6-fold higher bioavailability in comparison with the equivalent oily solution. In this trial, after a median followup of 46 months, we observed a significant difference in the frequency of second primaries (12% vs 21%) and total cancer failures (37% vs 48%) in favour of the treatment arm [16]. Despite our initial concerns and a very intense monitoring of side-effects in the pilot phase of the study, the toxicity and tolerability profile of high dose retinol palmitate was excellent. A high proportion of patients presented typical side-effects such as skin desquamation or dryness of mucosae, but in the treatment had to be discontinued in only very few patients because of toxicity [17].

The high frequency of easily detectable-side effects convinced us to avoid a double-blind placebo-controlled design. In our opinion, the use of placebo would have been feasible and convenient only with a much lower dose, below the threshold of clinical toxicity. As for other adjuvant trials in cancer patients, placebo control may not be necessary if the efficacy of intervention is being assessed with hard endpoints such as recurrence, second primary or death. However, the use of placebo becomes essential if soft endpoints such as intermediate biomarkers are chosen, or chemoprevention is being offered to healthy individuals.

Based on these favourable pilot experiments, a series of trials has been designed with the purpose of preventing new primary malignancies after curative resection. The EUROSCAN cooperative study was set up in 1988 as a joint venture of the E.O.R.T.C. Lung Cancer and Head and Neck Cancer Cooperative Groups [18], to test the efficacy of retinol palmitate and NAC, given for two years with a 2×2 factorial design to patients with previous cancer of the larynx, oral cavity and lung (NSCLC). The accrual was closed in 1994, with 2,595 patients entered, and the preliminary analysis is planned for the end of 1996. Another chemoprevention trial on resected stage I NSCLC was started by the U.S. Intergroup in 1992. This study is expected to enter over 600 patients per arm, to be treated with oral 13-*cis*-retinoic acid at the dose of 30 mg/day.

9. Biological Markers and Chemoprevention

The identification of specific biomarkers of lung carcinogenesis has become one of the crucial aspects in the development of chemoprevention, not only to select the best candidates for specific intervention programmes, but also to monitor the results in the short and intermediate term [19].

In fact, to increase the cost/benefit ratio of intervention plans, specific subpopulations of very high risk individuals should be identified on the basis of constitutive or acquired abnormalities detectable in the target tissues. Moreover, biologically intermediate endpoints will became essential in the near future to monitor the efficacy of preventive strategies, before the actual occurrence of invasive cancer [20–22].

A number of genetic abnormalities have been consistently observed in lung cancer, premalignant lesions, and normal bronchial mucosa, and represent potential biomarkers for chemoprevention (Table 3).

In practical terms, it is now conceivable to use a panel of specific markers (3p deletion, p53, EGFR, K-*ras*, MSI) to select candidates for chemoprevention. In fact, with the present developments research technology, such as immunocytochemistry, fluorescence in situ hybridisation (FISH) and PCR, even small samples collected through bronchoscopic biopsies, brushing or sputum cytology will become suitable for systematic screening of high risk individuals [23].

A large effort will be required in the coming years to test and validate such a large group of biomarkers through purpose-designed, small-scale, controlled studies. To justify their systematic use, intermediate endpoints will have to prove specific for the process of carcinogenesis under study, correlate quantitatively or qualitatively with the degree of tumour progression, and be modulated by the selected preventive agent. In addition, such biomarkers should be easily measurable on small specimens and the process of sampling tolerable at repeated intervals.

Table 3. Intermediate biomarkers in lung cancer chemoprevention

Genetic markers	Micronuclei
	Ploidy and DNA content
	Chromosome deletions/translocations
	Microsatellite instability (MSI)
	p53
	K-*ras*
	Neu
Differentiation markers	Squamous markers (keratins, involucrin)
	Mucin gene expression
	Blood group antigens
Proliferation markers	Proliferating cell nuclear antigen (PCNA)
	Thymidine labelling index (TLI)
	Retinoic acid receptors (RARβ)
	Epidermal growth factor receptor (EGFR)
	Transforming growth factor-β (TGF-β)
	Bombesine-like peptide receptors
	Tyrosine kinase receptor
	Bcl-2
	Angiogenesis

References

1. Greenwald P, Stern HR (1992) Role of biology and prevention in aerodigestive tract cancers. *J Natl Cancer Inst Monogr* 13: 3–14.
2. Greenwald P, Sondik E, Lynch BS (1986) Diet and chemoprevention in NCI's research strategy to achieve national cancer control objectives. *Annu Rev Public Health* 7: 267–291.
3. Sporn MB, Newton DL (1979) Chemoprevention of cancer with retinoids. *Fed Proc* 38: 2528–2534.
4. Lotan R (1980) Effects of vitamin A and its analogs (retinoids) on normal and neoplastic cells. *Biochim Biophys Acta* 605: 33–91.
5. Lotan R, Clifford JL (1990) Nuclear receptors for retinoids: mediators of retinoid effects on normal and malignant cells. *Biomed Pharmacother* 45: 145–156.
6. De Flora S, Izzotti A, D'Agostini F, Balansky R, Cesarone CF (1992) Chemopreventive properties of *N*-acetylcysteine and other thiols. *In:* Wattenberg L, Lipkin M, Boone CW, Kelloff GJ (eds): *Cancer Chemoprevention,* CRC Press, Boca Raton, FL, pp 183–194.
7. Lippman SM, Kessler JF, Meyskens FL (1987) Retinoids as preventive and therapeutic anticancer agents (part II). *Cancer Tr Rep* 71: 493–515.
8. Kelloff GJ, Boone CW, Crowell JA, et al. (1994) Chemopreventive drug development: Perspectives and progress. *Cancer Epidemiol Biomarkers Prev* 3: 85–98.
9. The alpha-tocopherol, beta-carotene cancer prevention study group. The effect of vitamin E and beta-carotene on the incidence of lung cancer and other cancers in male smokers. *N Engl J Med* 330: 1029–1035.
10. Omenn GS, Goodman GE, Thornquist MD, Balmes J, Cullen MR, Glass A, et al. (1996) Effects of a combination of beta-carotene and vitamin A on lung cancer and cardiovascular disease. *N Engl J Med* 334: 1150–1155.
11. Hennekens CH, Buring JE, Manson JE, Stampfer M, Rosner B, Cook NR, et al. (1996) Lack of effect of long-term supplementation with beta-carotene on the incidence of malignant neoplasms and cardiovascular disease. *N Engl J Med* 334: 1145–1149.
12. Arnold AM, Browman GP, Levine MN, D'Souza T, Johnstone B, Skingsley P, Turner-Smith L, Cayco R, Booker L, Newhouse M, Hryniuk WM (1992) The effect of the synthetic retinoid etretinate on sputum cytology: results from a randomised trial. *Br J Cancer* 65: 737–743.
13. Lee JS, Benner SE, Lippman SM, Lee JJ, Ro JY, Lukeman JM, Morice RC, Peters EJ, Pang AC, Hittelman HM, Hong WK (1993) A randomised placebo-controlled chemoprevention trial of 13-cis-retinoic acid (cRA) in bronchial squamous metaplasia. *Proc ASCO* 13: 1117.
14. Hong WK, Lippman JM, Itri L, et al. (1990) Prevention of second primary tumors with isotretinoin in squamous cell carcinoma of the head and neck. *N Engl J Med* 323: 795–801.
15. Pastorino U, Soresi E, Clerici M, Chiesa G, Belloni PA, Ongari M, Valente M, Ravasi G (1988) Lung Cancer Chemoprevention With Retinol Palmitate. *Acta Oncologica* 27: 773–782.
16. Pastorino U, Infante I, Maioli, M, Chiesa G, Buyse M, Firket P, Rosmentz N, Clerici M, Soresi E, Valente M, Belloni PA, Ravasi G (1993) Adjuvant treatment of stage I lung cancer with high dose vitamin A. *J Clin Oncol* 11: 1216–1222.
17. Pastorino U, Chiesa G, Infante M, Soresi E, Clerici M, Valente M, Belloni PA, Ravasi G (1991) Safety of high-dose vitamin A. Randomized trial on lung cancer chemoprevention. *Oncology* 48: 131–137.
18. De Vries N, Van Zandwijk N, Pastorino U (1991) The EUROSCAN Study. *Br J Cancer* 64: 985–989.
19. Lee JS, Lippman SM, Hong WK, Ro JY, Kim SY, Lotan R, Hittelman WN (1992) Determination of biomarkers for intermediate end points in chemoprevention trials. *Cancer Res* 52(9 Suppl): 2707s–2710s.
20. Sozzi G, Miozzo M, Tagliabue E, Calderone C, Lombardi L, Pilotti S, Pastorino U, Pierotti MA, Della Porta G (1991) Cytogenetic abnormalities and overexpression of receptors for growth factors in normal bronchial epithelium and tumor samples of lung cancer patients. *Cancer Res* 51: 400–404.
21. Sundaresan V, Ganly P, Hasleton P, Rudd R, Sinha G, Bleehen NM, Rabbitts P (1992) p53 and chromosome 3 abnormalities, characteristic of malignant lung tumours, are detectable in preinvasive lesions of the bronchus. *Oncogene* 7: 1989–1997.

22. Sozzi G, Veronese ML, Negrini M, Baffa R, Cotticelli MG, Inoue H, Tornielli S, Pilotti S, De Gregorio L, Pastorino U, Pierotti MA, Ohta M, Huebner K, Croce CM (1996) The FHIT gene at 3p14.2 is abnormal in lung cancer. *Cell* 85: 117–126.
23. Miozzo M, Sozzi G, Musso K, Pilotti S, Incarbone M, Pastorino U, Pierotti MA (1996) Microsatellite alterations in bronchial and sputum specimens of lung cancer patients. *Cancer Res* 56: 2285–2288.

Clinical and Biological Basis of Lung Cancer Prevention
ed. by Y. Martinet, F.R. Hirsch, N. Martinet, J.-M. Vignaud
and J.L. Mulshine

CHAPTER 24
Regional Delivery of Retinoids: A New Approach to Early Lung Cancer Intervention

James L. Mulshine[1], Luigi M. De Luca[2] and Robert L. Dedrick[3]

[1] *Intervention Section, Cell and Cancer Biology Department, Medicine Branch, Division of Clinical Sciences, National Cancer Institute, Rockville, Maryland, USA*
[2] *Laboratory of Cellular Carcinogenesis and Tumor Promotion, Division of Basic Science, National Cancer Institute, Bethesda, Maryland, USA*
[3] *Biomedical Engineering and Instrumentation Program, National Center for Research Resources, National Institutes of Health, Bethesda, Maryland, USA*

1. Synopsis

Currently, most new lung cancers are found only after symptoms or signs reflect the occurrence of regional or distant metastases. Delayed awareness of lung cancer accounts for its 87% five year mortality rate. New insights may lead to improved methods of early lung cancer detection. Experimental intervention proposed for early cancer management generally entails the oral administration of chemoprevention agents. In this chapter, we discuss an alternative delivery strategy using direct aerosol delivery. The model chemoprevention agents for this discussion are the vitamin A analogues. Preliminary clinical reports suggest benefit in reducing the frequency of new lung cancers for previously resected non-small cell lung cancer patients as well as treated head and neck cancer patients. Chronic oral administration of retinoids is problematic due to the frequency of debilitating side effects. Alternatively, by delivering retinoids directly to the airways as an aerosol, the first-pass drug exposure is to the target cell population and the amount of drug available to the systemic circulation may be greatly reduced. We hypothesize that this approach to retinoid delivery will result in a significantly greater therapeutic index. Direct delivery of the drug to epithelial surfaces afflicted by early cancer may also be a general strategy for improving the therapeutic index with other chemoprevention agents.

2. Introduction

In 1996, lung cancer will account for more than 157,000 deaths in the United States alone and this will also be the most frequently fatal malignancy in the world [1]. Increasing use of tobacco worldwide means even greater lung cancer mortality in years to come [2]. Despite smoking cessation, the risk of lung cancer remains high since lung cancer may take more than a decade to evolve from an initiated cell to a clinically evident cancer. The latency period for the 94,000,000 current and former smokers in the United States alone assures that a high rate of lung cancer will persist for decades [3]. The limited survival benefit from current approaches to lung cancer management dictates a need to identify new clinical management approaches [4]. Rational analysis of the biological basis for lung cancer suggests new options for lung cancer care [5–8].

Tobacco smoke can cause carcinogenic transformation anywhere in the smoker's respiratory tract, so diverse normal pulmonary cell populations exposed to tobacco smoke account for the wide range of histological types of lung cancer [9]. Conventional approaches to early lung cancer detection fail to improve survival significantly. The National Cancer Institute sponsored a study in the late 1970s at Sloan Kettering, Johns Hopkins and the Mayo Clinic evaluating the addition of conventional sputum cytology to chest X-ray. The result of that 30,000 subject trial was consistent with a lead-time bias. The screening arms were associated with a better rate of case detection, early stage and resectable cancers, but the longterm followup failed to show any significant reduction in lung cancer mortality [10–14]. This outcome emphasizes the difficulty in detecting early lung cancer.

Using a sputum immunocytochemical technique, we reported a dual antibody immunocytochemistry assay which identified the majority of lung cancer cases about two years in advance of clinically evident lung disease [15]. This correlational analysis was possible due to existence of an archive of stored serial sputa which had been prospectively acquired on an annual basis from the smokers enrolled during the previously discussed early lung cancer detection trial and stored at Johns Hopkins [13]. The long term clinical followup of that patient population revealed who went on to develop cancer and who remained cancer-free. So the sputum archive is an invaluable resource for early lung cancer markers. Two new ongoing clinical trials may also independently confirm the initial positive early detection report [16].

Over the last several years, improvements in diagnostic technology, as well as increased understanding of tumor biology brighten the prospect of early detection of lung cancer [5, 7, 8, 17, 18]. For example, the Johns Hopkins sputum archive material was also used to validate that mutations in *ras* and *p53* or microsatellite alterations could be detected in morphologically normal sputum specimens up to one year prior to clinical lung cancer [19, 20]. As biomarker technology continues to develop, further clues to the key sequence of events leading to epithelial cancer will emerge. Cautious optimism about the success of molecular detection of lung cancer also implies that increasing numbers of preinvasive (or airway-confined) lung cancer will come to medical attention. Recent experience with increased detection of early prostate cancer related to the use of prostate-specific antigen screening suggests that elucidating clinical management options for early lung cancer that do not involve morbid complications would be highly desirable [21]. If these new epithelial-directed diagnostics provide the ability to detect the preinvasive phase of lung cancer, then improved chemoprevention approaches will be required.

3. Retinoids as a Model for Direct Epithelial Delivery

The leading candidates for short-term application as lung cancer chemoprevention agents are vitamin A analogues. A wealth of clinical and experimental information has established retinoids as potent regulators of epithelial cell growth with reported benefit in the prevention and treatment of a number of neoplastic conditions [22–24]. The MD Anderson group has recently summarized the field of clinical trials for cancer chemoprevention [25]. Their investigations of retinoids in the chemoprevention of head and neck cancer and of lung cancer are provocative, since both diseases are generally related to tobacco exposure [25–28]. Though the precise mechanisms are not yet known, retinoids interact with nuclear receptors which are thought to control cell division and differentiation for a range of epithelial cells. Recently, Lotan and colleagues demonstrated that a number of retinoids can upregulate programmed cell death *in vitro* [29]. This important observation will be discussed later in more detail.

Despite the growing body of information beyond the published reports of Hong and coworkers suggesting the benefit of oral retinoids as chemoprevention agents [25], the side effects associated with chronic ingestion of currently available retinoids are a significant problem. Although the optimal duration of chemoprevention has not yet been defined, it appears likely that longterm delivery may be required [26]. The ideal situation for intervention in early lung cancer is to have a chemoprevention option that is well tolerated, so that poor compliance will not excessively compromise clinical benefit. New retinoids are in early clinical evaluation, and it remains to be established if this next generation of analogues will represent a major improvement with regard to side effect profile. In the setting of lung cancer prevention with a vast at-risk population, cost also represents a significant variable. An alternative pharmacological approach to oral retinoid delivery that preserves its chemoprevention effect but reduces side effects would constitute a major advance for lung cancer chemoprevention.

4. Rationale for Direct Epithelial Delivery

The complex pharmacology in attempting to control the evolution of carcinogenesis on the bronchial epithelial surface with oral delivery of retinoids is summarized in Figure 1. Oral administration is shown in the bottom panel. As reviewed by the group from the University of Arizona, absorption of 13-*cis*-retinoic acid is variable and incomplete following oral administration, the retinoid binds almost exclusively to albumin in the plasma (up to 99.9%) and appears not to be displaced by high metabolite concentration [30]. The presence of albumin reduces the functional bio-availability of retinoid. The net effect is that only a minute fraction of the administered retinoid dose is actually available to the respiratory epithelium.

Based on the success of the MD Anderson group in using 13-*cis*-retinoic acid as a chemoprevention agent for lung cancer [25–28], we have been interested in the effects of retinoids on epithelial cancers and have evaluated the antiproliferative effects of 13-*cis*-retinoic acid [31]. In contrast to previous studies, when defined serum-free medium is used, a broad range of cancer cell lines are significantly growth inhibited. This observation

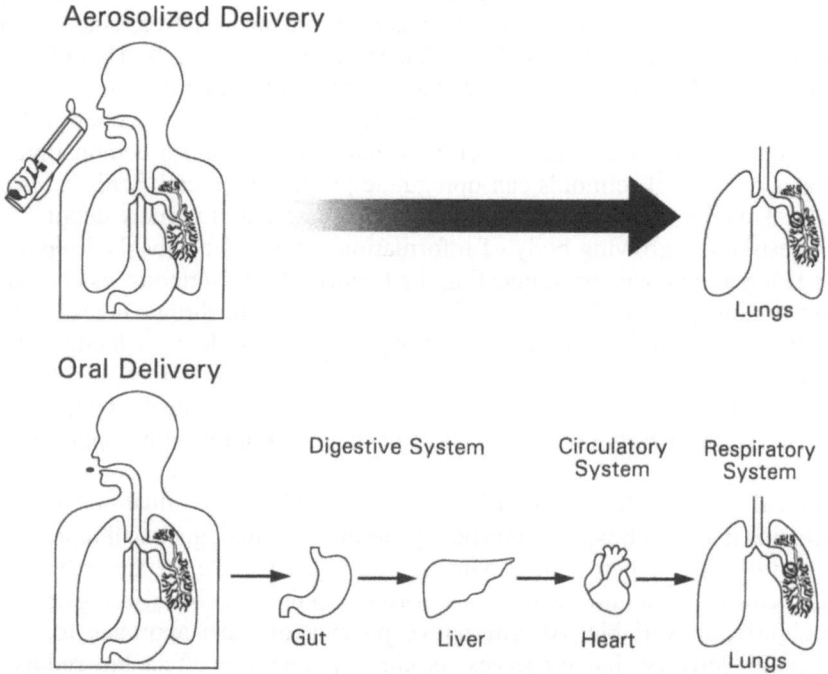

Figure 1. Schematic outlining the issues with either oral or aerosolized delivery of a chemo-prevention agent.

began a line of investigation that could lead to a new and more effective delivery for this important class of regulatory molecules.

Since the loss of retinoid regulation of growth observed *in vitro* with cancer cells can be blocked by preabsorbing albumin with high concentrations of free fatty acids, the issue of retinoid-protein interaction may be relevant in the airway in which the concentration of albumin in bronchial fluid is generally less than that in the plasma [32].

We and others have speculated that epithelial-directed drug delivery approaches may greatly improve the prospects for controlling early lung cancer [31, 33]. Direct aerosolization of the retinoid as shown schematically in the top half of Figure 1 may result in a significantly greater fraction of the administered dose reaching the target tissue in the lung. Enhancement in bronchial epithelial targeting might provide the required concentration of drug to activate retinoid receptors with a substantially reduced systemic dose. If successful, this delivery approach would permit the desired growth inhibition of the transformed respiratory epithelial cells without the debilitating systemic toxicity associated with oral retinoid administration. The goal of more targeted drug delivery is to provide the kind of "benign" chemoprevention option that would make participation in a population-based early cancer screening program more attractive to an individual at risk of developing lung cancer.

5. Status of the Development of Aerosol Delivery Systems

Many of the functional responses of the lung to exogenously administered drugs have been elucidated by investigators working on asthma or infectious disease therapies [32, 34–37]. The body of information about aerosolized drug delivery from this work is of direct relevance to the development of local therapies in the lung for chemoprevention. Current aerosolized delivery capability is a result of an enhanced understanding in several areas. Details of lung anatomy and physiology have better defined the target and its predictable biological responses [32]. The physical chemistry of drug formulation to achieve greater biostability, specific targeting and bioavailability have also recently improved [34, 35]. A range of delivery devices have been employed, and the evolution of this technology has resulted in significantly more efficient delivery systems [36, 37].

The gross anatomy of the lung's conducting airway, involving 23 levels of arborization, and its relationship to tobacco injury has long been known [32, 38]. The identity of all the numerous cell types in the lung has been more recently established. Each cell type performs different specialized functions such as gas exchange and detoxification of toxins as well as a range of endocrine and other metabolic functions [32]. All respiratory epithelial cells can potentially be a target for the carcinogenic action of tobacco smoke, so that the aerosolization of the retinoid must deliver effective dose concentrations to the entire epithelial surface. Without describing all of these cell types and their functions, it is of fundamental importance to determine the chronic effect of a new drug or delivery technique on the wellbeing of normal cell populations. Concerns about the tolerance of normal airway components to aerosolized retinoid are partly addressed by *in vitro* work of De Luca and coworkers which showed that hamster tracheal cultures of normal airway cells were quite tolerant of high ambient concentrations of retinoid, and grew without evident ill consequence [23, 24]. Despite favorable results with rodent models, careful preclinical evaluation of the precise formulation proposed for human administration is required. The experience with antibiotics provides a basis for optimism. With aerosolized antibiotics, an increase of effective pulmonary tissue drug levels 10 to 40 times that achieved with parenteral delivery, without increase in clinically evident toxicity, was found [39].

6. Use of Pharmacological Models to Refine Epithelial-Directed Interventions

The development of pharmacological models has allowed for much more predictable progress in drug development. The theoretical description of regional chemotherapy for intra-arterial and intracavitary drug administration is a relatively mature discipline with powerful predictive capability [40]. A simple equation permits the estimation of the pharmacokinetic advantage that can be obtained in a particular setting:

$$R_d = 1 + CL_{TB}/K(1 - E) \tag{1}$$

where R_d is the pharmacokinetic advantage (defined as the ratio of the tissue exposure to the systemic exposure following regional drug delivery divided by the same ratio following systemic delivery), CL_{TB} is the total body clearance following intravenous drug administration, K is the intercompartment transport parameter, and E is the irreversible extraction of drug by the target region. Exposure may be measured by the area under the concentration vs time curve (AUC) of plasma that would be in equilibrium with the tissue. If there is no extraction by the region (E = 0), Equation (1) becomes simply:

$$R_d = 1 + CL_{TB}/K \tag{2}$$

The advantage of regional delivery derives from the first pass of the drug through the compartment containing the target epithelial cell population; absorbed drug acts as a systemic dose. Equation (2) shows that the pharmacokinetic advantage depends on the ratio of CL_{TB} to K. If K were the same for two drugs, then the agent with the larger clearance from the body would be kinetically preferred.

A number of assumptions are required in the derivation of the basic equation for pharmacokinetic advantage. These include: (1) constant CL_{TB}

and K, (2) linearity of the underlying biological processes such as metabolism, binding and transport, and (3) a uniform concentration of drug in
the target region. All of these assumptions raise questions or pose difficulties to the application of the simple theory to aerosol delivery to the lung.
The total body clearance of retinoids in human subjects has generally not
been measured because of the unavailability of intravenous formulations;
however, approximate estimates may be possible for some from oral data
[41–43]. Careful kinetic studies of absorption of drugs and other chemicals
from the lung of several species are available following both intratracheal
and aerosolized delivery [44]. These provide considerable insight into the
effect of molecular size and lipid solubility, but the rate is expressed as a
first-order rate constant (min^{-1}), and conversion to the transport parameter
K (ml/min) is not immediately obvious because the effective volume is not
known. We are not aware of any work reporting the rate of absorption of
retinoids from the lung. Studies of a variety of retinoids in rodents have
established that most tissues, including the lung, can track the plasma
concentration quite closely [45–48]. The brain and testes appear to have a
small barrier. Linearity of the biological processes is not established and is
unlikely to be correct at all relevant concentrations. Application of the
model is confused by the spatial distribution of the drug within the airways,
and by concentration gradients that exist during drug absorption from the
airway surfaces. In principle, we would like to know the (free) drug
concentration at the epithelial sites of action and its variation with time.
Definition of the pharmacokinetic advantage in terms of the AUC may not
adequately address the biological effect (pharmacodynamics) of retinoids.
The effect may depend both on concentration and duration of exposure and
not simply on their integral as expressed by the area under the concentration curve.

This analytical approach suggests that a critical feature with direct
epithelial delivery will be the first-pass concentration of the drug. From
this perspective using a rapidly cleared retinoid such as all-*trans*-retinoic acid
[42] may be comparable to a more slowly cleared drug such as fenretinide
if they have similar values of CL_{TB} and K. The only data for apparent
clearance of retinoids is after oral administration in humans [43]. Yet from a
biological perspective, we might argue for the use of fenretinide because it
seems to be more potent in stimulating apoptosis [29]. The concept of
programmed cell death or apoptosis has been catapulted to critical attention
in the cancer biology community in recognition of the central importance
of this regulatory mechanism to the pathogenesis of cancer [49, 50]. This
prominence is reflected in Figure 2 which schematically demonstrates the
central regulatory influence of apoptosis in maintaining normal differentiation. While apoptosis can be modulated by retinoids [29], many other drugs
are also capable of enhancing this action [49–52]. The prospective evaluation of such complex leads will help define the most critical variables to
derive a predictive pharmacological equation for aerosolized intervention

CARCINOGENESIS:

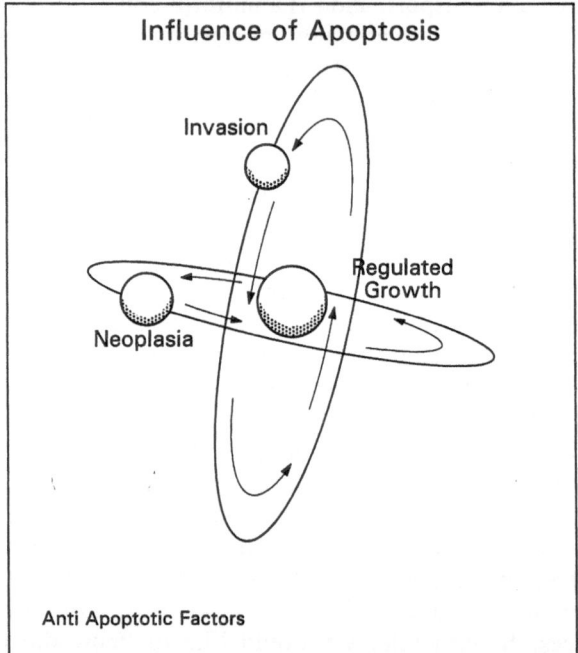

Figure 2. Schematic representation of the influence of apoptosis in maintaining normal differentiation by suppressing clonal emergence of populations capable of invasion or metastasis.

delivery. The experience with retinoids may guide the general development of subsequent epithelial-directed intervention approaches for other chemoprevention agents. Other approaches to aerosol delivery modelling can be evaluated [53] to determine which is the most predictive and would be applicable to other chemoprevention agents being considered for aerosolized delivery. In the future, if we determine that a proposed intervention agent such as the lipoxygenase inhibitor must be aerosolized [52], then an established development path will be much clearer. A large number of drugs could find application in this setting.

The possibility of aerosolizing retinoids has considerable intuitive appeal in the clinical community, so that if preliminary clinical evaluation validated the benefit of aerosolized retinoids, this approach may be rapidly expanded. Despite the strong potential of using epithelial-directed chemoprevention strategies, the pharmaceutical industry may not be interested in developing these agents. A NCI Working Group on Chemoprevention Development found that the drug development cost and longterm risk of side effects functionally excluded the pharmaceutical industry from developing chemoprevention agents [54]. Aerosolized delivery could improve this situation as the anticipated dose to protect the airway could be much less than the oral dose so that the potential for systemic side effects is greatly reduced. This also means that patient expense is reduced. If this change in delivery strategy results in more enthusiastic participation of the pharmaceutical and biotechnology industry, this field will develop at a much faster rate.

7. Conclusion

Developments in the field of molecular diagnostics provide a basis for cautious optimism about progress in population-based early lung cancer screening. Parallel developments are clearly needed refine the range of therapeutic intervention for early cancer management. Successful early diagnostic approaches will routinely identify individuals with carcinogenic involvement restricted to the airway. Compounds such as retinoids provide important models to evaluate for local benefit with early cancer. The most efficient route to deliver agents to arrest the development of the early cancer may be via the airway. Refinements in aerosolized drug delivery over the last decade have resulted in a greatly improved ability to deliver drugs to the respiratory epithelium. This chapter reviews the prospects for development of new approaches to cancer care.

References

1. Parker, SL, Tong T, Bolden S, Wingo PA (1996) Cancer statistics. *CA Cancer J Clin* 65: 5–27.
2. Peto R, Lopez AD, Boreham J, et al. (1992) Mortality from tobacco in developed countries: Indirect estimation from national vital statistics. *Lancet* 339: 1268–1278.
3. Gaffney M, Altshuler B (1988) Examination of the role of cigarette smoke in lung carcinogenesis. *J Natl Cancer Inst* 80: 925–931.
4. Beardsley T (1994) The war not won. *Sci Am* 1: 130–138.
5. Ames BN, Gold LS, Willett WC (1995) The causes and prevention of cancer. *Proc Natl Acad Sci* 92: 5258–5265.
6. Mulshine JL, Treston Am, Scott FM, Avis I, Boland C, Phelps R, Kasprzyk PG, Nakanishi Y, Cuttitta F (1990) New approach to the management of lung cancer: Rational strategies for early detection and intervention. *Oncol* 5: 25–32.
7. Mulshine JL, Magnani J, Linnoila RI (1991) Applications of monoclonal antibodies in the treatment of solid tumors. *In:* DeVita V, Hellman S, Rosenberg S (eds): *Biologic Therapy of Cancer,* pp 563–588.
8. Mulshine JL, Shaw GL, Cuttitta F, Scott F, Avis I, Treston AM, Linnoila RI, Birrer M, Brown P, Gupta PK et al. (1993) Applications of Biomarkers for Lung Cancer Early Detection. *In:* Fortner J, Rhoads J (eds): *Accomplishments in Cancer Research*, Lippincott Co, Philadelphia, pp 204–216.
9. Linnoila RI, Aisner SC (1995) Pathology of Lung Cancer: An Exercise in Classification. *In:* Johnson BE and Johnson DH (eds): *Lung Cancer*. Wiley-Liss, New York, pp 73–95.
10. Bailar JC (1984) Early lung cancer cooperative study group: Early lung cancer detection. Summary and conclusion. *Am Rev Respir Dis* 130: 565–570.
11. Bailar JC (1984) Editorial, Screening for lung cancer – where are we now? *Am Rev Respir Dis* 130: 541–542.

12. Tockman MS, Becklake MR, Clausen JL, Cox PM, Fontana RS, O'Brien RJ, Permutt S, Petty TL, Reed C, Reichman LB, et al. (1983) Screening for adult respiratory disease: The official ATS statement. *Am Rev Respir Dis* 128: 768–774.
13. Tockman MS, Levin ML, Frost JK, Ball WC Jr, Marsh BR (1985) Screening and detection of lung cancer. *In:* Aisner J (ed): *Lung Cancer.* New York, Churchill Livingstone, p 25–40.
14. Szabo E, Mulshine JL (1996) Lung cancer prevention: historical and future perspectives. *In:* Aisner J, Arrigada R, Green MR, Martini N, Perry MC (eds): *Comprehensive Textbook of Thoracic Oncology.* Baltimore, Williams and Wilkins, p 90–104.
15. Tockman MS, Gupta PK, Myers JD, Frost JK, Baylin SB, Gold EB, Mulshine JL (1988) Sensitive and Specific Monoclonal Antibody Recognition of Human Lung Cancer Antigen on Preserved Sputum Cells: A New Approach to Early Lung Cancer Detection. *J Clin Oncol* 6: 1685–1693.
16. Tockman MS, Erozan, YS, Gupta P, Piantadosi S, Mulshine JL, Ruckdeschel JC, LCEDWG Investigators (1994) The early detection of second primary lung cancers by sputum immunostaining. LCEDWG investigators. Lung cancer early detection working group. *Chest Suppl* 106: 385S–390S.
17. Zhou J, Mulshine JL, Unsworth, Avis I, Cuttitta F, Treston A (1996) Purification and characterization of a protein which permits early detection of lung cancer: identification of heterogeneous nuclear ribonucleoprotein-A2/B1 as the antigen for monoclonal antibody, 703D4. *J Biol Chem* 271: 10760–10766.
18. Zhou J, Jensen SM, Steinberg, Mulshine J, Linnoila RI (1996) Expression of early lung cancer detection marker P31 in neoplastic and non-neoplastic respiratory epithelium. *Lung Cancer* 14: 85–97.
19. Mao L, Hruban RH, Boyle JO, Tockman MS, Sidransky D (1994) Detection of oncogene mutation in sputum precedes the diagnosis of lung cancer. *Cancer Res* 54: 1634–1637.
20. Mao L., Lee DJ, Tockman MS, Erozan JA, Askin F, Sidransky D (1994) Microsatellite alterations as clonal markers in the detection of human cancer. *Proc Natl Acad Sci* 91: 9871–9875.
21. Woolf SH (1995) Screening for prostate cancer with prostate-specific antigen. *N Engl J Med* 333: 1401–1405.
22. Moon RC, McCormick DL, Mehta RG (1983) Inhibition of carcinogenesis by retinoids. *Cancer Res* 43: 24696–24755.
23. DeLuca LM (1991) Retinoids and their receptors in differentiation, embryogenesis and neoplasia. *FASEB J* 5: 2924–2933.
24. McDowell EM, Ben T, Coleman B, Chang S, Newkirk C, DeLuca LM (1987) Effects on retinoid acid on the growth and morphology of hamster tracheal epithelia cells in primary culture. *Virchows Arch B* 54: 38–51.
25. Lippman S, Benner S, Hong W (1994) Cancer Chemoprevention. *J Clin Oncol* 12: 851–873.
26. Benner SE, Pajak TF, Lippman SM, Early C, Hong WK (1994) Prevention of second primary tumors with isotretinoin in patients with squamous carcinoma of the head and neck: long-term follow-up. *J Natl Cancer Inst* 86: 140–141.
27. Hong WK, Lippman SM, Itri LM, Karp DD, Lee JS, Byer RM, Shantz SP, Kramer AM, Lotan R, Peters LJ (1990) Prevention of second primary tumors in squamous cell carcinoma of the head and neck with 13-*cis*-retinoic acid, *N Engl J Med* 323: 795–801.
28. Lee JS, Lippman SM, Benner SE, Lee JJ, Ro JY, Lukeman JM, Morice RC, Peters EJ, Pang AC, Fritsche HA Jr, Hong WK (1994) Randomized placebo-controlled trial of isotretinoin in chemoprevention of bronchial squamous metaplasia. *J Clin Oncol* 12: 5; 937–945.
29. Oridate N, Lotan D, Xu X-C, Hong WK, Lotan R (1996) Differential induction of apoptosis by all-*trans*-retinoic acid and N-(4-hydroxyphenyl)retinamide in head and neck squamous cell carcinoma cell lines. *Clin Cancer Res* 2: 855–863.
30. Meyskens FL, Goodman GE, Alberts DS (1985) 13-*cis*-retinoic acid: Pharmacology, toxicology and clinical application for the prevention and treatment of human cancer. *Crit Rev Oncol Hematol* 3 :75–101.
31. Avis I, Mathias A, Unsworth EJ, Miller MJ, Cuttitta F, Mulshine JL, Jakowlew SB (1995) Analysis of small cell lung cancer growth inhibition by 13-*cis*-retinoic acid: importance of bioavailability. *Cell Growth Diff* 6: 485–492.
32. Altiere RJ, Thompson DC (1996) Physiology and Pharmacology of the Airways. *In:* Hickey AJ (eds): *Inhalation Aerosols.* M. Dekker, New York, pp 85–138.

33. Tong WP, Benedetti F, Brooks A, et al. (1996) Inhaled retinoids for prevention of epithelial cancers of the respiratory tract. *Proc Am Soc Clin Oncol* 15: 173.
34. Ma JKH, Bhat M, Rojanasakul Y (1996) Drug metabolism and enzyme kinetics in the lung. *In:* Hickey AJ (eds): *Inhalation Aerosols*. M. Dekker, New York, pp 155–198.
35. Newman SP (1996) Delievery of drugs to the respiratory tract. *In:* Chung KF, Barnes PJ (eds): *Pharmacology of the respiratory tract*. M. Dekker, New York, pp 701–720.
36. Adjei AL, Qiu Y, Gupta PK (1996) Bioavailability and pharmacokinetics of inhaled drugs. *In:* Hickey AJ (eds): *Inhalation aerosols*. M. Dekker, New York, pp 197–228.
37. Patton JS (1996) Mechanisms of macromolecule absorption by the lung. *J Advanced Drug Delivery Rev* 19: 3–36.
38. Auerbach O (1979) Changes in the bronchial epithelium in relation to cigarette smoking. *N Engl J Med* 300: 381–385.
39. Pascal S, Diot P, Lemarie E (1992) Antibiotics in aerosols. *Rev Mal Respir* 9: 145–153.
40. Dedrick RL (1986) Interspecies scaling of regional drug delivery. *J Pharm Sci* 75: 1047–1052.
41. Colburn WA, Vane FM, Bugge CJL, Carter DE, Bressler R, Ehmann CW (1985) Pharmacokinetics of ^{14}C-isotretinoin in healthy volunteers and volunteers with biliary T-tube drainage. *Drug Metab Disposition* 13: 327–332.
42. Muindi JRF, Frankel SR, Huselton C, DeGrazia F, Garland WA, Young CW, Warrell RP Jr (1992) Clinical pharmacology of oral all-*trans* retinoic acid in patients with acute promyelocytic leukemia. *Cancer Res* 52: 2138–2142.
43. Peng Y-M, Dalton WS, Alberts DS, Xu M-J, Lim H, Meyskens FL (1989) Pharmacokinetics of N-4-hydroxyphenylretinamide and the effect of its oral administration on plasma retinol concentrations in cancer patients. *Int J Cancer* 43: 22–26.
44. Schanker LS, Mitchell EW, Brown RA Jr (1986) Species comparison of drug absorption from the lung after aerosol inhalation or intratracheal injection. *Drug Metab Disposition* 14: 79–88.
45. Kalin JR, Starling ME, Hill DL (1981) Disposition of all-*trans*-retinoic acid in mice following oral doses. *Drug Metab Disposition* 9: 196–201.
46. Swanson BN, Zaharevitz DW, Sporn MB (1980) Pharmacokinetics of N-(4-hydroxyphenyl)-all-*trans*-retinamide in rats. *Drug Metab Disposition* 8: 168–172.
47. Tzimas G, Collins MD, Nau H (1995) Developmental stage-associated differences in the transplacental distribution of 13-*cis*- and all-*trans*-retinoic acid as well as their glucuronides in rats and mice. *Toxicol Appl Pharmacol* 133: 91–101.
48. Wang C-C. Campbell S, Furner RL, Hill DL (1980) Disposition of all-*trans*- and 13-*cis*-retinoic acids and N-hydroxyethylretinamide in mice after intravenous administration. *Drug Metab Disposition* 8: 8–11.
49. White E. Life (1996) Death and the pursuit of apoptosis. *Genes Devel* 10: 1–15.
50. Thompson C (1995) Apoptosis in the pathogenesis and treatment of disease. *Science* 267: 1456–1457.
51. Morin PJ, Vogelstein B, Kinzler KW (1996) Apoptosis and APC in colorectal tumorigenesis. *Proc Natl Acad Sci* 93: 7950–7954.
52. Avis I, Jett M, Boyle T, Treston A, Scott F, Mulshine JL (1996) Growth control of lung cancer by interruption of the 5-lipoxygenase-mediated growth factor signaling. *J Clin Invest* 97: 806–813.
53. Swift DL (1996) Use of mathematical aerosol deposition models in predicting the distribution of inhaled therapeutic aerosols. *In:* Hickey AJ (eds): *Inhalation aerosols*. M. Dekker, New York, pp 51–78.
54. Mulshine JL (1995) Fostering chemoprevention agent development: How to proceed? *J Cell Biochem* 22S: 254–259.

Clinical and Biological Basis of Lung Cancer Prevention
ed. by Y. Martinet, F. R. Hirsch, N. Martinet, J.-M. Vignaud
and J. L. Mulshine

CHAPTER 25
Natural Inhibitors of Carcinogenesis

Hirota Fujiki, Masami Suganuma, Atsumasa Komori, Sachiko Okabe, Eisaburo Sueoka, Naoko Sueoka, Tomoko Kozu and Yukiko Tada

Saitama Cancer Center Research Institute, Ina, Kitaadachi-gun, Saitama, Japan

1. Introduction

For the purpose of finding nontoxic cancer preventive agents, we studied natural products derived from marine and plant sources. The following compounds inhibited tumor promotion on mouse skin in two-stage carcinogenesis experiments: two marine natural products and four plant natural products. Among these natural inhibitors, we suggest green tea as a cancer preventive in humans. This chapter reviews our basic study on cancer preventive agents derived from natural sources.

1. Marine natural products (Figure 1)

    a) Sarcophytol A, isolated from a soft coral, *Sarcophyton glaucum*, a cembrane-type diterpene [1]

    b) Canventol, a synthetic compound derived from the structure of sarcophytol A [1]

    c) Discodermin A, isolated from a marine sponge, *Discodermia kiiensis*, a peptide [2]

2. Plant natural products (Figure 1)

    a) (–)-Epigallocatechin gallate (EGCG), isolated from green tea, *Camellia sinensis*, a tea polyphenol [1, 3]

    b) Penta-*O*-galloyl-β-D-glucose (5GG), which is obtained by hydrolysis of tannic acid, isolated from a gall, *Schisandrae fructus*, a polyphenol [3]

    c) Morusin, isolated from the root bark of the mulberry tree, *Morus alba* L., an isoprenylated flavone [4]

    d) Cryptoporic acid E, isolated from a fungus, *Cryptoporus volvatus*, a dimer of drimane sesquiterpene isocitric acid [5].

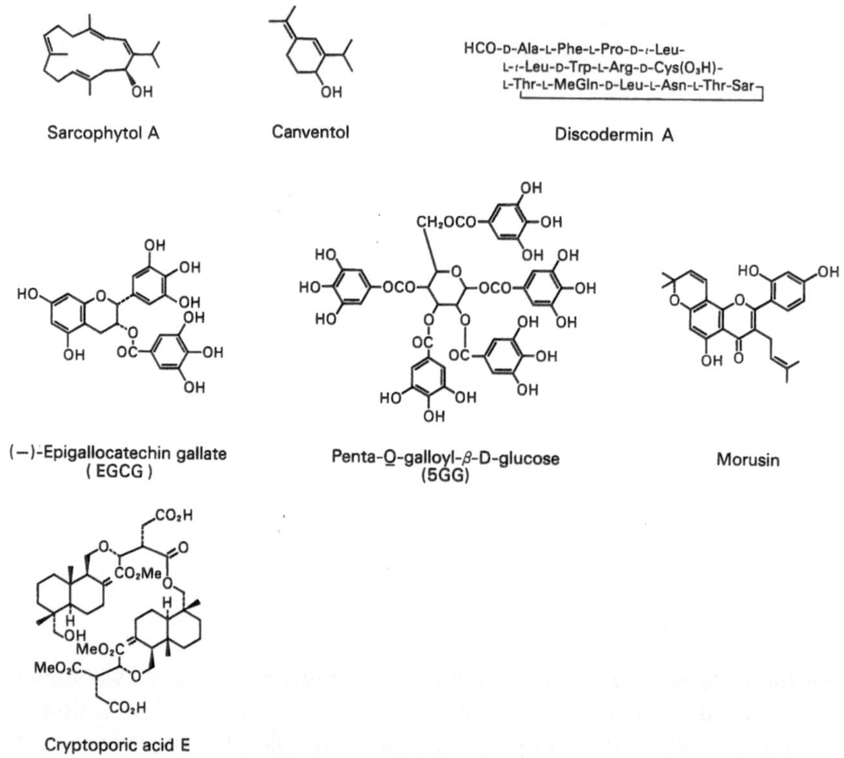

Sarcophytol A   Canventol

HCO-D-Ala-L-Phe-L-Pro-D-ı-Leu-
L-ı-Leu-D-Trp-L-Arg-D-Cys(O₃H)-
L-Thr-L-MeGln-D-Leu-L-Asn-L-Thr-Sar⌐

Discodermin A

(−)-Epigallocatechin gallate
(EGCG)

Penta-O-galloyl-β-D-glucose
(5GG)

Morusin

Cryptoporic acid E

Figure 1. Structures of sarcophytol A, canventol, discodermin A, EGCG, 5GG, morusin and cryptoporic acid E.

2. Inhibitory Potency of Tumor Promotion

It is relatively easy to find various inhibitors, when compounds are subjected to two-stage carcinogenesis experiments on mouse skin initiated with 7,12-dimethylbenz(a)anthracene (DMBA) plus a tumor promoter, either teleocidin (one of the 12-O-tetradecanoylphorbol-13-acetate (TPA)-type tumor promoters), or okadaic acid. Table 1 shows inhibitory potency of tumor promotion by various compounds. This assay system has numerous advantages as a tumor model, because it is rapid, quantitative and has been well investigated [1]. As for mechanisms of action, the compounds inhibit clonal growth of the initiated cells containing mutations in the second nucleotide of codon 61 of the c-Harvey-ras protooncogene induced by DMBA.

3. Canventol

In addition to inhibition of tumor promotion, sarcophytol A in the diet inhibited carcinogenesis of the colon, bladder, pancreas, liver, breast and lung

Table 1. Inhibition of tumor promotion by various compounds

Inhibitors	Tumor promoter	Reduction of tumor-bearing mice (%)	Reduction of average number of tumors/mouse	Ref.
Sarcophytol A	Teleocidin	53.0 → 7.1	2.1 → 0.1	[1]
	Okadaic acid	86.7 → 46.7	4.7 → 1.5	[1]
Canventol	Okadaic acid	86.7 → 20.0	4.7 → 0.5	[1]
Discodermin A	Okadaic acid	86.7 → 46.7	4.7 → 1.1	[2]
EGCG	Teleocidin	53.0 → 13.0	2.1 → 0.1	[3]
	Okadaic acid	73.0 → 0	4.2 → 0	[1]
5GG	Teleocidin	100.0 → 53.0	3.3 → 0.9	[3]
Morusin	Teleocidin	100.0 → 60.0	5.3 → 1.1	[4]
Cryptoporic acid E	Okadaic acid	73.3 → 20.0	4.2 → 0.5	[1]

Initiation on mouse skin was achieved by a single application of DMBA in all these experiments.

in rodents. However, we had difficulty continuing the experiments with sarcophytol A, due to a shortage of the compound [1].

Dr. Marcus A. Tius at Department of Chemistry, University of Hawaii has synthesized a compound associated with a simpler structure than sarco-phytol A (Fig. 1). The compound, named canventol, inhibited tumor promotion by okadaic acid on mouse skin more strongly than sarcophytol A did (Table 1) [1].

Dr. Vernon E. Steele at the National Cancer Institute subjected canventol to his multiple experimental preclinical system consisting of six bio-chemical assays [6]. Canventol affected four assays: it inhibited TPA-induced ornithine decarboxylase in rat tracheal epithelial cells; it inhibit-ed benzo(a)pyrene-DNA binding in human bronchial epithelial cells; it induced reduced glutathione in buffalo rat liver cells; and it induced NADPH-quinone reductase. We also found that canventol inhibits both protein isoprenylation in the cells and release of tumor necrosis factor-α (TNF-α) from BALB/3T3 cells induced by okadaic acid [1]. We think canventol has potential as a possible cancer preventive agent in various organs.

4. EGCG and Green Tea

One of the most important advantages of EGCG and green tea as cancer preventives in humans is nontoxicity. Japanese drink green tea every day and Western people drink black tea, which is originally derived from the same plant, *Camellia sinensis*. As Table 2 shows, EGCG in drinking water inhibited carcinogenesis in rat glandular stomach, mouse duodenum, rat colon and mouse liver [1]. Green tea extract (GTE) in drinking water, which corresponds to green tea itself, inhibited both lung carcinogenesis in mice induced by a nicotine-derived nitrosamine, 4-(methylnitrosamino)-1-

Table 2. Inhibition of carcinogenesis with EGCG and green tea extract

Organs	Species	Carcinogens	Inhibitors	Reduction of tumor incidence (%)	Ref.
Glandular stomach	Rat	MNNG	EGCG	62.0 → 31.0	[1]
Duodenum	Mouse C57BL/6	ENNG	EGCG	63.0 → 20.0	[1]
Colon	Rat	AOM	EGCG	77.3 → 38.1	[1]
	Rat	MNU	GTE	67.0 → 33.0	[1]
Liver	Mouse C3H/HeN	Spontaneous	EGCG	83.3 → 52.2	[1]
Lung	Mouse A/J	NNK	GTE	96.3 → 65.5	[7]
Pancreas	Hamster	BOP	GTE	54.0 → 33.0	[1]
Skin	Mouse SKH-1	UVB	GTE	67.0 → 7.0	[8]

MNNG: N-methyl-N'-nitro-N-nitrosoguanidine; ENNG: N-ethyl-N'-nitro-N-nitrosoguanidine; AOM: azoxymethane; MNU: methylnitrosourea; NNK: 4-(methylnitrosoamine)-1-(3-pyridyl)-1-butanone; and BOP: N-nitrosobis-(2-oxopropyl)amine.

(3-pyridyl)-1-butanone (NNK) [7], and tumor development on mouse skin induced by either UVB light or UVB light plus TPA [8].

^{3}H-EGCG administered by a p.o. intubation into mouse stomach is distributed into various organs. Radioactivity was found after 24 hours in the digestive tract, liver, lung, brain and skin [9]. EGCG and green tea extract had previously shown inhibition of carcinogenesis in most of the organs.

The cohort study of the town of Yoshimi in the Saitama prefecture, which was conducted by Drs. Kei Nakachi and Kazue Imai at the Division of Epidemiology of our Research Institute, revealed that cancer onset of patients who had consumed more than 10 cups of green tea per day was 8.7 years later among females, and 2.5 years later among males, than that of patients who had consumed fewer than three cups per day [10]. Looking at the numbers of lung cancer patients among the 164 women, the results indicated that drinking green tea prevents development of lung cancer in humans [10].

5. A New Process of Cancer Prevention

We have studied the mechanisms involved in tumor promotion, that is, the process of clonal growth of the initiated cells. Based on evidence that a tumor promoter, okadaic acid, mimics TNF-α/interleukin-1 (IL-1) in inducing phosphorylation of proteins and expression of early response genes in human fibroblasts, as well as activation of NF-κB in Jurkat cells, we have demonstrated that TNF-α acts both as a tumor promoter and a central mediator of tumor promotion [1].

Pretreatment with the inhibitors mentioned above (such as sarcophytol A, canventol and EGCG), commonly inhibited TNF-α mRNA expression and TNF-α release in BALB/3T3 cells induced by okadaic acid, whereas it enhanced the expression of early response genes, rather than inhibiting them. Thus, inhibition of TNF-α mRNA expression along with inhibition of TNF-α release is a new process of cancer prevention [11].

Recent investigation has revealed that TNF-α is involved in various diseases, such as rheumatoid arthritis, Crohn's disease, multiple sclerosis, graft versus host disease, HIV, malaria, sepsis, and cachexia associated with cancer. It is reasonable to conclude that specific inhibitors of TNF-α production will almost certainly be effective not only in cancer prevention but also in the therapy and prevention of these other diseases.

6. Summary

We have reviewed our contributions in finding natural inhibitors of carcinogenesis. Green tea is now an acknowledged cancer preventive in Japan and will possibly soon be recognized as such in other countries. Moreover, green tea has advantages over other cancer chemopreventive agents, as it is also effective against cardiovascular and liver disease. It is apparent that natural products are rich sources of new inhibitors of various diseases.

Acknowledgements

This work was supported by Grants-in-Aid for Cancer Research, Overseas Scientific Research Program (Cancer Program) from the Ministry of Education, Science and Culture, a grant from the Ministry of Health and Welfare for the Second Term of Comprehensive 10-Year Strategy for Cancer Control, Japan; grants from the Foundation for Promotion of Cancer Research; the Princess Takamatsu Cancer Research Fund; the Smoking Research Fund; the Uehara Memorial Life Science Foundation; The MOA Health Science Foundation; Suzuken Memorial Foundation; the Asahi Glass Foundation, and the Plant Science Research Foundation of the Faculty of Agriculture of Kyoto University.

References

1. Fujiki H, Komori A, Suganuma M (1997) Chemoprevention of Cancer. *In:* Bowden TG, Fischer SM (eds): *Comprehensive Toxicology*, Vol. 12, pp 453–471.
2. Yatsunami J, Fujiki H, Komori A, Suganuma M, Nishiwaki S, Okabe S, Nishiwaki-Matsushima R, Ohta T, Matsunaga S, Fusetani N et al. (1992) Marine natural products against tumor development. *In:* Kobayashi T (ed): *Proceedings of the 1st International Congress on Vitamins and Biofactors in Life Science,* pp 333–336.
3. Yoshizawa S, Horiuchi T, Suganuma M, Nishiwaki S, Yatsunami J, Okabe S, Okada T, Muto Y, Frankel K, Troll W et al. (1992) Penta-*O*-galloyl-β-D-glucose and (–)-epigallocatechin gallate, cancer preventive agents. *In:* Huang M-T, Ho C-T, Lee CY (eds): *Phenolic Compounds in Food and Their Effects on Health II*, American Chemical Society, Washington, DC, pp 316–325.
4. Nomura T, Fukai T, Hano Y, Yoshizawa S, Suganuma M, Fujiki H (1988) Chemistry and antitumor promoting activity of *Morus* flavonoids. *In:* Cody V, Middleton E Jr, Harborne JB, Berets A (eds): *Plant Flavonoids in Biology and Medicine*, Alan R. Liss, New York, pp 267–281.

5. Hashimoto T, Tori M, Mizuno Y, Asakawa Y, Fukazawa Y (1989) The superoxide release inhibitors, cryptoporic acids C, D, and E; dimeric drimane sesquiterpenoid ethers of iso-citric acid from the fungus *Cryptoporus volvatus*. *J Chem Soc Chem Commun* 258–259.
6. Sharma S, Stutzman JD, Kelloff GJ, Steele VE (1994) Screening of potential chemopre-ventive agents using biochemical markers of carcinogenesis. *Cancer Res* 54: 5848–5855.
7. Wang Z-Y, Hong J-Y, Huang M-T, Reuhl K, Conney AH, Yang CS (1992) Inhibition of N-nitrosodiethylamine- and 4-(methylnitrosamino)-1-(3-pyridyl)-1-butanone-induced tu-morigenesis in A/J mice by green tea and black tea. *Cancer Res* 52: 1943–1947.
8. Wang Z-Y, Huang M-T, Ferraro T, Wong C-Q, Lou Y-R, Reuhl KR, Iatropoulos M, Yang CS, Conney AH (1992) Inhibitory effect of green tea in the drinking water on tumorigenesis by ultraviolet light and 12-*O*-tetradecanoylphorbol-13-acetate in the skin of SKH-1 mice. *Cancer Res* 52: 1162–1170.
9. Suganuma M, Okabe S, Oniyama M, Sueoka N, Kozu T, Komori A, Sueoka E, Hara E, Fujiki H (1997) Mechanisms of (–)-epigallocatechin gallate (EGCG) and green tea in inhi-bition of carcinogenesis. *In:* Ohigashi H, Osawa T, Terao J, Watanabe S, Yoshikawa T (eds): *Food Factors for Cancer Prevention,* Springer, Tokyo, pp 127–129.
10. Nakachi K, Imai K, Suga K (1997) Epidemiological evidences for prevention of cancer and cardiovascular diseases by drinking green tea. *In:* Ohigashi H, Osawa T, Terao J, Watanabe S, Yoshikawa T (eds): *Food Factors for Cancer Prevention*, Springer, Tokyo, pp 105–108.
11. Suganuma M, Okabe S, Sueoka E, Iida N, Komori A, Kim S-J, Fujiki H (1996) A new process of cancer prevention mediated through inhibition of tumor necrosis factor α ex-pression. *Cancer Res* 56: 3711–3715.

CHAPTER 26
Gene Delivery to Airways

Christian Schatz and Andrea Pavirani

Transgène S. A., Strasbourg, France

1. Introduction

Experimental evidence for introducing functional genes into tissues and organs has opened new therapeutic approaches to reverse genetic or acquired pathologies. Gene therapy strategies applied to airway disorders (such as cystic fibrosis (CF), cancer and α1-antitrypsin (α1-AT) deficiency) have recently been implemented. At present the direct delivery of beneficial genes to diseased airway cells is accomplished using either replication defective viral vectors, based on the adenovirus, adeno-associated virus (AAV), retrovirus genome, or nonviral synthetic vectors, such as cationic lipids complexing plasmid DNA (for review see [1]). Virus-based vectors efficiently transfer foreign genes to different target airway cells. However, safety considerations and limitations, such as host immune response, may limit their application to certain diseases. On the other hand, synthetic vectors are interesting candidates owing to their putative immunotolerance and low toxicity. However, their gene transfer efficiency needs to be increased. Several clinical protocols involving patients with cystic fibrosis, α1AT deficiency and lung cancer have been approved and conducted in the USA and in Europe. The vast majority involves CF patients.

2. Cystic Fibrosis

Mutations in the cystic fibrosis transmembrane conductance regulator (*CFTR*) gene are responsible for cystic fibrosis, one of the most common autosomal recessive diseases in the Caucasian population (approximately 1/2500 live births). The major affected organs are the lungs, the pancreas and the gastrointestinal tract, but complications in lungs are the major cause of morbidity and mortality [2]. At present there is no efficient longterm therapy available for cystic fibrosis, so CFTR gene delivery to airways may represent an alternative to correct or alleviate the respiratory manifestations [3, 4]. The first clinical protocols involving replication-deficient adenovirus- or AAV-based vectors or plasmid/cationic lipid complexes expressing the CFTR cDNA started in 1993 [5, 6], 1995 and 1994 [7], respectively, and since then many other trials have been conducted (Table 1). The goal of these trials has been to demonstrate the absence of toxicity at a vector dose that may induce potential clinical efficiency. Moreover, since the vectors currently employed do not permanently transfer a recombinant CFTR gene to the airway epithelium, repeat administrations are envisaged. Thus no inflammatory or immune response should be associated with vector delivery.

The first results have shown CFTR transfer and expression to the nasal and pulmonary epithelium of patients using both adenovirus and synthetic vectors. Partial and transitory correction of the nasal epithelial potential differences was observed [5–10, 12]. In particular, Crystal et al. [5] reported expression of CFTR mRNA (up to 9 days) and protein (up to 4 days) in nasal and bronchial cells after adenovirus instillation into the nose and bronchi of a few patients. Zabner et al. [6] and Knowles et al. [8] have also shown transitory presence of CFTR mRNA after nasal instillation of a recombinant adenovirus. However CFTR transfer and expression was not demonstrated in all patients. Adenovirus vectors carrying the CFTR cDNA were shown to correct the CF nasal epithelium electrophysiologically by reducing the basal potential differences and by increasing the potential differences in the presence of β-agonists after administration to the nose [6, 9, 10]. Partial and variable Cl$^-$ transport corrections have been reported after repeated nasal instillations, which were probably due to an observed immune response against adenovirus [10]. In the Knowles study [8] no correction in Cl$^-$ and Na$^+$ nasal epithelia transport was demonstrated using a recombinant adenovirus. After cationic lipid-mediated instillation of a CFTR-expressing plasmid, partial electrophysiological correction was observed in some nasal epithelia [7].

In terms of safety, gene transfer to CF patients has been well tolerated with only a few exceptions. In the study by Crystal et al. [5] one patient receiving 2×10^9 plaque forming units (pfu) of a recombinant CFTR adenovirus (20 ml volume) in a lung lobe showed a transient systemic and pulmonary syndrome possibly mediated by interleukin (IL)-6 [11]. At the nasal level, inflammation and increase in albumin, IL-6 and IL-8 in the nasal lavage have been reported by Knowles et al. [8] in two out of three patients treated with 2×10^{10} pfu of recombinant adenovirus. Shedding and spreading of recombinant adenovirus were seldom found and no novel infectious virus was generated by possible genomic recombination.

Table 1. Clinical protocols involving CF patients (as of June 1996)

Principal investigator	Vector (promoter)	Dose (min–max)	Site of administration (Mode)	Number of administered subjects	Reported results (Ref.)
Unique dose					
Crystal	Ad5 (MLP2)	$2\times10^5 - 2\times10^9$ pfu	Nose and lung (bronchoscopy)	9	[5, 9, 11]
Welsh	Ad2 (E1a)	$2\times10^6 - 5\times10^7$ pfu	Nose	3	[6]
Wilson	Ad5 (CMV/β actin)	$7\times10^5 - 2{,}1\times10^7$ pfu	Lung (bronchoscopy)	8	–
Boucher/Knowles	Ad5 (CMV/β actin)	$2\times10^7 - 2\times10^{10}$ pfu	Nose	12	[8]
Wilmott/Whitsett	Ad5 (RSV)	$1\times10^5 - 5.1\times10^8$ pfu	Nose and lung (bronchoscopy)	2	–
Bellon	Ad5 (MLP2)	$1\times10^5 - 5.4\times10^8$ pfu	Nose and lung (aerosol)	6	[12]
Dorkin/Lapey	Ad2 (PGK)	$8\times10^6 - 2.5\times10^9$ pfu	Lung (bronchoscopy and aerosol)	14	–
Geddes/Alton	DC-Chol : DOPE (SV40)	10–300 µg DNA/placebo	Nose	9/6	[7]
Higgins	DC-Chol : DOPE (SV40)	40–400 µg DNA/placebo	Nose	8/4	–
Porteous	DOTAP (CMV)	400 µg DNA/placebo	Nose	8/8	–
Zabner	GL67:DOPE (CMV)	0.8–4 mg DNA	Nose	9	–
Sorscher/Logan	DMRIE : DOPE (SV40)	100–400 µg DNA	Nose	2	–
Flotte	AAV2 (ITR)	$1\times10^6 - 1\times10^{10}$ total particles	Nose and lung (bronchoscopy)	6	–
Gardner	AAV2 (ITR)	$10^2 - 5\times10^4$ infectious particles	Maxillary sinus	7	–
Repeat doses					
Welsh	Ad2 (PGK)	$2\times10^7 - 1\times10^{10}$ infectious units	Nose	6	[10]
Crystal	Ad5 (CMV)	$3\times10^6 - 3\times10^9$ pfu	Lung (bronchoscopy)	12	–

Ad5, Ad2: adenovirus type 5, 2; MLP2: adenovirus type 2 major late promoter; E1a: adenovirus early region 1a; CMV: cytomegalovirus; RSV: Rous sarcoma virus; PGK: phosphoglycerate kinase; DC-Chol: DOPE: dimethylaminoethane-carbamoyl cholesterol: dioleoyl phosphatidylethanolamine; SV40: simian virus 40; DMRIE: dimyristyloxypropyl-3-dimethylhydroxyethylammonium bromide: DOTAP: 1,2-dioleoyl-3-trimethylammonium-propane; ITR: inverted terminal repeat.

The first clinical trial involving aerosolization of an adenoviral vector expressing CFTR was performed by Bellon et al. [12] on six CF patients. The results indicate that doses of up to 10^8 and 5.4×10^8 pfu in the nose and lungs, respectively, are well tolerated. No significant deviations in immunological and inflammatory parameters were seen in serum and bronchoalveolar lavage (BAL). Following aerosol administration no antibodies against adenovirus were found in BAL of all patients. CFTR expression in the lung was demonstrated by reverse transcriptase-polymerase chain reaction (RT-PCR) at a dose of 10^7 pfu and by immunocytochemistry starting from 10^8 pfu. CFTR mRNA expression lasted for 15 days after aerosolization. In the nose, CFTR mRNA and protein expression was seen in all patients and lasted up to 15 days.

3. Lung Cancer

Gene therapy has opened new avenues for directly destroying tumour cells or suppressing their growth. Two types of approach are currently under investigation: the introduction of tumour suppressor genes into tumour cells and the use of cytokine genes to induce immune response to tumours. Roth et al. [13] have injected a retrovirus expressing the wildtype p53 protein directly into the tumours of nine patients with non-small cell lung cancer (NSCLC). No appreciable vector-related toxicity was seen and gene transfer was confirmed in post-treatment biopsies. Regression of tumour size was observed in three patients and stabilization of tumour growth in three others. Another clinical protocol from the same group, in which a recombinant adenovirus expressing the wildtype p53 is injected into tumour of patients with NSCLC, has been approved in the USA [14].

Another approach for lung cancer gene therapy has been pursued by T. Tursz (Institut Gustave Roussy, Paris, France) utilizing recombinant adenovirus vectors expressing cytokines such as IL-2. The feasibility of the approach has been tested by injecting a recombinant adenovirus expressing *E. coli* β-galactosidase as a marker gene product directly into lung tumours of 12 inoperable patients [15]. At present 9 out of 12 patients have been treated using a fiberoptic bronchoscope. Doses ranged between 10^7 to 10^9 pfu. Vector delivery was well tolerated by patients. Vector DNA was detected by PCR in tumour biopsies for up to 84 days after virus administration and β-galactosidase expression was monitored in six out of nine patients for more than 30 days.

4. α1-Antitrypsin Deficiency

A clinical gene therapy protocol (K. Brigham, Vanderbilt University, Nashville, TN, USA) for the transfer of α1-AT cDNA into nasal and lower respiratory cells of patients with α1-AT deficiency and with adult respiratory distress syndrome (ARDS) has been approved by the US authorities. In lung, α1-AT neutralizes the effect of damaging proteolytic enzymes. Patients who inherit a defective $\alpha1$-AT gene develop emphysema at an early age due to lack of the active protein, while patients with ARDS release high levels of proteases, as a result of trauma, infection etc., which overwhelm the protective effect of α1-AT. The vector to be employed in the clinical setting consists of cationic lipids complexing plasmid DNA encoding α-AT.

5. Conclusion and Perspectives

There is compelling evidence that gene delivery to airway epithelium and lung tumours is feasible and can be well tolerated in CF and lung cancer patients. The large number of Phase I trials, especially those involving patients with CF, have however highlighted certain limitations of currently used gene transfer vectors. First, immune and inflammatory responses to the so-called "first generation" adenovirus vectors were observed at high doses and may limit their repeated use. Second, there is a general consensus when it comes to efficiency of gene transfer and expression, which is relatively low in the case of synthetic vectors. By capitalizing on the first clinical results, new research into virus biology and in vector construction has been initiated. These studies should enable the generation of novel vector systems with an improved safety and efficiency. The next years will be fundamental to translate gene delivery to airways into an established and valid therapeutic strategy.

Acknowledgements

The authors thank Bruce Acres for critical reading of the manuscript, and Noëlle Monfrini for excellent secretarial assistance.

References

1. Curiel DT, Pilewski JM, Albelda SM (1996) Gene therapy approaches for inherited and acquired lung diseases. *Am J Respir Cell Mol Biol* 14: 1–18.
2. Boat TF, Welsh MJ, Beaudet AL (1989) Cystic fibrosis. *In:* Scriver CR, Beaudet AL, Sly WS, Valle D (eds): *The Metabolic Basis of Inherited Disease.* McGraw-Hill Inc, New York, pp 2649–2680.
3. O'Neal WK, Beaudet AL (1994) Somatic gene therapy for cystic fibrosis. *Hum Molec Genet* 3: 1497–1502.
4. Crystal RG (1995) Transfer of genes to humans: early lessons and obstacles to success. *Science* 270: 404–410.
5. Crystal RG, McElvaney NG, Rosenfeld MA, Chu C-S, Mastrangeli A, Hay JG, Brody SL, Jaffe AH, Eissa NT, Danel C (1994) Administration of an adenovirus containing the human CFTR cDNA to the respiratory tract of individuals with cystic fibrosis. *Nature Genet* 8: 42–51.

6. Zabner J, Couture LA, Gregory RJ, Graham SM, Smith AE, Welsh MJ (1993) Adenovirus-mediated gene transfer transiently corrects the chloride transport defect in nasal epithelia of patients with cystic fibrosis. *Cell* 75: 207–216.
7. Caplen NJ, Alton EWFW, Middleton PG, Dorin JR, Stevenson BJ, Gao X, Durham SR, Jeffrey PK, Hodson ME, Coutelle C, et al. (1995) Liposome-mediated CFTR gene transfer to the nasal epithelium of patients with cystic fibrosis. *Nature Med* 1: 39–46.
8. Knowles MR, Hohneker K, Zhou Z, Olsen JC, Noah TL, Hu PC, Leigh MW, Engelhardt JF, Edwards LJ, Jones KR, et al. (1995) A controlled study of adenoviral-vector-mediated gene transfer in the nasal epithelium of patients with cystic fibrosis. *N Engl J Med* 333: 823–831.
9. Hay JG, McElvaney NG, Herena J, Crystal RG (1995) Modification of nasal epithelial potential differences of individuals with cystic fibrosis consequent to local administration of a normal CFTR cDNA adenovirus gene tranfer vector. *Hum Gene Ther* 6: 1487–1496.
10. Zabner J, Ramsey BW, Meeker DP, Aitken ML, Balfour RP, Gibson RL, Launspach, Moscicki RA, Richards SM, Standaert TA, et al. (1996) Repeat administration of an adenovirus vector encoding cystic fibrosis transmembrane conductance regulator to the nasal epithelium of patients with cystic fibrosis. *J Clin Invest* 97: 1504–1511.
11. McElvaney NG, Crystal RG (1995) IL-6 release and airway administration of human CFTR cDNA adenovirus vector. *Nature Med* 1: 182–184.
12. Bellon G, Michel-Calmard L, Thouvenot D, Jagneaux V, Poitevin F, Malcus C, Accart N, Layani M-P, Aymard M, Bernon H, et al. Aerosol administration of a recombinant adenovirus expressing CFTR to cystic fibrosis patients: a phase I clinical trial. *Hum Gene Ther* 8: 15–25.
13. Roth JA, Nguyen D, Lawrence DD, Kemp BL, Carrasco CH, Ferson DZ et al. (1996) Retrovirus-mediated wild-type p53 gene transfer to tumors of patients with lung cancer. *Nature Med* 2: 985–991.
14. Roth JA (1996) Modification of tumor suppressor gene expression and induction of apoptosis in non-small cell lung cancer (NSCLC) with an adenovirus vector expressing wildtype p53 and cisplatin. *Hum Gene Ther* 7: 1013–1030.
15. Tursz T, Le Cesne A, Baldeyrou P, Gautier E, Opolon P, Schatz C, Pavirani A, Courtney M, Lamy D, Ragot T, et al. Recombinant adenoviral-mediated gene transfer: preliminary report of a phase I study in lung cancer patients. *J Natl Cancer Inst* 88: 1857–1863.

Clinical and Biological Basis of Lung Cancer Prevention
ed. by Y. Martinet, F.R. Hirsch, N. Martinet, J.-M. Vignaud
and J. L. Mulshine
© 1998 Birkhäuser Verlag Basel/Switzerland

CHAPTER 27
Lung Cancer Prevention: The Point of View of a Public Health Epidemiologist

Annie J. Sasco

Programme of Epidemiology for Cancer Prevention, International Agency for Research on Cancer, World Health Organization, Institut National de la Santé et de la Recherche Médicale, Lyon, France

1. Lung Cancer Epidemiology

1.1. Descriptive Epidemiology

Lung cancer is the most frequent cancer in the world, with more than one million new cancer cases occurring each year. When the world cancer burden was last estimated in 1985, it was calculated that 896,000 cases were diagnosed in that year, 677,000 in men and 219,000 in women [1]. This represented a clear increase compared to estimations for preceding years. In 1980 lung cancer ranked second to stomach cancer both in mortality and incidence worldwide [2].

Very large variations exist across countries in terms of either proportional share of lung cancer mortality among all cancer deaths (from less than 1% to more than 15% among men), or in terms of incidence rate (from less than 10 new cases/100,000 man-years to more than 100, age-standardized to the world population). There are also large discrepancies among women [3].

In France, cancer is the main cause of death among men (86,166 deaths per year) and the second among women (55,665 deaths per year) [4]. In men, lung is the leading cancer site with more than 19,000 deaths, whereas in women the figure is around 3,000. This situation is the result of a dramatic rise in male lung cancer mortality from 1950 to today. Among women, lung cancer mortality is still low, but a sharp increase is predicted [5].

1.2. Etiological Epidemiology

1.2.1. Tobacco: We cannot discuss lung cancer without mentioning tobacco. It is currently estimated that tobacco kills three million people per year throughout the world, not only from lung cancer but from all tobacco-related ailments such as cancers of the upper aerodigestive tract, bladder, kidney, pancreas and cervix, cardio- and cerebrovascular diseases, chronic respiratory diseases and yet other pathologies. By the year 2025, tobacco will kill ten million people per year.

The association between lung cancer and tobacco use has been the testing ground for the methodology of chronic disease epidemiology. Although some astute clinicians had already suspected such an association during the last century and the first half of this one, notably in Germany, it has mainly been from 1950 onwards that data have accumulated. The two pioneering studies on this topic were published in the United Kingdom [6] and the USA [7]. The first was a prospective study conducted among medical practitioners which is still ongoing and for which the results of forty years of followup have been published [8]. The second study was the first of a long series of case-control studies [7]. This was closely followed by two similar studies in the United Kingdom [9] and in France [10] which played a highly educational role. Today, hundreds of studies are available using different methodological approaches, with a larger number of case-control studies rather than cohort studies conducted in many populations of the world by a multitude of research teams.

So much information has accumulated that tobacco has been officially recognized as a carcinogen, both as smokeless tobacco [11] and tobacco smoking [12]. Tobacco therefore constitutes the most widespread carcinogenic agent in the world and is generally recognized as such.

1.2.2. Other lung carcinogens: Given the fact that up to 85% of lung cancers are due to tobacco in men and at least 60% in women [13], the determination of other etiological factors is problematic and may have been substantially delayed. It is difficult to identify the role both of rare exposures, for example in the workplace, and of low exposures, as in the general environment. The problem is compounded by the fact that in general only small risks are expected, therefore making even harder the separation of true causal effects from potential biases. Nevertheless, a list of confirmed or probable lung carcinogens has been compiled and is fairly lengthy; most of these have been identified in an occupational setting [14]. It includes, among others, asbestos, arsenic and its compounds, beryllium and its compounds, bis-chloromethylether, chloromethylether of technical quality, cadmium and its compounds, chromium and its compounds (hexavalent), mustard gas, nickel and its compounds, vinylchloride, talc-containing asbestos fibres, toluene chloride, dimethylsulphate, aflatoxins, acrylonitrile, soot, tars and some mineral oils, rubber products, radon and its derivatives, and most recently, silica.

2. Methodology for Research on Lung Cancer

2.1. The Traditional Epidemiological Approach

Although much is already known about lung cancer etiology, significant discoveries may still take place using long-established epidemiological methods [15]. Rare, well-defined exposures will lead to the setting up of cohort studies which, depending on available means, may either be retrospective if data bases already exist, or prospective if the importance of the problem warrants the cost. Frequent exposures, sometimes not well defined, will be evaluated through case-control studies using traditional or more innovative approaches [16]. Newer methods, sometimes called hybrid, may also be used such as case-control studies nested within cohorts or case-cohort and related designs. The latter use different sampling schemes based on the source population of non-cases.

2.2. Molecular Epidemiology

This new development has been presented as the "magical" tool which will be able to estimate whatever cannot be measured by questionnaires and will quantify both exposure and effect validly and accurately. In other words, it will give us the definitive answer. In reality, we are not yet there. However, molecular biology has potentially a powerful contribution to make to cancer research by allowing for a more precise definition of a set of events between exposure and disease. Biology will give us the tools to identify and measure series of exposure markers, markers of disease and also markers of susceptibility. This will make apparent and quantifiable many intermediate points in the causal links between exposure and disease. It will also, hopefully, give us better means for adequate prevention [17].

2.2.1. Exposure markers: Tobacco is an excellent example of an exposure which may at the same time be extremely easy to measure in the domain of active smoking, and much more difficult when dealing with environmental tobacco smoke.

Tobacco consumption is usually estimated both in terms of daily quantity of tobacco and number of years of smoking, the latter being by far the most relevant in cancer etiology. By contrast, the evaluation of exposure to tobacco in the environment is a more delicate, although attainable, goal. It is within this context that molecular epidemiology can contribute considerably.

Rather than just measuring an external dose, we can now attempt to estimate the internal dose. This corresponds to measurements in the biological fluids of either the agent itself or its metabolite. With regard to tobacco, we can for example measure cotinine or N-nitrosoproline, or carry out a general test of the mutagenicity of urine. These methods come closer to measuring the actual exposure of the individual than simple measurements of external dose.

Even more relevant to the etiology of disease is the evaluation of the biologically active dose, which reflects not only the external agent becoming internal, but also the interaction with the host at the most fundamental level, leading to the appearance of DNA or protein adducts. The list of specific examples in the modelling of exposure to tobacco is long: N-3-(2-hydroxyethyl)-histidine, N-(2-hydroxy-ethyl)-valine, 4-amino-hemoglobin, various DNA adducts, in particular with polycyclic aromatic hydrocarbons (PAH), as well as protein adducts for the same PAH, and specific compounds such as nornitrosonicotine-hemoglobin adducts or nornitrosocotinine.

2.2.2. Disease markers: These should be more correctly termed biological markers of effect as they reveal an impact of the agent or exposure on the host, not immediately resulting in pathology, but already having a measurable effect. Early preclinical effects include, at the subcellular level, gene mutation, oncogene activation or inactivation of tumour suppressor genes. More advanced effects lead to sister chromatid exchange or even chromosomal damage.

If the exposure continues and nothing is done to prevent neoplastic change, progression to functional or structural modifications preceding the occurrence of clinical disease will take place. Even at this late stage, after the appearance of symptoms, the evolution towards death will be conditioned by a number of factors with prognostic significance.

2.2.3. Susceptibility markers: This last series of markers is of paramount importance as they act throughout, from exposure to disease and death. At each step, from the exposure agent's action to reaction of the cell and the host in general, as well as disease progression, development will be conditioned by susceptibility phenomena, some of which can be measured.

Two fields of research have grown considerably in recent years. The domain of enzymatic activity was the first to be developed via studies of specific P450 cytochromes. Examples of such topics include the CYP2D6 involved in debrisoquin metabolism, in which intense metabolizers have six times the risk of getting lung cancer as slow metabolizers; P450 2D6 protein and NNK metabolism; inducibility of CYP1A1 (arylcarbohydrate hydroxylase activity in relation to PAHs) where once again a higher inducibility is associated with a greater risk. On a more general level, enzymes may be involved either in metabolic activation or in detoxification and excretion as they are both potentially relevant to carcinogenesis.

In the field of genetic predisposition to cancer, growing importance is being given to inherited mutations of tumour suppressor genes, including recessive forms, the role of *p53* in carcinogenesis, as well as acquired genetic mutations, in particular at the HPRT locus.

Finally, other elements have to be included under the influence of nutritional, as well as immune, status which clearly condition cancer susceptibility.

2.2.4. Strategies for future studies related to lung cancer prevention: These should address the continuum of states from exposure to death and the issue of separation between risk factor and pathological process. Two types of study can be envisaged [17].

2.2.4.1. Transitional studies. The first step corresponds to biomarker development studies which have to assess issues of reliability of markers, along with considerations of collection and treatment of samples. The second generation deals with biomarker characterization studies which can be cross-sectional or longitudinal studies.

2.2.4.2. Etiological and intervention studies. Observational studies can be either simply descriptive, or aiming at etiology (and therefore analytical). All study designs can be used: cross-sectional, cohort or longitudinal, as well as case-control. More and more hybrid research designs are added, such as case-control studies nested within cohorts, case-cohort and related studies using different sampling schemes based on non-cases. Intervention studies can bring useful information on the influence of modification of risk factors and screening, in particular using sensitive methods for the evaluation of susceptibility in large populations of former smokers and of course in treatment, including the delicate area of pharmacoprevention.

2.2.5. Statistical methodology: Software enabling almost everyone to use complex multivariate models is now available. This has promising potential but also presents a great hazard, as the likelihood of misuse increases exponentially. Issues to be dealt with are many: calculation of the power of a study, specification of sensitivity and specificity, evaluation and quantification of random or differential misclassification, evaluation of interaction, antagonism or synergism, use of multiple markers, repeated measurements and data correlated over time, and need for transformation to satisfy statistical assumptions [17].

2.2.5.1. Molecular biology issues. Validation of measurements has to be addressed first, in terms of internal and external validity, as well as selection of markers. In practice, variability within and between laboratories will also have to be evaluated in terms of quality assurance and quality control. Biomonitoring and pharmacokinetic modelling may be used to estimate doses, taking into account biological marker kinetics as well as pharmacokinetic models and molecule-host interactions, with regard to practical applications.

A related issue is the question of biological banking of specimens. These may have many uses but this domain is not free from problems such as measurement error, selection bias and confounding. In addition, it is crucial to keep in mind ethical and legal considerations.

3. Prevention of Lung Cancer

3.1. Population-Based Prevention

It is clear that throughout the world today the absolute priority is the fight against tobacco. If we could eliminate tobacco, we could save millions of lives in years to come. This goal is particularly important for developing countries, where we should be attempting to halt the progression of the tobacco epidemic. In addition, the elimination of tobacco should also be an aim for children and adolescents in all societies of the world, and last but not least for women.

3.2. Chemoprevention

Preliminary attempts at chemoprevention have not proven particularly successful. For example, the Finnish study on β-carotene and α-tocopherol did not yield the expected results [18] and therefore the following question can be asked: "β-carotene, helpful or harmful?" [19].

Issues to consider before launching such studies include possible iatrogenicity of these products, which would limit their use in healthy subjects [20]. On the other hand, their potential could be great, in particular for addressing the needs of large populations of former smokers where intervention to control the late stages of tumour promotion could be envisaged.

3.3. Research Agenda for the Future

Information should be sought on quantitative rather than purely qualitative risk assessment, issues of identification and monitoring of genetically predisposed subjects and possibly newer generations of cancer screening studies. Plenty of questions remain to be answered.

4. Conclusion

The domain of lung cancer prevention offers scope for everyone. Action can and should be immediate, strong and continuous in order to fight tobacco use. This will be the role of public health leaders, but even more so of people in the field and the population at large. This is complementary to the research effort which has to be pursued within the scientific community. Through better communication between public health experts and researchers, as well as between epidemiologists and laboratory scientists, a better world can be built.

References

1. Pisani P, Parkin DM, Ferlay J (1993) Estimates of the worldwide mortality for eighteen major cancers in 1985. Implications for prevention and projections of future burden. *Int J Cancer* 55: 891–903.
2. Parkin DM, Läärä E, Muir CS (1988) Estimates of the worldwide frequency of sixteen major cancers in 1980. *Int J Cancer* 41: 184–197.
3. Parkin DM, Muir CS, Whelan SL, Gao YT, Ferlay J, Powell J, (eds) (1992): *Cancer incidence in five continents, Vol VI, IARC Scientific Pub 120,* International Agency for Research on Cancer, Lyon.
4. Lion J, Hatton F, Magnin P, Maujol L (1993) Statistiques de santé. Statistiques des causes médicales de décès 1990. Paris: *éditions INSERM.*
5. Hill C, Koscielny S, Doyon F, Benhamou E (1993) Evolution de la mortalité par cancer en France 1950–1990. Mise à jour 1986–1990. Paris: *éditions INSERM.*
6. Doll R, Hill AB (1954) The mortality of doctors in relation to their smoking habits. A preliminary report. *Br Med J* 1: 1451–1455.
7. Wynder EL, Graham EA (1950) Tobacco smoking as a possible etiologic factor in bronchiogenic carcinoma. A study of six hundred and eighty four proven cases. *J Am Med Ass* 143: 329–336.
8. Doll R, Peto R, Wheatley K, Gray R, Sutherland I (1994) Mortality in relation to smoking: 40 years' observations on male British doctors. *Br Med J* 309: 901–911.
9. Doll R, Hill AB (1952) A study of the aetiology of carcinoma of the lung. *Br Med J* ii: 1271–1286.
10. Schwartz D, Flamant R, Lellouch J, Denoix PF (1961) Results of a French survey on the role of tobacco, particularly inhalation in different cancer sites. *J Natl Cancer Inst* 26: 1085–1108.
11. International Agency for Research on Cancer. IARC Monographs on the evaluation of carcinogenic risk of chemicals to humans. Vol 37. Tobacco Habits other than Smoking; Betel-Quid and Areca-Nut Chewing; and Some Related Nitrosamines. Lyon: International Agency for Research on Cancer, 1985.
12. International Agency for Research on Cancer. IARC Monographs on the evaluation of carcinogenic risk of chemicals to humans. Vol. 38. Tobacco Smoking. Lyon: International Agency for Research on Cancer, 1986.
13. Parkin DM, Sasco AJ (1993) Lung cancer: worldwide variation in occurrence and proportion attributable to tobacco use. *Lung Cancer* 9: 1–16.
14. Merletti F, Heseltine E, Saracci R, Simonato L, Vainio H, Wilbourn J (1984) Target organs for carcinogenicity of chemicals and industrial exposures in humans: a review of results in IARC Monographs on the evaluation of carcinogenic risk of chemicals to humans. *Cancer Res* 44: 2244–2250.

15. Sasco AJ (1997) Validiy issues in study designs. *In:* Stellmann J (ed): *ILO Encyclopaedia of Occupational Health and Safety.* International Labour Office, section 28.19, Geneva (in press).
16. Liu Q, Sasco AJ, Riboli E, Hu MX (1993) Indoor air pollution and lung cancer risk in Guangzhou, People's Republic of China. *Am J Epidemiol* 137: 145–154.
17. Schulte PA, Perera FP (1993) Molecular epidemiology. Principles and practice. San Diego: *Academic Press, Inc.*
18. The Alpha-Tocopherol, Beta-Carotene Cancer Prevention Study Group. The effect of vitamin E and beta-carotene on the incidence of lung cancer and other cancers in male smokers. *N Engl J Med* 1994; 330: 1029–1035.
19. Nowak R (1994) Beta-carotene: helpful or harmful? *Science* 264: 500–501.
20. Sasco AJ (1995) Epidémiologie et prévention des cancers: Quelques réflexions sur l'éthique des démarches de santé publique. *Bull Acad Natle Méd* 179: 987–1007.

Clinical and Biological Basis of Lung Cancer Prevention
ed. by Y. Martinet, F. R. Hirsch, N. Martinet, J.-M. Vignaud
and J. L. Mulshine
© 1998 Birkhäuser Verlag Basel/Switzerland

CHAPTER 28
Biomarkers as Intermediate Endpoints in Chemoprevention Trials: Biological Basis of Lung Cancer Prevention

Vali A. Papadimitrakopoulou and Waun K. Hong

*The University of Texas. Department of Thoracic/Head and Neck Medical Oncology,
M. D. Anderson Cancer Center, Houston, Texas, USA*

1. Introduction

Lung cancer remains a common cause of mortality throughout the world; in the U.S. alone, 177000 new cases were predicted for 1996 and an estimated 158000 Americans died of lung cancer [1]. The impact of improvements in multimodality therapy on lung cancer mortality remains modest [2]. Although substantial reduction in adult smoking has been achieved in the U.S. (50% of adults are former smokers) [3], many new lung cancers are being diagnosed among former smokers [4, 5]. Data analysis from both M.D. Anderson Cancer Center and Harvard-affiliated hospitals showed that more than 50% of lung cancer cases occur in former smokers. From the current smoking trends, it appears that former smokers will account for a growing percentage of all lung cancer patients. We must therefore examine which former smokers are at high risk for lung cancer.

Strategies extending beyond smoking cessation to direct preventive intervention in order to inhibit and reverse the carcinogenesis process (i.e. chemoprevention), are clearly needed and have the potential to reduce lung cancer incidence and mortality. Well-focused, comprehensive programs of integrated clinical and laboratory studies providing the opportunity to analyse biological and genetic parameters of successful retinoid intervention at the bronchial tissue level are currently underway. These programs are based on recent clinical evidence for the feasibility and effectiveness of retinoids in oral leukoplakia reversal [6], and in prevention of second primary tumors (SPTs) in the high risk group of previously treated head and neck cancer patients [7]. Well-characterized agents, suitable cohorts and reliable intermediate markers of risk and efficacy that would replace cancer incidence as an endpoint are three critical aspects of successful chemoprevention trials [8]. Another critical issue in the development of effective prevention strategies is understanding the early sequences of cancer: critical genetic events or critical levels of event accumulation that lead to the emergence of malignant clones. Intraepithelial neoplasia has long been identified as an intermediate step in the causal pathway to cancer, but the use of recently available molecular tools is providing the basis for identification of cellular and molecular biomarkers that can be used as surrogate endpoints for cancer incidence in chemoprevention trials, and for increased risk cohort selection for such trials. Careful application of the most accurate and sensitive of these biomarkers, along with risk factors (genetic or lifestyle) and exposure biomarkers (measures of carcinogen exposure such as carcinogen-DNA adducts), can accelerate the pace of intervention research progress.

2. Field Cancerization and Multistep Carcinogenesis

The use of chemoprevention strategies in lung cancer is based on a great and still growing body of information that implicates several initiating and promoting factors in the carcinogenesis process, and on the two seminal concepts of field cancerization and multistep carcinogenesis. Field cancerization, a term proposed by Slaughter et al. [9], predicts a diffuse response to carcinogenic injury throughout the exposed field and is manifested by the frequent occurrence of premalignant lesions, leukoplakia, squamous metaplasia/dysplasia, and multiple primary tumors within the lungs and the upper aerodigestive tract. Multiple lung primary tumor formation (a clinical manifestation of field cancerization) is common; individuals with lung cancer have a 15 to 20% chance of developing a second primary at a rate of 2 to 3% a year [10]. Carcinogen exposure produces a series of genetic changes that eventually lead to cancer development. These changes vary in their rate of accumulation, depending upon the individual's inherent susceptibility to carcinogenic exposure. This multistep process is histologically evidenced as bronchial metaplasia or dysplasia. The extent of these histological changes in smokers reflects their smoking history [11], although it is unclear which of these changes will eventually transform into cancer. Thus, premalignant histology may not be the most definitive surrogate marker for cancer risk or tissue response. New markers, ideally reflecting cellular responses to the actions of chemopreventive agents, are needed. Detection of molecular changes in bronchial washings and sputum samples is one potential method of screening patients for the presence of premalignant or malignant cells, in particular with the use of the new PCR-based technology, which has sensitivity far exceeding that of standard cytological techniques [12].

3. Genetic Biomarkers

It is now apparent that multiple genetic changes and molecular events (including mutations, deletions, gene amplifications or translocations), occur during the multistep molecular pathogenesis of lung cancer. A molecular analysis of changes present in apparently nontumorous lung tissue in the field of the lung tumor may give insight into the risk of a particular individual for developing an SPT. In situ hybridization, which allows the visualization of chromosomes in nondividing cells, applied on tissue biopsies from the field at risk, demonstrated that genomic instability (as manifested by chromosome polysomy) was associated with the extent of histological progression and appeared highest in individuals who subsequently developed cancer [13, 14].

Allelotype analysis provides another way to estimate the degree of genomic instability that is linked to the multistep process of tumorigenesis, by identifying commonly deleted chromosomal segments in tumors; these often harbor genes that function as tumor suppressors in the tissue. Analysis of frequently observed allelic losses in premalignant lesions of the lung might yield a higher sensitivity for clonal outgrowth, which can act as an additional risk factor beyond generalized genomic instability. Several groups have molecularly characterized premalignant lesions or second primary tumors distant from primary lung tumors and have demonstrated that these lesions can exhibit evidence of clonal outgrowth, as marked by genetic changes frequently observed in the primary lung cancer [15, 16]. These changes are often distinct from those in the primary lung tumor, which supports the idea that the tumorigenesis process is ongoing at many sites in the carcinogen-exposed lungs. Sozzi et al. found evidence for chromosomal rearrangements, including 3p and 17p deletions and overexpression of growth factors receptors, by examining short-term cultures of "normal" lung cells from patients with lung tumors [17] with a significantly higher frequency of changes in patients with multiple tumors of the upper aerodigestive tract [18].

The loss of chromosome 9p21 represents one of the most common genetic changes in lung cancer [19]. Mapping studies on chromosome 9p21 identified *p16* and characterized it as a cdk inhibitor involved in the G1/S transition of the cell cycle [20], and functional studies have demonstrated its tumor suppression function [21]. The paucity of point mutations in *p16* in many tumor types [22] pointed to alternative mechanisms of *p16* inactivation, including homozygous deletions which are frequent in lung cancers [23] and methylation of a 5′ CpG island leading to transcriptional inactivation [24, 25]. Furthermore, loss of chromosome 9p is now known to occur early in the progression of lung cancer. Kishimoto et al. identified loss of heterozygosity (LOH) at the 9p locus in 38% of hyperplastic foci, 80% of dysplastic foci, and 100% of carcinoma in situ (CIS) lesions in bronchial epithelium from patients with non-small cell lung cancer (NSCLC) [26]. Loss of the identical allele in preneoplastic lesions and the corresponding tumor was seen in all cases, which supports the field cancerization theory. In the same tissue specimens, LOH at 3p occurred in 76% of hyperplasias, 86% of dysplasias, and 100% of CIS [27]. Loss of genetic material on chromosome 3p is one of the most common changes in these tumors. Chromosome 3p involves at least three distinct regions (3p25, 3p21.3 and 3p14-cen) that presumably harbor undiscovered tumor suppressor genes, inactivation of which may be critical for the development of lung cancer [28]. Deletions of 3p in preinvasive bronchial lesions have also been previously described [15, 27, 29] as occurring in an incremental fashion following histological progression from hyperplasia to invasive cancer, which further supports the theory of accumulation of genetic damage during the multistep lung carcinogenesis process, and demonstrates the potential value of such alterations as risk markers for the subsequent development of invasive cancer [29].

Our group has performed molecular analyses to determine the nature of genetic damage in the bronchial epithelium of smokers at several chromosomal loci, and analysed microsatellite alterations at three loci (3p14, 9p21 and 17p13) in bronchial biopsies from current and former smokers [30]. LOH was found in 75%, 59%, and 18% of informative cases for 3p14, 9p21, and 17p13, respectively. Higher LOH frequency was observed in current versus former smokers and in those with metaplasia index $\geq 15\%$ versus those with $< 15\%$. These data demonstrate the high prevalence of genetic alterations in the bronchial epithelium of smokers, and the persistence of these alterations even after smoking cessation. Individuals harboring such changes could benefit from chemopreventive intervention.

As stated above, 17p loss is another frequent finding in preinvasive lesions and lung cancer. The *p53* gene in this region has the highest frequency of mutations of any gene yet identified in human cancers [31]; the frequency of *p53* mutations in lung cancer is estimated to be 56% (90% in small cell lung cancer and about 55% in NSCLC) [32]. During lung carcinogenesis, *p53* mutations occur at the interface between severe dysplasia and CIS [15, 17]. In fact, immunohistochemical study of premalignant lesions contiguous to head and neck tumors conducted by our group has shown a correlation of accumulated p53 protein levels with histological progression [33] and that p53 positivity correlated with higher levels of polysomy, a correlation that was more pronounced in dysplastic and cancer lesions [34]. In addition, abnormal p53 expression in these lesions is associated with refractoriness to retinoids [35] and with lack of RAR-β upregulation following treatment with 13-*cis*-retinoic acid. Furthermore, p53 abnormalities in the initial head and neck tumor predict increased incidence of second primary tumors, as well as recurrences of the primary tumor [36]. Our ability to detect clonal populations of *p53* mutation-containing cells could help us to select the population of patients who would benefit most from chemopreventive approaches and novel biological approaches such as gene therapy [37].

4. Retinoid Biology and Chemoprevention

The use of retinoids in lung cancer chemoprevention is based on evidence that vitamin A deficiency leads to squamous metaplasia and keratinization of the mucosal epithelium of the airways that can be reversed by retinoids, and on the suppression of experimental lung carcinogenesis in animals. Retinoids exert their actions through activation of the nuclear retinoid receptors that act as transcription factors for genes that influence cell growth and differentiation; therefore, changes in their expression may cause aberrations in the response of cells to retinoids, and alterations in growth and differentiation regulation. It was found that RARβ expression is suppressed in many lung cancer cell lines [38], a finding that suggests implication of a selective suppression of RARβ in malignant transformation. Selective suppression of RARβ in the early stages of carcinogenesis in the oral cavity and marked upregulation of RARβ after retinoid treatment [39] associated with clinical response have been confirmed, thus giving RARβ excellent potential as an intermediate biomarker. A pilot study of RARβ expression in specimens from a previous chemoprevention trial in bronchial metaplasia revealed that only 55% expressed RARβ before treatment and some upregulation of RARβ expression was noted after retinoid treatment. Retinoid receptor expression was compared in specimens from normal and malignant lung tissue. All receptors were expressed in at least 89% of control normal bronchial tissue specimens from patients without a primary lung cancer and distant normal bronchus specimens from NSCLC patients. RARα, RXRα, and RARγ were expressed in >95% of the 79 NSCLC specimens, in contrast to RARβ, RARγ, and RXRβ expression, which was detected in only 42%, 72%, and 76% of NSCLC specimens, respectively [40]. These findings provide further evidence for implication of RARβ, and possibly RARγ and RXRβ, in lung carcinogenesis.

5. Conclusions

The challenge of serious prevention research for lung cancer is still great, but the advances already made, especially in the characterization of the molecular events occurring during tumorigenesis, justify the optimism of investigators in this field. Ahead of us remain years of, hopefully, fruitful collaboration between basic scientists, epidemiologists, pathologists and clinicians in an attempt to delineate definitively the parameters of successful preventive intervention.

Acknowledgement

This work was supported in part by NCI CA52051, NCI CA94022, and NCI CA16772.

References

1. Parker SL, Tong T, Bolden S, Wingo PA (1996) Cancer Statistics 1996. *CA Cancer J Clin* 46: 5–28.
2. Minna JD, Pass H, Glatstein E, Ihde DC (1989) Lung cancer. *In:* DeVita VT, Rosenberg S, and Hillman S (eds): *Principles and Practice of Oncology,* Lippincott, Philadelphia, pp 591–705.
3. Pierce JT, Frome MC, Novotny TE, Hatziandreu EJ, Davis RM (1989) Trends in cigarette smoking in the United States. Projections to the year 2000. *J Am Med Assoc* 261: 61–65.
4. Halpern MT, Gillespie BW, Warner KE (1993) Patterns of absolute risk of lung cancer mortality in former smokers. *J Natl Cancer Inst* 85: 457–464.
5. Lubin JH, Blot WJ (1993) Lung cancer and smoking cessation: patterns of risk. *J Natl Cancer Inst* 85: 422–423.
6. Hong WK, Endicott J, Itri L, Doos W, Batsakis JG, Bell R, Fofonoff S, Byers R, Atkinson EN, Vaughan C, et al. (1986) 13-cis retinoic acid in the treatment of oral leukoplakia. *N Engl J Med* 315: 1501–1505.
7. Hong WK, Lippman SM, Itri LM, Karp DD, Lee JS, Byers R, Schantz SP, Kramer AM, Lotan R, Peters LJ, et al. (1990) Prevention of second primary tumors with isotretinoin in squamous cell carcinoma of the head and neck. *N Engl J Med* 323: 795–801.
8. Zelen M (1988) Are primary cancer prevention trials feasible? *J Natl Cancer Inst* 80: 1442–1444.
9. Slaughter DP, Southwick HW, Smejkal W (1953) Field cancerization in oral stratified squamous epithelium: Clinical implications of multicentric origin. *Cancer* 6: 963–968.
10. Fontana RS, Sanderson DR, Woolner LB, Taylor WF, Miller WE, Muhm JR (1986) Lung cancer screening: The Mayo program. *J Occ Med* 28: 746–750.
11. Auerbach O, Hammond EC, Garfinkel L (1979) Changes in bronchial epithelium in relation to cigarette smoking, 1955–1960 vs 1970–1977. *N Engl J Med* 300: 381–386.
12. Mao L, Hruban RH, Boyle JO, Tockman M, Sidransky D (1994) Detection of oncogene mutations in sputum precedes diagnosis of lung cancer. *Cancer Res* 54: 1634–1637.
13. Lee JS, Kim SY, Hong WK, Lippman SM, Ro JY, Gay ML, Hittelman WN (1993) Detection of chromosomal polysomy in oral leukoplakia, a premalignant lesion. *J Natl Cancer Inst* 85: 1951–1954.
14. Voravud N, Shin DM, Ro JY, Lee JS, Hong WK, Hittelman WN (1993) Increased polysomies of chromosomes 7 and 17 during head and neck multistage tumorigenesis. *Cancer Res* 53: 2784–2883.
15. Sundaresan V, Ganly P, Hasleton P, Rudd R, Sinha G, Bleehen NM, Rabbits P (1992) p53 and chromosome 3 abnormalities, characteristic of malignant lung tumors, are detectable in preinvasive lesions of the bronchus. *Oncogene* 7: 1989–1997.
16. Gazdar AF (1994) Molecular changes preceding the onset of invasive lung cancers. *Lung Cancer* 11 (suppl 2): 16–17.
17. Sozzi G, Miozzo M, Donghi R, Pilotti S, Cariani CT, Pastorino U, Della Porta G, Pierotti MA (1992) Deletions of 17p and p53 mutations in preneoplastic lesions of the lung. *Cancer Res* 52: 6079–6082.
18. Sozzi G, Miozzo M, Pastorino U, Tagliabue E, Donghi R, Maneti G, Minoletti F, Pilotti S, Ravasi G, Pierotti MA (1994) Genetic elements in the multi-step lung carcinogenesis. *Lung Cancer* 11 (suppl 1): 20.
19. Olopade OI, Buchhagen DL, Malik K, Sherman J, Nobori T, Bader S, Nau MM, Gazdar AF, Minna JD, Diaz MO (1993) Homozygous loss of the interferon genes defines the critical region on 9p that is deleted in lung cancers. *Cancer Res* 53: 2410–2415.
20. Serrano M, Hannon G, Beach D (1993) A new regulatory motif in cell cycle control causing specific inhibition of cyclin D/CDK4. *Nature* 366–704.

21. Lukas J, Parry D, Aagard L, Mann DJ, Bartkova J, Strauss M, Peters G, Bartek J (1995) Retinoblastoma-protein-dependent cell-cycle inhibition by the tumour suppressor p16. *Nature* 375: 503–506.

22. Cairns P, Mao L, Merlo A, Lee DJ, Schwab D, Eby Y, Tokino K, van der Riet P, Blaugrund JE, Sidransky D (1994) Low rate of p16 (MTS1) mutations in primary tumors with 9p loss. *Science* 265–415

23. Cairns P, Polascik TJ, Eby Y, Tokino K, Califano J, Merlo A, Mao L, Herath J, Jenkins R, Westra W, et al. (1995) High frequency of homozygous deletion at p16/CDKN2 in primary human tumors. *Nature Genet* 11: 210–212.

24. Merlo A, Herman JG, Mao L, Lee DJ, Gabrielson E, Burger PC, Baylin SB, Sidransky D (1995) Methylation of the tumour suppressor p16(CDKN2) in human cancers. *Nature Med* 7: 686–692.

25. Shapiro GI, Park JE, Edwards CD, Mao L, Merlo A, Sidransky D, Ewen ME, Rollins BJ (1995) Multiple mechanisms of p16[INK4A] inactivation in non-small cell lung cancer. *Cancer Res* 55: 6200–6209.

26. Kishimoto Y, Sugio K, Hung JY, Virmani AK, McIntire DD, Minna JD, Gazdar AF (1995) Allele-specific loss in chromosome 9p loci in preneoplastic lesions accompanying non-small cell lung cancer. *J Natl Cancer Inst* 87: 1224–1229.

27. Hung J, Kishimoto Y, Sugio K, Virmani A, McIntire DD, Minna JD, Gazdar AF (1995) Allele-specific chromosome 3p deletions occur at an early stage in the pathogenesis of lung carcinoma. *JAMA* 273: 558–563.

28. Hibi K, Takahashi T, Yamakawa K, Ueda R, Sekido Y, Ariyoshi Y, Suyama M, Takagi H, Nakamura Y, Takahashi T (1992) Three distinct regions involved in 3p deletion in human lung cancer. *Oncogene* 7: 445–449.

29. Thiberville L, Payne P, Vielkinds J, LeRiche J, Horsman D, Nouvet G, Palcic B, Lam S (1995) Evidence of cumulative gene losses with progression of premalignant epithelial lesions to carcinoma of the bronchus. *Cancer Res* 55: 5133–5139.

30. Mao L, Lee JS, Kurie JM, Fan YH, Lippman SM, Lee JJ, Ro JY, Broxson A, Yu R, Morice RC, et al. (1997) Clonal Genetic Alterations in the Lungs of Current and Former Smokers. *J Natl Cancer Inst* 89: 857–862.

31. Hollstein M, Sidransky D, Vogelstein B, Harris CC (1991) p53 mutations in human cancers. *Science* 253: 49–53.

32. Harris CC (1996) Tumor suppressor gene: From basic research laboratory to the clinic – an abridged historical perspective. *Carcinogenesis* 17: 1187–1198.

33. Shin DM, Kim J, Ro JY, Hittelman J, Roth JA, Hong WK, Hittelman WN (1994) Activation of p53 gene expression in premalignant lesions during head and neck tumorigenesis. *Cancer Res* 54: 321–326.

34. Shin DM, Ro JY, Shah T, Hong WK, Hittelman WN (1994) p53 expression and genetic instability in head and neck multistep tumorigenesis. *Proc Am Assoc Cancer Res* 35: 158 [abstract].

35. Lippman SM, Shin DM, Lee JJ, Batsakis JG, Lotan R, Tainsky MA, Hittelman WN, Hong WK (1995) p53 and retinoid chemoprevention of oral carcinogenesis. *Cancer Res* 55: 16–19.

36. Shin DM, Lee JS, Lippman SM, Lee JJ, Tu ZN, Choi G, Heyne K, Shin HJ, Ro JY, Goepfert H, et al. (1996) p53 expression: predicting recurrence and second primary tumors in head and neck squamous cell carcinoma. *J Natl Cancer Inst* 88: 519–529.

37. Roth JA, Nguyen D, Lawrence DD, Kemp BL, Carrasco CH, Ferson DZ, Hong WK, Komaki R, Lee JJ, Nesbitt JC, et al. (1996) Retrovirus-mediated wild-type p53 gene transfer to tumors of patients with lung cancer. *Nat Med* 2: 985–991.

38. Nervi C, Vollberg TM, George MD, Chambon P, Jetten AM (1991) Expression of nuclear retinoic acid receptors in normal tracheobronchial cells and in lung carcinoma cells. *Exp Cell Res* 195: 163–170.

39. Lotan R, Xu X-C, Lippman SM, Ro JY, Lee JS, Lee JJ, Hong WK (1995) Suppression of retinoic acid receptor β in premalignant oral lesions and its upregulation by isotretinoin. *N Engl J Med* 332: 1405–1410.

40. Xu X-C, Lee JS, Sozzi G, Ro J, Pastorino U, Hong WK, Lotan R (1995) Differential expression of retinoid acid receptors in non-small cell lung carcinomas and in bronchial epithelia. *Proc Am Assoc Cancer Res* 36: 3579B [abstract].

Clinical and Biological Basis of Lung Cancer Prevention
ed. by Y. Martinet, F. R. Hirsch, N. Martinet, J.-M. Vignaud
and J. L. Mulshine
© 1998 Birkhäuser Verlag Basel/Switzerland

CHAPTER 29
Biological Tools for Mass Screening

Nadine Martinet* and Michael Hogan

* INSERM U14, Plateau de Brabois, CD 10, Nancy, France

1. Introduction

It was felt that huge advancement has been made in achieving an under-standing of lung cancer in terms of somatic mutation and the alteration of tumor gene expression during the past ten years. At the same time, techni-cal advances have been made in the areas of automated PCR, *in situ* hybridization, flow cytometry, immuno-histochemistry and array-based hybridization methods.

The general consensus which has emerged is that, although it is as yet unclear which molecular biomarkers should be employed, the knowledge base and the technology in hand have made the mass screening of risk and early lung cancer diagnosis a realistic possibility during the next five years. In that context, several specific considerations were discussed.

2. The Concept of a Decision Making Hierarchy

It was suggested that mass screening should be considered in terms of a spectrum of molecular tests, from the most easily implemented and least expensive to the most detailed, costly and presumably most informative in terms of molecular detail.

At the least costly extreme, it was proposed that blood-based screening should be more thoroughly investigated, with the study of bloodborne anti-p53 antibodies being an excellent recent lead in this area.

Sputum and BAL analysis was viewed as the most promising example of analysis at the intermediate level of sophistication, especially in view of its noninvasive character and recent efforts to establish staged, archival sputum and BAL libraries. Continued development of PCR, *in situ* PCR, *in situ* hybridization, computer assisted immuno-histochemistry and array hybridization methods were discussed as warranting more vigorous study for the analysis of such samples.

Finally, at the most complicated extreme, continued development of endobronchial biopsy was encouraged, especially in those instances where blood, sputum or BAL analysis have indicated unusual risk factors. Although this method of sample accumulation is clearly more expensive, the relative purity of the biopsy material is most conductive to the advanced methods of molecular analysis.

For blood, sputum, BAL and endobronchial biopsy, a general conclusion was drawn that individual biomarkers are not likely to be as valuable as panels of biomarkers, chosen in the context of recent advancements in the understanding of initiation and promotional biology of lung tumorigenesis. Thus, based upon current advancement in multiplexed-PCR, SSP, multi-probe microscopy and flow cytometry and the microarray hybridization methods, efforts should be focused on development of integrated bio-marker sets, to analyse mutation and expressional markers concurrently.

Such sets could entail expressional biomarkers associated with xeno-biotic inactivation, DNA repair, cellular proliferation and apoptosis. Muta-tional endpoints such as k-*ras* and *p53*, more generalized LOH and others should also be evaluated in such analyses.

The challenge remaining is the determination of the combination of expressional and mutational biomarkers which provides the most useful risk or diagnostic information, at the earliest possible step in the disease process. In parallel, significant work needs to be done in order to extend the technologies of the day, so that such highly detailed information can be readily obtained at low cost in large populations.

3. Hardware and Software

Several technologies which seem most promising for large scale biomarker screening involve the use of electrophoresis, flow cytometry, and 2D imaging methods via digital microscopy, phosphorimagers, CCD cameras or proximal imaging. Although many of these methods are currently employed in the practice of pathology, it is felt that to be employed for large scale screening they must be coupled to methods of automated sample pre-paration and data analysis, thereby maximizing speed and minimizing (costly) human intervention.

Implementation of advanced concepts for large-scale sample analysis, especially for relatively complex sets of biomarkers, may become simpli-fied by the general availability of sample preparation robotics (hardware) and data analysis software which should be robust enough to accommodate large populations, with minimal human input.

These sample preparation and automation difficulties are still significant and must be addressed as soon as possible.

4. Ethical Questions

The concept of low-cost, multiparameter biomarker analysis of early lung cancer risk is emerging as a practical technical possibility. In spite of the huge potential for such technology, significant questions were raised as to the ethical application of such mass screening methods.

First, concern was raised that, in the absence of validated chemopreventative or curative treatment protocols for lung cancer, technology for early risk and diagnostic screening would provide little practical benefit to the patient population, beyond an additional rationale to terminate smoking.

More importantly, fears were raised that such very early risk information could be used as the basis for the withholding of medical or life insurance to high risk individuals, especially in countries such as the USA which lack universal health care coverage.

5. Direct Coupling of Early Risk Assessment and Therapeutics

In a more positive light, it was generally concluded that the short-term ethical problems associated with these new technologies may be worth the risk, in that the development of very high throughput, multiple biomarker technologies for population-based screening are likely to fuel expansion of our current understanding of lung tumor biology, and more directly, become a set of tools to be used in the development of chemopreventative therapy.

Current Phase I/II studies in the use of retinoids as chemopreventive agents were cited as a good preliminary example. Current molecular biology suggests that development of such retinoid therapies would greatly benefit if the pool of available patients could be prescreened with respect to a relatively complete set of expression biomarkers in the lung which might be important to an understanding of drug activity (P450 levels, retinoic acid receptor (RAR) expression, expression of related genes in the RAR signaling pathway, etc.).

The nature of early-stage drug intervention is that, by definition, tumor tissue and symptoms associated with tumor invasion have not yet appeared. Therefore, in short-term trials, it is not possible to use traditional indicators of progression or remission to evaluate the efficacy of such chemopreventative agents. The general availability of molecular biomarker panels is viewed as a powerful new set of tools to evaluate the short- and long-term efficacy of such novel chemopreventative agents, at the level of molecular physiology, and to direct the design and implementation of improved drug candidates.

6. Summary

At present, the molecular understanding of lung cancer etiology and the technologies which would implement such knowledge are not well-enough developed to initiate large-scale populations-based risk assessment or disease diagnosis.

However, advances in cancer molecular biology and analytical methodology have been very rapid over the past five years. When paired with the enormous input of information from the Human Genome Project, it is felt that we are on the "doorstep" of an era where large-scale population-based screening of risk and diagnosis can be envisaged, based on the analysis of very large biomarker panels, with endpoints which include biomarkers of expression and mutation in the same set.

A challenge for the next five years should be systematic efforts to co-ordinate research and development programs of molecular genetics, biotechnology and clinical research, with the goal of developing these very high throughput technologies.

On the engineering side, new research and development efforts should be directed to search for improved hardware and software for fully automated sample preparation, new physical methods for detecting mutation and gene expression at the RNA and protein level, new automated solutions for very high throughput sample handling, and finally informatics which can compile the massive expression data sets which would be generated.

On the biological side, emphasis should be placed on multiple biomarker analysis (the markers being chosen on the basis of molecular genetics) while keeping a simultaneous focus on the application of such technology to programs of chemopreventative drug discovery. For example, new basic research efforts should be directed towards the search for mutation and patterns of gene directed towards the search for mutation and patterns of gene expression that could serve as the biomarker set to screen populations for a predisposition towards tobacco-induced chemical carcinogenesis. A candidate gene set of that kind might include most or all of the P450s, along with the several glutathione transferases.

Simultaneous effort should be made to evaluate the cost/benefit ratio to be obtained form such advanced methods, along with the many ethical implications. In the final analysis, the greatest value to be obtained from the new technologies for mass screening of populations, will be their ability to identify members of the population at greatest risk of lung cancer and *simultaneously* to drive the discovery of new therapies which can be used to treat that high risk sub-population. The goal will be to detect the disease process and to intervene medically at a point which is so early in tumor progression that we can realistically begin to consider a cure for lung cancer, rather than being limited to the management of its late stage and generally fatal symptoms.

Clinical and Biological Basis of Lung Cancer Prevention
ed. by Y. Martinet, F.R. Hirsch, N. Martinet, J.-M. Vignaud
and J.L. Mulshine
© 1998 Birkhäuser Verlag Basel/Switzerland

CHAPTER 30
Optimization of the Use of Biological Samples for the Prospective Evaluation of Preneoplastic Lesions: Summary of Breakout Session

R. Gemmill, Elisabeth Brambilla, J.P. Martin and Ugo Pastorino*

*Thoracic Survery, Royal Brompton Hospital, London, UK

The participants in this joint session had a wide-ranging discussion about these issues and came up with specific recommendations, since sample availability is such a major issue of prospective evaluation. Questions discussed included:

1. What truly constitutes a neuroendocrine tumor?
2. What events characterize distal preneoplasias?
3. Is there a precursor lesion for small cell lung cancer?
4. What are the best markers to use for preneoplasias, especially considering the limited materials available?

Suggestions included p53 which was felt to be an excellent marker to predict future development of invasive carcinoma. At the same time, we have only a poor idea of the total spectrum of genetic changes present in preneoplastic lesions. Another suggested marker is the HNRNP A2/B1 epitope detected by antibody 703D4.

In light of the fact that the WHO is developing a new histological classification for lung tumors, and that for the first time this classification will include preneoplastic lesions, now is the time to define the constellation of genetic changes that characterize these lesions. This will permit genetic changes to be correlated with phenotype wherever possible. To achieve this goal, the participants made several specific suggestions:

1. Encourage histopathologists and molecular pathologists or molecular geneticists to work together on the same lesions.
2. Encourage investigators to cast a wide net for discovery of more genetic changes. Techniques could include comparative genomic hybridization, representational difference analysis, methylated CpG island detection, high density cDNA arrays.
3. Request that the IASLC sponsor a workshop within one year to focus on correlating histopathology and molecular genetic changes in preneoplasia.

4. Establish a WWW site to foster communication among groups looking at genetic lesions in preneoplasias. Initially, this site should include names, addresses, genes and markers being examined. With time, it could be used as a forum to share tools and protocols so that results are comparable, by allowing and stimulating standardization. The site could also provide a forum for reporting problems with techniques. It is not intended that people necessarily share samples, since these are very limited.

It is hoped that these recommendations will hasten the time when the definition of a preneoplastic lesion will include both histology and genetic/molecular pathology and that this combination will give us a much better predictor for risk of progression.

Index

D. Raeburn, *Rhône-Poulenc Rorer Ltd, Dagenham, UK*
M.A. Giembycz, *Royal Brompton National Heart and Lung Institute, London, UK (Eds)*

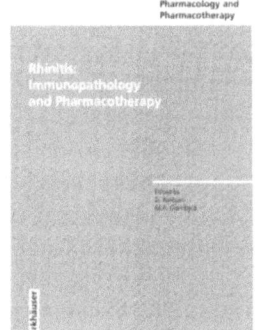

Rhinitis: Immunopathology and Pharmacotherapy

1997. 248 pages. Hardcover • ISBN 3-7643-5301-5

Continuing the Respiratory Pharmacology and Pharmacotherapy series, this volume explores the pathophysiology and therapy of rhinitis. The volume is introduced by a chapter describing the normal anatomy and physiology of the nose and sinuses. Against this background the contributing authors describe and discuss the immunological and pathological changes which occur in rhinitis. The various causes and the types of rhinitis – such as allergic, vasomotor, and infectious – are considered as are the treatments available (pharmacotherapy, immuno-therapy, surgery). The book concludes with a description of the animal models of rhinitis which are now available. This book will be indispensable to bench scientists and clinicians alike.

From the contents:
V. Lund: Anatomy and Physiology of the Nasal Cavity and Paranasal Sinuses
J.G. Widdicombe: Pathophysiology of the Nose in Rhinitis
G.K. Scadding: Immunology of the Nose
M. Andersson, C. Svensson, L. Greiff, J. Erjefält and C.G.A. Persson: Inflammation in Rhinitis
R.J. Davies and M.A. Calderon: Allergic Rhinitis
J. Krasnick and R. Patterson: Vasomotor Rhinitis
S. Criscione and E. Porro: Infectious agent-induced Rhinitis
J. Bousquet, P. Demoly and F.-B. Michel: Specific Immunotherapy in Allergic Rhinitis
J.A. Cook: Surgery of Rhinitis
K.L.S. Chen: Animal models of Rhinitis

For detailed information please see
http://www.birkhauser.ch
or mail to
sales@birkhauser.ch

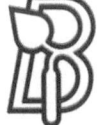

Birkhäuser Verlag • Basel • Boston • Berlin

D.F. Rogers, National Heart and Lung Institute, London, UK /
M.I. Lethem, Univ. of Brighton, UK (Eds)

Airway Mucus: Basic Mechanisms and Clinical Perspectives

1997. 400 pages. Hardcover. ISBN 3-7643-5691-X
(Respiratory Pharmacology and Pharmacotherapy)

Conceptually unsavoury, airway mucus is nevertheless vital to homeostasis in the respiratory tract. In contrast, when abnormal, mucus contributes significantly to the pathophysiology of a number of severe bronchial diseases, including asthma, chronic bronchitis and cystic fibrosis. This volume provides wide-ranging and in depth coverage of the scientific and clinical aspects of airway mucus.

Discussion of the scientific aspects of airway mucus commences with chapters which address the biochemical and molecular biological basis of airway mucus and is extended by chapters which provide comprehensive coverage of the various physiological and rheological aspects of respiratory secretions. The clinical aspects of the topic are then considered in chapters discussing the involvement of mucus secretions in bacterial infections and the role of mucus in hypersecretory diseases of the airway. The volume concludes with a discussion of the therapeutic aspects of the topic, both in terms of the possible approaches to the treatment of mucus hypersecretion and of the interaction of drugs used in respiratory disease with airway mucus.

Contents:
1. Airway Surface Liquid: Concepts and Measurements
2. Structure and Biochemistry of Human Respiratory Mucins
3. Airway Mucin Genes and Gene Products
4. The Microanatomy of Airway Mucus Secretion
5. Mechanisms Controlling Airway Ciliary Activity
6. Rheological Properties and Hydration of Airway Mucus
7. Goblet Cells: Physiology and Pharmacology
8. Airway Submucosal Glands: Physiology and Pharmacology
9. Mucus–Bacteria Interactions
10. Experimental Induction of Goblet Cell Hyperplasia *In Vivo*
11. Mucus Hypersecretion and Its Role in the Airway Obstruction of Asthma and Chronic Obstructive Pulmonary Disease
12. Mucus and Airway Epithelium Alterations in Cystic Fibrosis
13. Drug–Mucus Interactions
14. Therapeutic Approaches to the Lung Problems in Cystic Fibrosis
15. Therapeutic Approaches to Airway Mucous Hypersecretion

For detailed information please see
http://www.birkhauser.ch
or mail to
sales@birkhauser.ch

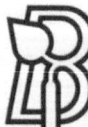

Birkhäuser Verlag • Basel • Boston • Berlin

R.W. Wilmott,
Children's Hospital Medical Center, Cincinnati, OH, USA (Ed.)

The Pediatric Lung

1997. 352 pages. Hardcover • ISBN 3-7643-5703-7
Respiratory Pharmacology and Pharmacotherapy (RPP)

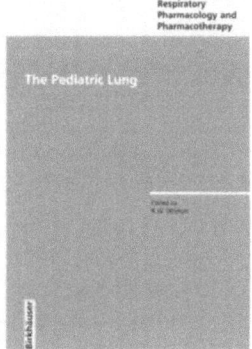

Focussed specifically on children and pediatric respiratory diseases, *The Pediatric Lung* reviews the current status of pharmacological therapy for asthma, viral pneumonia, cystic fibrosis, bronchopulmonary dysplasia and acute respiratory failure. A review of aerosol delivery systems in children and an up-to-date treatise on mucolytic agents is also included.

The chapters are written by leading specialists in the field and summarize the latest developments in pediatric pulmonology, as well as covering a comprehensive range of respiratory diseases in children.

Pediatric pulmonologists, allergologists, intensivists, neonatologists and general pediatricians will find *The Pediatric Lung* an invaluable source of reference. Clinicians will be particularly interested in the new information concerning aerosol delivery systems, gene therapy for cystic fibrosis, new modalities of therapy for asthma, the emerging role of nitric oxide and a treatise on modern mycolytic agents.

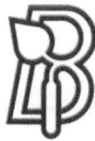

Birkhäuser Verlag • Basel • Boston • Berlin

D.A. Isenberg, University College, London, UK /
S.G. Spiro, Middlesex Hospital, London, UK (Eds)

Autoimmune Aspects of Lung Disease

1997. Approx. 280 pages. Hardcover • ISBN 3-7643-5719-3
(Respiratory Pharmacology and Pharmacotherapy)

The lung forms an integral part of the body's immune system and is subject to a range of diseases which are either autoimmune in nature or have clear-cut immunological abnormalities. *Autoimmune Aspects of Lung Disease* provides a concise review of the lung's role in the immune system and a detailed account of both primary and secondary lung diseases which are characterised by immunological perturbation or frank autoimmunity.

The volume presents a detailed, up-to-date account of disorders ranging from infection to neoplasia and is written in both an informative and stimulating style by a prestigious group of authors. The chapters are extensively referenced and provide numerous insights into the aetiopathogenesis and clinical features and treatment of immunologically-linked pulmonary disease.

The book is intended as both an overview for physicians and scientists with an established interest in diseases of the lung, immunologists seeking to learn more about relevant disorders in the lung and general physicians, whether specialists or in training, seeking to enrich their knowledge of the links between the pulmonary and immune systems.

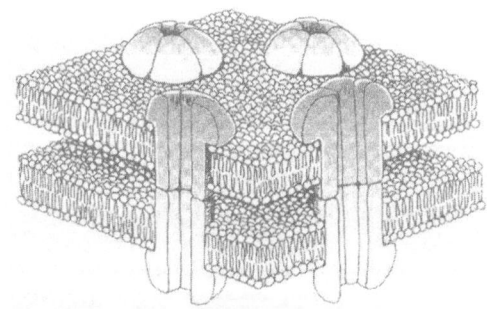

For detailed information please see
http://www.birkhauser.ch
or mail to
sales@birkhauser.ch

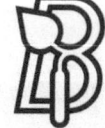

Birkhäuser Verlag • Basel • Boston • Berlin